Clinical Pharmacology for Nurses

We have made every effort to ensure that the information and drug dosages in this book are correct at the time of publication but mistakes may have occurred and therapeutic regimes may have been altered. Where there is any doubt, dosage should be checked against the manufacturer's data sheet or some other authoritative source of information.

For Churchill Livingstone

Publisher: Mary Law
Project Editor: Dinah Thom
Production Controller: Neil A. Dickson
Sales Promotion Executive: Hilary Brown

Clinical Pharmacology for Nurses

John Trounce MD FRCP

Professor Emeritus of Clinical Pharmacology, Guy's Hospital Medical School,
and Physician Emeritus, Guy's Hospital, London, UK

Nursing Adviser

Dinah Gould BSc MPhil DipN RGN RNT

Lecturer in Nursing Studies, King's College, London, UK

FOURTEENTH EDITION

CHURCHILL LIVINGSTONE
EDINBURGH LONDON MADRID MELBOURNE NEW YORK AND TOKYO 1994

CHURCHILL LIVINGSTONE
Medical Division of Longman Group UK Limited

Distributed in the United States of America by Churchill
Livingstone Inc., 650 Avenue of the Americas, New York,
N.Y. 10011, and by associated companies, branches and
representatives throughout the world.

First Edition 1958
Second Edition 1961
Third Edition 1964
Fourth Edition 1967
Fifth Edition 1970
Sixth Edition 1973
Seventh Edition 1977

Eighth Edition 1979
Ninth Edition 1981
Tenth Edition 1983
Eleventh Edition 1985
Twelfth Edition 1988
Thirteenth Edition 1990
Fourteenth Edition 1994
Reprinted 1994

ISBN 0-443-04888-6

British Library Cataloguing in Publication Data
A CIP catalogue record for this book is available from the
British Library.

Library of Congress Cataloging in Publication Data
Trounce, J. R. (John Reginald)
    Clinical pharmacology for nurses / John Trounce; nursing adviser,
Dinah Gould. — 14th ed.
        p.   cm.
    Includes bibliographical references and index.
    ISBN 0-443-04888-6
    1. Pharmacology.   2. Nursing.   I. Gould, Dinah.   II. Title.
    [DNLM: 1. Pharmacology, Clinical–nurses' instruction. QV4 T861p
1993]
RM300.T75   1993
615'.1'024613–dc20
DNLM/DLC
for Library of Congress

The
publisher's
policy is to use
**paper manufactured
from sustainable forests**

Produced by Longman Singapore Publishers Pte Ltd
Printed in Singapore

Contents

Contributors

Chapter on Anaesthetic drugs by

M.B. Barnett MB BS FRC Anaes
Consultant Anaesthetist,
Guy's Hospital

Chapter on the Nurse and the pharmaceutical
service by

R.W. Horne MSc BPharm MPS
Director of Pharmacy,
Guy's Hospital

Chapter on Drugs and the eye

D.M. Watson MB BS FRCS
Consulting Ophthalmic Surgeon,
Guy's Hospital

Contributing to the chapter on Local
application of drugs

Lynette Stone BA RGN RM (NSW) DMS
Clinical Nurse Manager,
St. John's Institute of Dermatology,
St. Thomas' Hospital, London

Preface to the Fourteenth Edition

Nurses have an increasingly important role in the use of drugs. Not only may they be responsible for administering them, recording the patient's response and keeping an eye open for adverse effects but they may soon be able, under certain circumstances, to prescribe. In addition to all this, patients often ask them for advice regarding drugs so they play a most necessary part in patient education. It is therefore important for them to understand both the actions and uses of the drugs they give to their patients. Administration or prescription without understanding can be dangerous.

This book has been extensively revised and gives an account of the drugs commonly used in medical practice. There is a chapter on general principles and another on details of administration and prescription. The problems of adverse effects, interactions and drug monitoring are discussed and there is a brief section on clinical trials. Each chapter ends with a list of suggested articles for further reading which, although not exhaustive, will enable nurses to start reading round a subject.

We are sorry that Dr Hall and Dr Wells cannot continue to contribute and we take this opportunity to thank them for their help over many years. In their place we welcome Miss Stone who brings a wealth of experience in teaching and writing about the nursing aspects of dermatology and Dr Barnett who helped with the anaesthetic section in the last edition and has now completely rewritten it.

We would like to thank our many colleagues in the nursing and medical professions for their advice and the Drug Information Unit, Guy's Hospital, who could always be relied upon to know the answer.

Finally, we would like to thank the staff of Churchill Livingstone for their unfailing help in the preparation of this edition.

London 1993

J. R. T.
D. J. G.

Acknowledgements

We would like to thank the following for permission to reproduce their illustrations:

Allen and Hanbury Ltd—Figure 3.8.
Becton Dickinson—Figures 2.1, 2.2, 2.3.
The European Resuscitation Council 1992 who hold the copyright for Figure 11.2.

MTP Press—Figures 3.6, 4.5, 4.6, 12.1, 14.1 from *Commonsense Use of Medicines* by J. Fry, J. Trounce and M. Godfrey.
Prentice Hall International—Figures 13.10, 13.12 from *Nursing Care of Women* by Dinah Gould.
Graseby Medical for permission to use their name in the illustration, Figure 8.3.

1

Introduction

Pharmacology may be defined as the study of drugs. This includes their origin, chemical structure, preparation, administration, actions, metabolism and excretion. The application of the action of drugs and other measures in the treatment of disease is called therapeutics.

Drugs have been used in treating disease for thousands of years. The writings of most of the ancient civilizations contain directions for the preparation and administration of drugs. Nearly all the remedies described had little if any effect but it is of interest that among the bizarre prescriptions containing such ingredients as fat of the hippopotamus and pig bile, can be found drugs which are still used today. The ancient Egyptians were familiar with the purging effect of castor oil, the Arabians used both opium and senna, and in more recent times the effects of digitalis on oedema were known to country people with no medical training. Nevertheless, the use of drugs in the treatment of disease remained entirely empirical and usually misdirected until the nineteenth century. This period saw the emergence of rational physiology and pathology and on this foundation it was possible to study the effect of drugs and their use in disease.

At first, investigation was confined to observation of the effect on the whole animal or human patient. With the rise of experimental physiology it became possible to investigate the action of drugs on isolated organs and thus obtain a much clearer picture of their effects and potential uses as therapeutic agents. These investigations have

1

brought into use such drugs as adrenaline and ergometrine.

While this work was progressing the chemical structure of many drugs was being unravelled and it thus proved practicable to relate the function of drugs to their chemical composition. This was an important advance for it meant that by altering slightly the structure of a drug it might be possible to enhance its useful action and get ride of any troublesome side-effects. This led to the introduction of many synthetic substances which have proved invaluable in the treatment of disease.

Although extensive experiments in animals led to many useful advances, it is now realized that there are important differences between the pharmacology of drugs in animals and man. Even in the relatively early stages of introducing a new drug, investigation of its action requires studies in humans. This has led to the emergence of *clinical pharmacology* which is essentially the study of drug action in man.

At the present time the frontiers of pharmacology are still being extended, and much work is now concerned with the actual effect of the drug on the complex chemical reactions which are continually occurring within the living cell. Much of this work is difficult, expensive and time consuming, but it is by such a methodical approach, occasionally illuminated by a flash of empirical genius, that pharmacology will advance and the therapeutic armoury of the nurse and doctor be enlarged.

PHARMACOLOGY

ABSORPTION AND METABOLISM OF DRUGS

Drugs may be given to a patient in various ways; they may be injected, absorbed from the gastrointestinal tract after oral or rectal administration or applied locally.

The term *bioavailability* is used to denote that proportion of the administered dose of a drug which reaches the circulation. If it is given intravenously then the bioavailability is obviously 100%, if it is swallowed then only a proportion may reach the circulation.

Oral administration is the commonest and easiest way to give a drug and the bioavailability by this route depends on several factors.

1. Absorption. This will depend on the physical properties of the drug which determine whether it will pass through the wall of the gut, and on the formulation of the drug by the manufacturer.

Absorption may be modified by the rate at which the stomach empties, the presence or absence of food in the stomach and, sometimes, interactions with other drugs or diseases of the gastrointestinal tract (p. 9).

2. First pass effect. When absorbed from the gastrointestinal tract drugs have to pass via the portal vein to the liver before reaching the general circulation (Fig. 1.1). This may be important as many drugs are metabolized (broken down) as they pass through the liver so that only a proportion of the amount absorbed actually reaches the circulation. This removal of the drug as it passes through the liver is called the first pass effect. Drugs which show a very large first pass effect are almost inactive if swallowed, examples being lignocaine and glyceryl trinitrate, and these have to be injected or, if absorbed from the oral mucosa, can be chewed or sucked thus by passing the liver.

After absorption, drugs enter the blood stream and are carried round the body. They may be in simple solution in the plasma, but many are poorly soluble and are partially bound to plasma

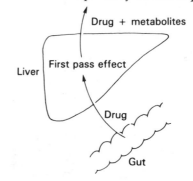

Fig. 1.1 First pass metabolism of a drug.

proteins which act as carriers. *It is important to realize that the fraction of a drug which is bound to protein is inactive and only the free unbound portion has any pharmacological action.*

The concentration of a drug in the blood stream is a good index of whether the correct dose is being given to produce a satisfactory therapeutic effect. Therefore, the nurse should know some-thing of the factors which govern the blood concentration.

1. *The dose.* It is obvious that the larger the dose, the higher the concentration achieved.

2. *The route of administration.* Intravenous injection produces a rapid rise in blood concentration whereas oral administration gives a slower rise and a lower peak concentration. Intramuscular injection rates lie between the two (Fig. 1.2).

3. *The distribution of the drug.* This is another important factor in determining the plasma concentration and also its activity and therapeutic usefulness (Fig. 1.3). Some drugs are confined to the blood stream, and this obviously limits their effect; for instance, an antibiotic which would not enter the tissues would be useless in treating most infections.

Other drugs diffuse out of the circulation into the tissue spaces and some enter the cells and spread through the total water of the body. A few drugs are actually concentrated in cells.

The average volume of the distribution space for an adult is:

Plasma	3 litres
Extracellular space	15 litres
Total body water	36 litres

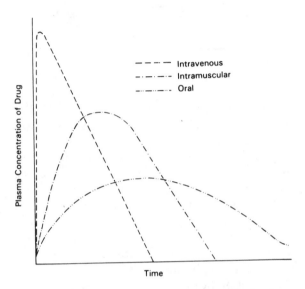

Fig. 1.2 The effect of the route of administration of a drug on the plasma concentrations after a single dose.

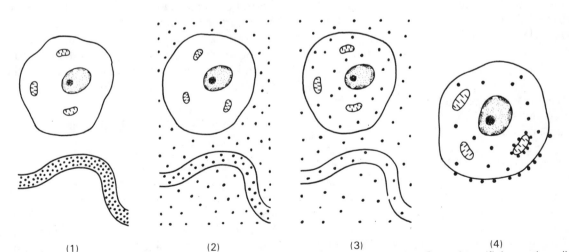

(1)
All drugs enter the blood stream first

(2)
Next they may diffuse into the extracellular fluid

(3)
Finally the drug may enter the cells

(4)
Some drugs 'fix' onto the cell membrane or other structures

Fig. 1.3 Distribution of drugs in the body.

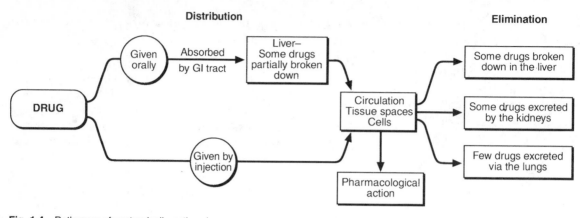

Fig. 1.4 Pathways of systemically-acting drugs.

It can be seen, therefore, that the more widely a drug diffuses, the lower will be the concentration produced by a given dose.

4. *The rate of elimination.* The faster the body breaks down or excretes a drug, the more rapidly will the blood level fall.

Drugs are usually eliminated in one or two ways (Fig. 1.4):

a. They may be broken down or combined with some other chemical so that they are no longer pharmacologically active. This usually occurs in the liver and is brought about by substances called enzymes. Enzymes have the property of promoting certain chemical reactions, and some of these are concerned with the inactivation of drugs. Therefore, if the liver cells are damaged by disease or the circulation to the liver reduced, as in cardiac failure, the inactivation process may be slower than normal. The activity of the liver enzymes can be increased or decreased by drugs and this has important implications in treating patients (see Drug Interactions, p. 266).

There are also genetically determined differences in the rate at which some drugs can be broken down by the body (see p. 6). Suxamethonium normally produces a transient paralysis of voluntary muscle, as it is broken down by an enzyme, but in certain families this enzyme is lacking and suxamethonium causes a prolonged paralysis.

With certain types of drug, if given repeatedly, the breakdown process becomes more effective.

Therefore, larger and larger doses are required to produce the same effect and this is known as *drug tolerance.*

b. Drugs or their breakdown products may be excreted through the kidneys, and if these are damaged by disease, excretion will be delayed and accumulation can occur. By the age of 80 years, kidney function is reduced to about half that of young adults, so with some drugs reduced dosage is required in the elderly. Rarely, drugs are excreted through the lungs and this route is important in the case of volatile anaesthetics.

The speed of elimination is the main factor in deciding the duration of action of a drug and is referred to as the *plasma half-life* ($t\frac{1}{2}$) of that drug. This figure is obtained experimentally by giving a single dose, usually intravenously, and measuring the plasma concentration at intervals. The time taken for this concentration to halve is the plasma or biological half-life (Fig. 1.5).

FACTORS INFLUENCING THE DOSAGE REGIME

Several factors must be considered when a drug is given to a patient. *The time it takes to act* is largely determined by the route of administration. *The blood level and therapeutic effectiveness* depend on the dose, distribution within the body and to some degree on the mode of administration and speed of elimination.

Rapidly excreted drugs with short half-lives will require frequent administration or even con-

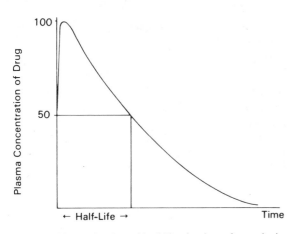

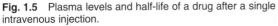

Fig. 1.5 Plasma levels and half-life of a drug after a single intravenous injection.

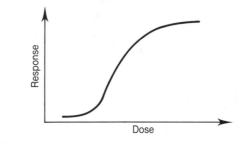

Fig. 1.7 Dose response curve.

tinuous infusion to maintain a fairly constant concentration in the body whilst those that are eliminated slowly can be given once or twice daily. With repeated dosing, the concentration in the plasma climbs until a more or less steady level is obtained. This is termed *steady state* (Fig. 1.6). The time taken to reach steady state is approximately five times the half-life of the drug. For example, the half-life of digoxin is 36 hours so steady state for digoxin given regularly will be reached in 36 x 5 = 180 hours.

It can be seen that the shorter the half-life (i.e. the quicker the elimination) of a drug, the more rapidly will it reach steady state. In order to hasten the achievement of steady state and full therapeutic effect with more slowly excreted

drugs, a large *loading dose* may be given followed by smaller maintenance doses (see Fig. 1.6).

Dose response

In general the response to a drug is related to the dose; an increased dose leads to a greater response. If the log of the dose is plotted against the response (Fig. 1.7) most drugs show a sigmoid curve.

With the majority of drugs, when used therapeutically, the dose/response is on the steep part of the curve, i.e. increased dose → increased effect. However, with some drugs, for example the analgesic buprenorphine, the dose/response is towards the upper end of the curve so that increasing the dose beyond a certain level does not enhance the therapeutic effect of the drug.

SOME FACTORS WHICH MAY MODIFY DRUG RESPONSE

There are a number of variables that can influence drug response. It is true that the pharmacological action of a drug rarely differs between subjects, but the intensity and duration of that action often differs considerably.

This may occur for two main reasons:

1. Because the concentration of the drug within the body, and thus its intensity of action, is subject to interindividual variation.
2. Because the sensitivity and responsiveness of receptor mechanisms involved in drug action may differ between subjects.

Although many of these interindividual differences in drug response are not large enough to be

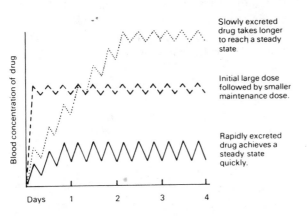

Fig. 1.6 Steady state concentrations of drugs.

of practical importance, with some drugs, particularly if there is only a narrow margin between toxicity and therapeutic effect, such variations in response may represent the difference between success and disaster and therefore some knowledge of the factors involved is useful to the nurse and they are discussed below.

Size of the patient

This can be expressed either in terms of body weight or body surface area. It is obvious that when a drug, after absorption, is distributed throughout the body, the larger that body (and thus the volume of distribution) the lower will be the concentration of a given dose of a drug and the less intense will be its actions.

In order to correct for variations due to differences in weight the dose may be expressed as:

Dose per kilogram weight of the patient.

Example: For a patient weighing 60 kilograms and the dose being 10 mg/kg

Dose = 60 x 10 = 600 mg

Even greater accuracy can be achieved by relating the dose to the surface area of the patient, this being derived from the patient's height and weight. The dose is then expressed as:

Dose per square metre of body surface area.

This removes as far as possible variation in response due to differences in patient size.

Age of the patient

There are considerable variations in response related to age, due to difference in patient size and to other factors and these are considered in Chapter 21, page 255.

Genetic factors

There are a number of inherited variations in drug response largely related to differences in drug elimination. Many drugs are broken down by enzymes (usually in the liver) and this terminates their actions. It is now believed that there are considerable interperson differences in the activity of these enzymes.

With certain drugs it is possible to distinguish between two populations of people: one group with a highly active enzyme system which is able to break down the drug rapidly and the other with a less active system and relatively slower breakdown of the drug. This type of genetic variation, where two populations can exist which differ in the metabolism of a drug, is known as *genetic polymorphism*.

Example

A number of important drugs including isoniazid (p. 205), sulphonamides (p. 197) and hydralazine (p. 58) are inactivated by acetylation, a process involving enzyme action. In the UK 40% of the population are fast acetylators (with highly active acetylator enzymes) and 60% are slow acetylators. This is an inherited characteristic and the ratio of fast/slow acetylators varies in different parts of the world—100% of Canadian Eskimos are rapid acetylators whereas 80% of Egyptians are slow acetylators.

Difference in acetylator status does not usually matter in the UK, except when high doses of the drugs are being used when there is a slightly increased risk of toxic effects in subjects who are slow acetylators. In the Third World where, for reasons of expense, very minimal doses may be necessary, for example, isoniazid in the treatment of tuberculosis, those who are rapid acetylators may suffer some falling-off of therapeutic efficacy.

Another example of genetic polymorphism is deficiency in the enzyme glucose 6 phosphate dehydrogenase (G6PD). This involves largely Africans and Indians affecting about 100 million people. It is due to an abnormal enzyme in the red blood cells and results in the breakdown of these cells when exposed to certain substances:

- quinine
- sulphonamides
- broad beans
- chloroquine
- chloramphenicol.

There are many other examples of inherited differences in response to drugs and some are still being discovered.

Nutritional factors

Frank malnutrition can modify response to drugs. Loss of body mass is one factor involved and reduction of enzyme activity which can occur as a result of protein lack, may result in slowed breakdown of drugs. Malnutrition as such is not usual in the UK, but prolonged illness associated perhaps with sepsis and fever can produce very much the same result. Under these circumstances the response to a drug may be greater than expected.

Example

Warfarin (see p. 69) is an anticoagulant which is broken down in the liver by enzymes. Its effect on coagulation is often greater in patients who have suffered a long illness and are in a poor nutritional state and they may require a smaller than usual dose.

Even without malnutrition diet can effect drug response. Vegetarians and heavy smokers both show several differences in enzyme activity which could modify drug response, although the changes are usually too small to cause serious problems.

Race and drug response

The increasing movement of populations means that the nurse may be looking after patients of several ethnic groups and it is becoming apparent that with some drugs different races may show differing sensitivities. For instance, it has been shown that in America the β blocker propranolol is less effective in lowering blood pressure in black than in white subjects. These differences could be due to:

1. Genetic differences in drug metabolizing enzymes leading to variations in the blood levels achieved.

2. Different lifestyles (e.g. diet) which could also alter the metabolizing enzymes.

3. Differences in the actual response to the drug.

At present very little is known about the problem and with many drugs it is probably unimportant, but it provides an interesting field for further research.

Intercurrent illness

This may both *modify drug elimination* and *affect receptor sensitivity* and is an important cause of altered response to a drug.

Most drugs are either broken down by the liver or excreted by the kidneys, so disease of these organs with diminished function can lead to accumulation of the drug with a more intense and prolonged action which can reach dangerous proportions.

Example

Morphine when given to a patient with cirrhosis of the liver has a more marked and prolonged effect than normal, and dangerous depression of respiration can develop.

Normally morphine is broken down in the liver; in cirrhosis distortion of the normal anatomy, so that blood bypasses the liver, and loss of liver cells both result in decreased enzyme activity, and thus accumulation of morphine.

It is not always necessary for there to be liver damage for drug metabolism to be altered. In heart failure the blood flow through the liver is reduced and this alone may be sufficient to reduce appreciably the breakdown of drugs.

Example

Lignocaine (p. 49) is used to treat cardiac arrhythmias, particularly after myocardial infarction; it is broken down by the liver. If it is given to patients with heart failure (a not uncommon happening) then its elimination is slowed and toxicity will result if the dose is not reduced.

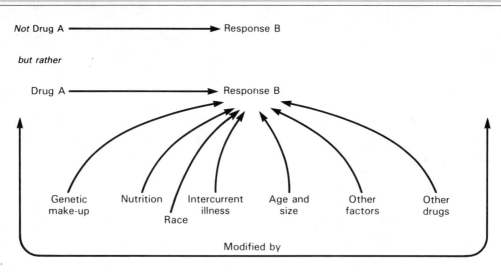

Fig. 1.8

Kidney function may also modify drug response.

Example

Gentamicin (see p. 204) is excreted by the kidneys and when renal function is reduced serious accumulation occurs with normal dosage. This is why careful monitoring of blood levels with subsequent modification of doses is required when gentamicin is given, particularly in renal disease.

Receptor sensitivity may also be affected by disease.

Example

In chronic respiratory disease, because the respiratory centre is chronically short of oxygen, it becomes very sensitive to the depressing effect of morphine and normal doses can result in severe respiratory depression.

Drug interactions

One drug can modify the response to another drug in a number of different ways. This is discussed on page 266.

Other factors including psychological ones may also be important in drug response. Expec-

tation of a successful outcome may appear to improve the results of treatment, for example analgesics are more effective if ignorance and fear are dispelled.

Thus the response of a patient to a particular drug should be looked at as shown in Figure 1.8.

Choosing and adjusting the dose

Most drugs are given in doses which have been found by experience to be satisfactory, although the dose may be modified by the factors discussed above. In the light of the clinical response some alterations may be needed (e.g. the dose of hypotensive drugs is adjusted until a satisfactory fall in blood pressure is achieved). With a few drugs e.g. phenytoin, lithium, the aminoglycoside antibiotics) *repeated measurements of the plasma concentration* are required and the dose is adjusted to obtain a safe and therapeutically effective level.

THE ADMINISTRATION OF DRUGS

Drugs are given in many ways and as this is often the duty of the nurse the methods are considered in detail (Fig. 1.9) and in Chapter 2.

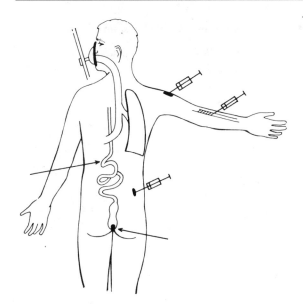

Fig. 1.9 Methods of administration of drugs.

ORALLY

The easiest and most usual way to give medicines is by mouth and there are many formulations for this purpose.

Tablets are prepared by mixing a drug with a base which binds it together. They are usually coated with sugar and some colouring material.

Capsules are made of gelatin or some similar substance and contain a drug which is liberated when the wall of the capsule is digested in the stomach or intestine.

The actual formulation of tablets and capsules is very important and determines how satisfactorily the drug is released. This governs its absorption and bioavailability. A great deal of care is taken in the manufacture of tablets to ensure the maximum bioavailability. It is also possible, by coating the tablets, by modifying the capsule or by binding the drug to some inert substance, to slow down the release of the active ingredient and thus prolong its absorption and effect.

Mixtures are liquids which contain several ingredients dissolved or diffused in water or some other solvent.

An emulsion is a mixture of two liquids in which one is dispersed through the other in a finely divided state.

A linctus is a liquid which contains some sweet syrupy substance used for its soothing effect on coughs.

When liquid medicines are prescribed they are accompanied by the British Standard oral syringe which should be used to draw up the fluid to achieve the exact dose. The use of the syringe reduces the risk of dosing errors which were common when such medicines were supplied with a standard 5 ml plastic spoon. The syringe is issued with a manufacturer's information leaflet advising on use and storage, but verbal explanations are still valuable, especially as liquid medicines are usually given to children and frequently administered by anxious parents. Families appreciate practical demonstrations of the use of the syringe provided by the nurse.

The absorption of oral medicines is affected by several factors other than drug formulation.

Food. If a drug is taken with or after a meal it is absorbed more slowly. This is due to delayed emptying of the stomach where little absorption occurs and because certain drugs become temporarily bound to food. When a rapid effect is required it should be given on an empty stomach. Drugs which may irritate the stomach should be given with food.

Rate of gastric emptying and drug interactions. Gastric emptying may be affected by drugs and this may modify absorption. For instance, atropine-like drugs delay gastric emptying whereas metoclopramide, which is often used for nausea, actually increases the speed of gastric emptying and thus the rate of absorption. If drugs are given together they may bind to each other and prevent absorption although this is a rare occurrence and, in practice, several different types of drug may be given at the same time.

BY INJECTION

Injections may be given *intravenously, intramuscularly, subcutaneously, intradermally* or into various body cavities such as the pleura or peritoneum, or into the spinal theca.

The intravenous route has the advantage of rapid action, complete bioavailability and it can be used for drugs too irritant to be given intramuscularly. However, it is technically more difficult and an inadvertent intra-arterial injection can cause arterial spasm with resulting tissue damage. Today, some drugs, particularly analgesics are given via an intravenous syringe-driver pump (see p. 101). These can be used by the patient at home as well as in hospital.

Intramuscular injection is easier. Absorption from the injection site is variable, being greatest from the deltoid and least from the buttock. It depends on muscle blood flow and is increased by exercise and rubbing the injection site and reduced in shock. Slow release formulations but available for a prolonged effect. Injection can be painful and 5 ml is the maximum acceptable volume. Rarely, it may result in abscess formation.

Subcutaneous injection is widely used. Absorption is lower than after intramuscular injection and is again influenced by local blood flow, being increased with exercise and decreased in shock. When a marked local effect is required (e.g. in local anaesthetics) a vasoconstrictor is added to the injection to prevent the drug being absorbed away from the injection site.

RECTALLY

Certain drugs are absorbed from the rectum and may be given as suppositories or enemata.

BY INHALATION

Drugs may be inhaled either to produce a local action on the respiratory tract or because they are absorbed via the lungs and produce a general effect.

BY LOCAL APPLICATION

Drugs are applied locally as *lotions, liniments, ointments* or *creams* (see p. 291) to the skin, mucous membranes and wound surfaces and produce their action at the site of application.

TRANSDERMAL APPLICATION

A number of drugs can be absorbed effectively via the skin. This is useful not only in the treatment of skin diseases but in some cases, where absorption is sufficient, in producing systemic actions.

The drug is applied to the skin as a plastic patch held in a container which releases it at a constant rate. There are regional variations in skin permeability: for example, the very thick skin of the palms or soles would not allow efficient absorption even if these were convenient locations. Patches are usually applied to clean, unbroken skin on the trunk or the post-auricular area (behind the ear) where good vascularity enhances uptake. Examples of drugs which can be administered in this way include:

1. Glyceryl trinitrate for angina
2. Hyoscine for motion sickness
3. Oestrogens for hormone replacement therapy.

Advantages. One patch may be effective for a relatively long period so replacement can be made infrequently.

Disadvantages. Absorption can be variable. Occasionally there may be skin reactions. If these occur, simply removing the patch will not halt the reaction immediately, as the drug that has been absorbed will continue to act for some time, depending on its nature and dose.

HOW ARE DRUGS OBTAINED?

Most drugs are made chemically in the laboratory or factory. Some, such as benzylpenicillin, are extracted from natural substances, though they may be modified chemically to make them more effective.

Certain substances which occur naturally (such as hormones) are proteins with a very complex structure. They are difficult to synthesize chemically and extraction from animals may be unsatisfactory and expensive and, in addition, if obtained from animal sources may not be identical to those found in man. This problem is now being solved by *genetic pharmacy*.

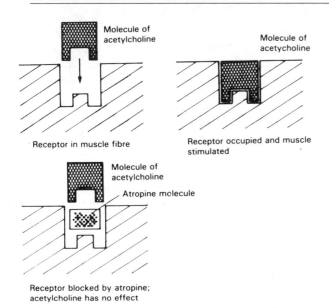

Fig. 1.10 Stimulation of muscle by acetylcholine showing occupation of the receptor by the drug. After atropine the receptor site is blocked and no stimulation occurs.

The gene responsible for the production of a complex protein is isolated from human cells and inserted into other vector (carrier) cells (such as the bacterium *Esch. coli*) which divide rapidly and are manipulated to produce the required protein in large quantities. This method is responsible for the production of several protein hormones such as human insulin and erythropoietin. Similar techniques offer great possibilities in the future.

HOW DO DRUGS WORK?

In spite of a great deal of research it is still not known how some drugs produce their effect but it is possible to describe the way in which some of them act.

1. The receptor theory. It is believed that the cells in certain tissues contain structures called receptors. These combine with substances which are produced naturally in the body and the cells are stimulated, the contraction of muscle fibres produced by acetylcholine being an example. The drug is thought to fit onto a receptor rather as a key fits a lock. It may then either stimulate the receptor and produce an effect similar to that of the naturally occurring substances or it may occupy the receptor without producing any effect by preventing any naturally occurring stimulation. The blocking of acetylcholine by atropine is a good example (Fig. 1.10).

2. Antimetabolites. These drugs closely resemble substances which are used by the cells for nutrition and when absorbed, the cells cannot use them and so fail to multiply. The sulphonamides which are used to stop the multiplication of bacteria are a good example. They are very similar in structure to para-aminobenzoic acid and certain bacteria cannot distinguish between them, and absorb the sulphonamides and stop multiplying.

3. Enzyme inhibitors. Enzymes are substances which speed up many chemical processes within the body. Some of these enzyme-activated processes are concerned with the transport of chemicals in and out of the cells. Certain drugs have the property of inhibiting their action and thus interfere with some of these processes. Diuretics are a good example as normally salt and water are transported out of the renal tubule back into the body, but this action requires enzymes and if they are inhibited by a diuretic, salt and water are not reabsorbed and pass out of the kidney with a resulting diuresis.

4. Action on cell membranes. The function of nerves and muscles depends on ions passing across the membranes surrounding these cells. Certain drugs interfere with the movement of these ions and thus prevent nerve or muscle function, as demonstrated by local anaesthetics which block impulses passing up a sensory nerve.

5. Replacement of deficiencies. In some diseases there is a deficiency of a substance which is necessary for the body to function normally. This may be a hormone (see p. 155) or some essential dietary factor such as a vitamin (see p. 235). By replacing the deficiency the disease can be controlled but the replacement drug will usually need to be taken for the rest of the patient's life.

6. Cytotoxic effect. Drugs may be used to kill bacteria or malignant cells without undue change to the patient's cells. The way this is brought about varies between drugs.

These are just a few of the ways in which drugs may work. It is probable that all drug action depends on their interference with cell activity, and when more is known about the processes within the cell, then more will be discovered about how they work.

FURTHER READING

Brodie M J 1988 Pharmacokinetics for the prescriber. Medicine International 59: 2408
Feeley J, Brodie M 1988 Practical clinical pharmacology. British Medical Journal 296: 1046
George C F 1984 Food, drugs and bioavailability. British Medical Journal 289: 1093
Holmes S 1986 Nutritional needs of medical patients. Nursing Times 82: 17, 34
Mucklow J C 1989 Accumulation. Prescribers Journal 29: 36
Rawlings M D 1988 Pharmacogenetics. Prescribers Journal 28: 64
Rogers H J, Spector R 1993 Aids to clinical pharmacology and therapeutics, 3rd edn. Churchill Livingstone, Edinburgh

2

The role of the nurse in drug administration

Drug therapy plays a major part in the treatment of patients and, although prescribed by the doctor, it is the responsibility of the nurse in hospital or the community to ensure safe and reliable administration and also to help with the monitoring of effects. The patient needs to understand the purpose of the therapy in order to comply and the nurse, by her regular contact, is in a unique position to help him/her achieve this.

The nurse must be aware that his or her responsibilities in giving drugs are governed by the Misuse of Drugs Act 1971, for Controlled Drugs, and the Medicines Act 1968, for Prescription Only Medicines, together with additional regulations formulated by individual Health Authorities. All health districts have their procedures and policies. The UKCC code of conduct, in laying down the general responsibilities of the nurse, stipulates that his or her actions should put the patient's safety and well-being first at all times.

In hospital, the custody and administration of drugs is the responsibility of the ward sister/charge nurse who may delegate this responsibility as instructed by the employing authority's policy. Although it is usual for a qualified nurse to give drugs, with a second nurse checking to prevent error, the UKCC takes the view that registered nurses should be seen as competent to administer drugs on their own and be responsible for their actions. Learner nurses will take part in drug administration and senior learner nurses who have shown competence may be allowed to act as the senior person giving drugs. Intravenous drugs must also be given by two nurses, the senior of whom must be qualified and certified to do so. Requirements will vary between employing authorities and if a qualified nurse moves she must obtain a certificate for the new district. The status of the person checking the drug will also be designated by the employing authority. Nurses' actions in relation to drug administration will be legally covered by the employing authority when the rules are followed.

The prescription

In hospital it is normal practice for all drugs to be prescribed. This enables the pharmacist to supply them and instruct the nurse in their administration. The prescription sheet which is a primary document in the case records must be headed with the patient's full name, age, number and ward. The prescription must be clearly and indelibly written and must contain the date, the approved name of the drug (preferably in block letters), the dose (using metric dosage), the route and frequency of administration with the validity period and signature of the medical practitioner. If any of these details are omitted the drug should not be given until amended. Frequency of dosage can be ordered by filling in allocated time spaces rather than using Latin abbreviations. Administration is recorded by initialling the relevant box on the prescription sheet. The exact format of this sheet will vary between districts, and nurses must familiarize themselves with documents in use when moving to a new district. On no account should a nurse write or alter a prescription.

Controlled drugs

In hospital Controlled Drugs (see p. 314) must always be given by two people and it is common practice for one to be a qualified nurse. Both nurses must sign the book following each administration *at the bedside* or *in the presence of the patient*. The prescription requires the number of doses in words and figures. An additional record is kept in a specially designed book so that every tablet or ampoule is accounted for when used, both nurses signing the book following each administration. The Controlled Drug Record Book is retained on the ward for 2 years after the date of the last entry. These are legal requirements for controlled drugs but some hospitals apply similar rules to other drugs liable to misuse.

Nursing aspects of administration

In the community most patients, or some member of the family, are responsible for drug administration although the district nurse or health visitor may have a role to play. Today, many people are discharged within a few days or hours of surgery while the average length of stay for medical patients has also been reduced. People returning home are often still taking drugs which until recently would have been given only within the confines of a hospital, so monitoring for adverse effects is an increasingly important aspect of the community nurse's role. The nurse must also be aware that some drugs, even if stopped before discharge, may still exert an action or cause side-effects.

The nurse is responsible for interpreting the prescription accurately, recording that the drug has been given and observing the patient's response. Prior to administration the nurse must know the reason for, action and usual dosage of the drug; this should enable her to recognize and question mistakes in prescribing. When in doubt about a prescription, advice should be sought and, if necessary, the doctor should be consulted. Observations should be made for therapeutic and adverse effects. The nurse should realize that the patient's condition may alter the effect of a drug and that there may be interactions with concurrent therapy. The nurse is greatly assisted in these circumstances by the ward pharmacist with whom a good working relationship will enhance safety of patient care.

The Committee on Safety of Medicines requests that adverse reactions be reported (yellow cards) and in addition, may require that a special watch be kept on certain preparations (see p. 269).

WARD ADMINISTRATION OF DRUGS

Drugs may be given to the whole ward by the same nurses or to a smaller group of patients by those directly involved in their care. The second method is preferable as timing is more accurate and the nurse will know the patients well and can cater for individual needs such as difficulty in swallowing medication. Time can be spent teaching patients about their medication and learner nurses can take part to gain experience in relating medication to the patient's condition. In some hospitals experimental schemes have involved patients being responsible for their own medication, particularly if they need to take the same drugs when they go home. On the whole these have been successful and provided valuable opportunities for patient education. Where members of the family will be giving drugs they can be invited to the ward at the appropriate time to practise a technique (such as giving an injection) or to ask about any anticipated problems. An innovative approach on some wards has been in the timing of drug rounds so that medicines can be given nearer the time patients would take them at home. Many people have taken their drugs at home for years and may be upset by altered timing in hospital. Many schemes have abolished the early morning drug round to give patients longer to sleep.

For a few drugs flexibility is not possible; antibiotics are more effective if doses are spread evenly throughout the day, and insulin must be given before meals. Others such as NSAIAs are best given with or after food.

Whichever approach is taken specific rules of drug administration must be followed to obviate error. The underlying principles, to give the correct dose of the prescribed drug to the right patient, by the right route, at the right time, require the nurse's undivided attention. When two nurses are involved, instructions should be read aloud.

1. Read the patient's full name from the prescription sheet.
2. Read the prescription, checking validity and time of last administration.
3. Read name of drug from label when removing container from shelf.
4. Check the label of the container for name, strength and dose of the drug, route of administration where relevant and expiry date against the prescription.
5. Measure or count the correct dose. Avoid contact with the drug as allergies can develop particularly if the hands are damp.

When measuring liquids, shake the bottle, hold the measure at eye level placing the thumbnail on the meniscus and pour from the back of the bottle to keep the label clean. A calibrated measure should be used. When a fractional dose is required calculations should be made independently before checking the dose.
6. Re-check the label before returning the container to the shelf.
7. Both nurses must verify the patient's identity by checking the details on the prescription sheet with the patient's identity bracelet. If this is absent, ask the patient to state his full name. If this is not possible identification must be confirmed by a member of his family or permanent staff.
8. Ensure the patient is in a fit state to receive the drug.
9. Give the dose and see that it has been swallowed.
10. Record the administration. Also record when a drug is not given and the reason.

Additional points. Patients who refuse to take a drug or show doubt or anxiety may have a good reason which will become apparent if the nurse takes time to listen to them.

Safety factors

- Do not leave the drug trolley unattended.
- Do not give drugs from memory, a prescription sheet must always be used.
- Do not give a drug from a container that is not correctly labelled.
- Do not give a drug prepared by anyone else.
- Do not return an unused dose to a stock bottle.
- Unused drugs may be returned to the pharmacy where they will be checked and used

for another patient. Drugs returned by out-patients should be destroyed.

Aids to taking oral drugs

Ensure the patient is sitting up whenever possible to facilitate swallowing.

Prepare a drink before giving the drug, and see that an adequate amount of fluid is taken with the drug to prevent oesophageal irritation/ulceration.

Liquid preparations are given via a British Standard oral syringe. Soluble tablets should be dissolved completely before presenting them. If a patient has difficulty holding a tablet it should be introduced on a spoon.

If a patient has difficulty swallowing a tablet, remove it, give a drink and try again. Many drugs can be prepared and given in liquid form if necessary.

If a drug tastes unpleasant it may be followed by a flavoured drink or mouthwash.

Although many drugs will be given orally the nurse will also administer them by the rectal and vaginal routes and by injection. In all cases the above rules must be followed.

Rectal drugs

These are given in suppository form using protective gloves and a small amount of lubricant to ease insertion. It is important that the method is explained to the patient beforehand and that correct positioning is used with the patient lying on the left side with hips and knees flexed. It has been shown that insertion of the blunt end of the suppository aids comfort and retention.

Long-term therapy may be given by this route in which case patients can be taught self-administration most effectively.

Vaginal drugs

Vaginal pessaries and creams are inserted with the patient lying on her side or back. Clean (rather than sterile) gloves are satisfactory except after delivery. A lubricant is used and the drug inserted into the posterior fornix of the vagina. In some circumstances a pad may be worn after insertion as leakage can occur. Again, patients can be instructed on self-medication by this method. Pessaries are best inserted last thing at night as they tend to become dislodged.

Injections

The nurse will be responsible for giving drugs by intradermal, subcutaneous and intramuscular routes. In certain circumstances trained nurses will give drugs intravenously through an established route. Fractional dosage may be required in these circumstances and careful calculation is vital as errors in dose measurement can occur, the danger of this being compounded by the more rapid action of drugs by injection. When giving injections, sterile equipment must be used and strict aseptic technique observed. Cleansing of the skin with an alcohol swab is still commonly used but the benefits of this are questionable. However, where the skin is contaminated or the balance of flora changed as in debilitated patients it may be necessary. If used, the alcohol should be allowed to dry before inserting the needle. In most circumstances the site is massaged after removing the needle to aid absorption of the drug.

Intradermal injection. The two most common reasons for giving intradermal injections are testing for sensitivity to allergens and immunization. In the former situation there is a risk of an anaphylactic reaction so adrenaline should be readily available. A very small amount of fluid (0.1 ml or less) is given using a 1 ml syringe graduated in 0.1 ml divisions through a short fine needle (26 gauge x $\frac{3}{8}$ in; see Fig. 2.1). This is introduced just under the skin at an angle of 10–15° which will raise a small weal. The area should not be massaged after removing the needle. The usual site of injection is the lightly pigmented area of the forearm where the reaction can be easily observed.

Subcutaneous injection. A subcutaneous injection is given into the fatty layer just under the

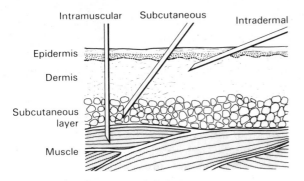

Fig. 2.1 The position of the needle for intramuscular, subcutaneous and intradermal injections.

skin (see Fig. 2.1). Small amounts of fluid are injected (0.5–2 ml) using a 25 gauge x $^{15}/_{16}$ inch needle. A fold of skin is raised between the thumb and forefinger and the needle is inserted at an angle of 45° (see Fig. 2.1). After insertion the plunger is withdrawn slightly to ensure a blood vessel has not been entered. If this occurs the needle should be removed, pressure applied to the area and a new injection prepared. For injections of heparin and insulin shorter needles are used. These may be the very short fine needles integral with insulin syringes or 25 gauge x $^{5}/_{8}$ needles. In these instances the needle enters the skin at 90°. The area is not massaged after withdrawing the needle but firm pressure is used to prevent haematoma formation when heparin is given and to ensure uniform absorption rates in diabetic patients. Other modifications which may be made when giving insulin are discussed on page 172.

The usual sites for subcutaneous injections are the outer aspect of the upper arm, the outer aspect of the upper thigh and the skin of the abdominal wall (Fig. 2.2).

Intramuscular injection. This is given into muscle so larger amounts can be injected, 1–5 ml (Fig. 2.3). The best site is the outer aspect of the thigh, locating the area in the middle third of the space between the knee and greater trochanter of the femur. The upper outer quadrant of the buttock is also used (Fig. 2.3). It is vital to determine the sites carefully to avoid damage to the sciatic nerve and major blood vessels. Alter-

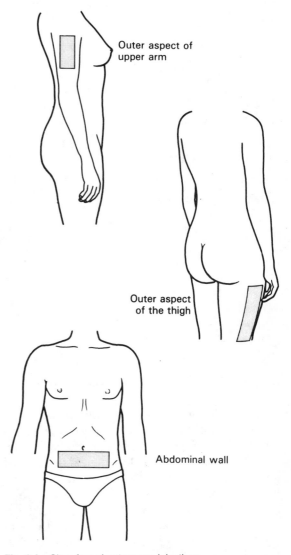

Fig. 2.2 Sites for subcutaneous injections.

natively the upper outer aspect of the arm may be used if the muscle is big enough. To aid relaxation the patient should be positioned comfortably; for buttock injections either lying on the abdomen with the toes turned in or lying on the side with the lower leg extended and the upper leg flexed. For thigh injections the limb should be slightly flexed and supported.

When preparing injections care should be taken to prevent skin contamination as contact dermatitis can occur. Gloves may be worn in

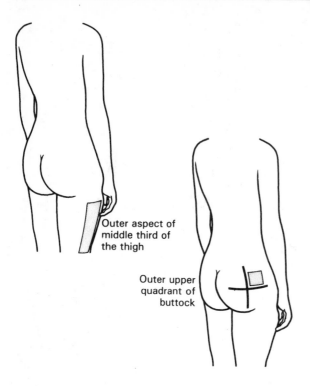

Outer aspect of
middle third of
the thigh

Outer upper
quadrant of
buttock

Fig. 2.3 Sites for intramuscular injections.

some circumstances and the hands washed thoroughly after completion of the procedure. Drugs which may cause this reaction are penicillin, the aminoglycosides and chlorpromazine. Special precautions are taken when using cytotoxic drugs (see p. 250). When giving an intramuscular injection the skin is held taut and a 21 gauge x $1\frac{1}{2}$ inch needle introduced at 90° (Fig. 2.1). As in the subcutaneous technique the plunger is withdrawn to check for inadvertent puncturing of a blood vessel. The fluid is then injected slowly, the needle withdrawn quickly, pressure applied initially and then the area massaged gently.

When injecting substances such as iron, which cause skin discoloration, the Z track method can be used. In this technique the skin is pulled to one side before inserting the needle, a few seconds are allowed to elapse before it is withdrawn, at which point the skin is released thus achieving the Z track.

Intravenous injections and additives. It has been estimated that 12% of patients have an intravenous infusion at some time during their stay in hospital usually for one or more of the following reasons: fluid replacement therapy, drug therapy, monitoring central venous pressure, hyperalimentation or to provide emergency access to a vein. Responsibility for drug administration by the intravenous route is now becoming part of the nurse's extended role, although in most health districts it is necessary to have attended a special training course and received a certificate of competence, which may not be valid in another institution. The intravenous route is most often used for heparin, cytotoxic agents and antibiotics. Individual drugs may be given as a bolus or added to the infusion fluid, in which case careful mixing and labelling are vital and it is important to check that drugs do not interact with each other in the infusion bottle. Intravenous drugs need very careful monitoring and the nurse requires an adequate knowledge of potential side-effects. It is therefore essential that learner nurses involved in checking and observing the effects of drugs given by this route are closely supervised. When the flow rate is mechanically controlled it is still necessary to check independently that the correct dose is being delivered. Any adjustment to dosage must only be undertaken by the trained nurse.

Infection is a known hazard of intravenous cannulation and is increased when drugs or additives are given because the apparatus will be handled more often. Patients must therefore be observed for signs of local infection at the site of the cannula and their temperature monitored carefully. Continuous infusion of drugs by an infusion apparatus is not very accurate although the use of a paediatric volume control administration device will render the flow rate more easily controllable.

60 microdrops (Soluset) = 1 ml
20 macrodrops (standard giving set) = 1 ml

For more satisfactory and accurate dosage an infusion pump should be used.

Giving drugs to children

Obtaining cooperation from children is very important and simple, honest explanation helps to achieve this. Children are more likely to take drugs from a familiar person and where appropriate, parents and relatives can actually give drugs observed by the nurses who have prepared the medication. As paediatric dosage is so different from that of adults it is important for nurses familiar with children's care to be involved in checking drugs, adhering to local policies. Fractional dosage is used and needs careful calculation to avoid error. Most drugs are given in liquid form. For very young children a medicine dispenser is useful. This is a special 1 ml syringe into which the required dosage is drawn via a special bottle adaptor. With the child sitting up, the dispenser is inserted into its mouth with the tip pointing to the inside of the cheek and the plunger is depressed slowly allowing the drug to be swallowed naturally. For older children a special graduated syringe is used. Medicines should not be given in milk or food and it is important to praise the child for taking them.

Giving drugs to the elderly

Many elderly patients dislike taking oral drugs and to overcome this, adequate time should be taken for simple explanation. If swallowing tablets proves difficult it may be possible to prescribe the drug in liquid form or to use semi-solids such as ice-cream as a vehicle for introducing medication. If there is doubt as to whether it has been swallowed, inspection of the mouth may be needed.

COMPLIANCE AND EDUCATION

In the past, giving drugs usually involved only passive participation by the patient with little information being offered unless it was requested. There is increasing evidence that adequate explanation to the patient increases the likelihood of adherence to a prescribed course of treatment. In order to comply, an understanding and acceptance of the treatment is vital; failure to do so may be unintentional due to lapse of memory or deliberate, when timing and dosage may be altered by the patient. Studies show that non-compliance is a major problem resulting in

omission or repetition of drug therapy which may require readmission to hospital. Unused drugs may be a potential danger to patients and relatives, increasing the risk of deliberate or accidental self-poisoning.

Education of the patient with regard to drug therapy is the responsibility of doctor, pharmacist and nurse. However, this also applies to educating other health care professionals such as social workers, occupational therapists, physiotherapists, non-professional carers and the general public in order to improve overall understanding of the significance of the proper use of drugs as a part of treatment.

In hospital the nurse is in an expedient position to fulfil this role by being the person primarily involved in drug administration and having continued contact with the patient. The aim of teaching is to help the patient to gain insight into the way drugs can be used to treat his/her condition. Implicit in this is the nurse's knowledge of the disease process and drug action. Answering patients' questions will impart a certain amount of information but this must be accompanied by a more structured approach.

Teaching begins on the patient's admission when an understanding of his/her present therapy should be established. Poor literacy or language difficulties impede comprehension and any problems elicited will need sensitive discussion. Anxiety about the harmful effects of chemicals and addiction to drugs may concern some patients and will hinder learning if not overcome it. It is also important to ascertain whether any regular self-medication is occurring as this may influence the action of prescribed drugs, e.g. the use of antacids concurrently with tetracycline reducing absorption rates.

At this time drugs brought in by the patient are seen by the doctor and permission gained, if possible, to dispose of them, explaining the dangers of error if a different regimen is prescribed on discharge. Teaching should continue during the hospital stay. It is common practice for the patient to be given brief, rather hurried instructions on drug therapy when being handed the bottles of drugs immediately before leaving the ward. At this time motivation and concentration may be low as the patient is more concerned with going home.

Teaching in preparation for discharge

People vary as to the amount of information they need so it must be tailored to individual requirements but should include the following:

1. The name and purpose of the drug stressing its positive effects.
2. Frequency and timing of administration according to home routine including advice about 'as required' medications.
3. Method of administration with special explanation and equipment for routes other than oral.
4. Proposed length of therapy—short- or long-term.
5. The importance of not stopping or starting drugs without advice and where to obtain that advice.
6. How to obtain further supplies and safely dispose of unwanted drugs.
7. Adverse effects to be reported and how to carry out special tests and observations to show if they are developing. The aim is to give adequate information without causing unnecessary alarm. Most drugs produce side-effects some of which are minor but others are potentially serious. In some cases it may be possible to advise on the relief of side-effects. If sufficient information is not given patients may just stop taking the drugs rather than report the adverse effects, or they may stop treatment when symptoms subside as perhaps in the case of antibiotic therapy. A well-informed patient able to participate in his/her own care will feel more in control and thus more responsible, contributing to compliance.

Teaching should continue during the stay in hospital and should *include members of the patient's family as appropriate*.

Some wards have experimented with schemes in which patients, under supervision, are responsible for their own drug administration. There is also evidence that a simple explanatory booklet given to patients on discharge reinforces teaching. Patients taking such drugs as steroids or anticoagulants should be given a card with information about dosage, etc.

Missed doses

The above discussion should have emphasized the importance of taking medicines in the correct dose, via the correct route and following particular instructions. It will also have highlighted the problem of non-compliance which continues to be a major stumbling block in therapeutics. In hospital the nurse is in a strong position to influence patient compliance and to provide explanations and allay anxieties as they occur. Time spent listening to patients' points of view and exploring their concerns is helpful to both nurses and patients.

In the community patients are more likely to be left alone to cope with their medication and, often, non-compliance occurs through forgetfulness or misunderstanding.

As nurse prescribing becomes a reality those in a position to influence which drugs and doses patients should take must remember:

1. It is sensible to choose medicines whose efficacy is unlikely to be affected by the occasional missed dose.
2. Drugs should not be used at the limits of their duration of action—a drug with an intermediate duration of action is more efficacious if taken twice daily rather than stretched to once daily by taking a higher dose.
3. Drugs that are eliminated slowly and accumulate in the body are least impaired by poor compliance.

Additional useful points

1. Drugs prescribed for others should not be taken even if the problems appear similar.
2. Drugs may deteriorate from moisture if kept in bathroom cabinets.
3. Different drugs should not be put in the same container as errors may occur. The drugs may interact chemically.
4. All drugs should be kept out of the reach of

children, preferably in a locked cupboard. They should never be referred to as 'sweets'.

Special problems of compliance may be found in patients with memory impairment, defects of sight or hearing and those with physical handicaps which interfere with mobility and dexterity. The elderly also form a group at particular risk as many of these problems may exist in one patient. Another group with special needs are those suffering from diabetes or other endocrine disorders, psychiatric disorders, hypertension and tuberculosis, for whom long-term therapy is necessary. Some of the drugs may be unpleasant to take, may affect the whole way of life of the patient or give rise to particularly unpleasant side-effects. In these situations on-going educational support is essential.

In all situations it is useful to have verbal information reinforced by written instruction as it is well known that anxiety limits retention of information. It is especially important that this is done where memory impairment is a feature. Instruction should be kept simple, memory aids such as tear-off calendars and recording cards can be of value. Special dose boxes, e.g. the Dosett pill dispenser, which hold up to 1 week's supply of drugs can be used but may be too complicated for some patients and still require another person to fill them.

Containers need to be labelled with adequate sized lettering and/or colour coding. Information on the label as to the purpose of the drug e.g. 'heart tablets', 'water tablets' may be helpful for the elderly. Braille labels can be used for the blind.

Drug manufacturers could also contribute to compliance by appropriate packaging and presentation of drugs. The container should be easy to open; child-resistant containers are used increasingly but are very difficult for the elderly and those suffering from arthritis to handle. Many people are unaware that ordinary screw-top bottles are available. Caps with wings can be supplied where necessary; the occupational therapist will be able to assess the patient's need and offer other helpful suggestions.

Despite these aids there will still be some patients who are unable to cope with drug ad-ministration independently. In these situations education of other family members, friends, neighbours or 'home-helps' will be necessary. A number of trials of self-administration of drugs in the elderly have been carried out in some parts of the country in preparation for discharge from hospital and to improve compliance. These programmes aim to identify individual patient problems well before discharge but require the total commitment of all staff involved and continued counselling and follow-up in the community. It appears that these programmes have proved useful in training elderly patients and it may be that special self-administration programmes could have a wider application.

NURSE PRESCRIBING

Legislation is going through Parliament which, from 1993, will allow nurses with district nursing or health visitor qualifications to prescribe a limited range of drugs (see Table 2.1); timing and dosage of medicines may be adjusted within a set patient-specific protocol, e.g. drugs for alleviating terminal pain. The medicines which a nurse will be able to prescribe will be detailed in a **Nurses' Formulary** and prescribing will take place in various community settings such as home, health centres and residential accommodation. Following a special training course, nurses may take responsibility for prescribing some over-the-counter drugs, wound and stoma care products and aids for patients with continence problems. Those most likely to benefit are the terminally ill cared for outside hospital, the elderly and disabled, especially those living in remote rural areas who would have to travel considerable distances to their general practitioners. Nurse prescribing is expected to reduce delays in obtaining medication and will increase efficiency by decreasing the administrative burden on GPs. It also has implications for the pharmacist. In many areas good links have been established between health centres and pharmacists and it is vital that these should be maintained and strengthened. An important issue is the practical consideration of information-sharing, records and referral mechanisms, as these involve all members of the health care team.

Breakdown of communication is possible after the patient is discharged from hospital and when

Table 2.1 Items to be included in the Nurses' Formulary

Gastrointestinal system
Laxatives
Isphagula granules
Sterculia
Bisacodyl suppositories
Glycerol suppositories
Lactulose
Phosphate enema
Sodium citrate enema

Stoma care products
Adhesives and adhesive removers
Deodorants
Skin protectives and cleaners

Analgesia
Aspirin
Paracetamol

Anthelmintics
Piperazine

Antifungal agents
Nystatin oral suspension and pastilles
Clotrimoxazole cream

ENT
Sodium hydrogen carbonate eardrops (removal of ear wax)

Urinary tract
Preparations for maintaining indwelling urinary catheters

Mouthwashes and gargles
Hexetidine
Povidone-iodine
Thymol

Skin care
Emollient and barrier creams
Emollient bath additives
Magnesium sulphate paste (for boils)
Skin disinfectants
—aqueous solution of 10% povidone-iodine
—silver nitrate
—sodium chloride
Desloughing agents
—iodosorb
—varidase topical

Anaesthesia
Lignocaine hydrochloride for topical use

Parasitical preparations
All British National Formulary items

medication may be prescribed by more than one person. The new prescribing–dispensing process will mean greater contact between the nurse and pharmacist, especially when problems arise. It has been recommended that prescribing records be stored in the patient's home as district nursing records are already kept. The prescribing record will contain details of previous and current medication, including any additional over-the-counter products and drug allergies. When prescribing, the nurse will need to consider psycho-social as well as physical factors and the need for patient education must be recognized. The record should monitor response to drugs and reasons for discontinuing their use.

Non-prescription drugs

For years social scientists have been interested in the 'sick role' phenomenon and the factors which cause people to decide they are ill and behave accordingly by taking medicines or going to bed. It has also become apparent that some people visit their doctors more frequently than others whilst some diagnose themselves as not ill enough to 'trouble' a doctor or nurse but, nevertheless, take some form of medication. Indeed, few households are without some mild form of analgesic or antiseptic, most people who travel abroad wisely purchase antidiarrhoeal agents and every year large numbers of people dose themselves for coughs, motion sickness and constipation. Health care professionals need to know what the patient is taking and this extends to over-the-counter as well as prescribed drugs. Aspirin is widely available but many people do not realize the full range and potency of its therapeutic effects. Paracetamol, another mild analgesic, can cause severe and fatal liver damage in overdose. Both these drugs are incorporated into numerous proprietary medicines, for example, several forms of Anadin are marketed containing different amounts of aspirin and in some cases paracetamol, with its implications in overdose or if prescribed drugs are needed. *When the nurse assesses the patient on hospital admission or the initial community visit he or she should not only enquire about prescribed drugs but any medication and, if possible, see it*. The commercial preparation 'Lomotil' for diarrhoea contains atropine, which in overdose may cause atropine toxicity or interact with other drugs. Some expectorants induce drowsiness and a few contain appreciable amounts of alcohol. Patients need to be aware of the likely side-effects and actions of these agents as much as of those which are prescribed.

With nurse-prescribing now a reality, a sound knowledge of non-prescription drugs is essential for all who provide care in hospital or the community.

FURTHER READING

Administration of Medicines 1986 United Kingdom Central Council, Advisor Paper, London

Bird C 1990 Drug administration; a prescription for self-help. Nursing Times 24(43): 54–57

Cousins S 1992 Rude awakening: the early drug round. Nursing Times 88(15): 24–28

Crooch J 1985 Medications to take home. The Professional Nurse 1: 15

Department of Health 1989 Report of the Advisory Group on Nurse Prescribing. DoH, London

Drug Administration 1988 A nursing responsibility, 2nd edn. Royal College of Nursing, London

Editorial 1991 Helping patients to make the best use of medicines. Drug and Therapeutics Bulletin 29(1): 1–2

Ernst M A, Buchanan A, Cox C 1991 Drug errors: a judgement of errors. Nursing Times 87(14): 26–30

Gould D 1988 Called to account. Nursing Times 84(12): 28–31

Hassall J 1991 Mutual benefits (drug self-administration). Nursing Times 89(18): 49–50

Hopps L A 1983 Care for patient teaching. Nursing Times 79(49): 42

Jeans A, Taylor D 1992 Stopping the drugs trolley—single nurse administration. Nursing Times 88(2): 27–29

Mathieson A 1986 Old people and drugs. Nursing Times 82(2): 22

Smith F, Ross F 1992 Nurse prescribing: principles of drug therapy. Community Outlook 2(2): 25–29

Walker R 1982 Suppository insertion. World Medicine 18: 58

3

The autonomic nervous system

The autonomic nervous system is that part of the nervous system which supplies the viscera as distinct from the voluntary muscles. The viscera include the gastrointestinal tract, the respiratory and urogenital systems, the heart and blood vessels, the intrinsic muscles of the eyes and various secretory glands.

The autonomic nervous system consists of two divisions and most viscera are supplied by nerves from both these divisions. They are called the *sympathetic* and *parasympathetic* systems and in general it may be said that they have opposite effects on the various viscera which they supply and that they also differ both in their anatomical arrangement and mechanism of function.

ANATOMY

The *sympathetic* system consists of the chain of ganglia lying on either side of the vertebral column and extending from the cervical to the lumbar vertebrae. Sympathetic nerve fibres after passing out from the spinal cord, leave the anterior nerve root and pass to one of these ganglia. Here they form a synapse or junction with further nerve cells whose fibres are distributed to the viscera. Some sympathetic fibres, after leaving the spinal cord pass through the ganglia and form their synapses in ganglia situated peripherally— the group of ganglia surrounding the coeliac artery being a good example of this arrangement.

The *parasympathetic* fibres leave the central nervous system and are distributed with certain

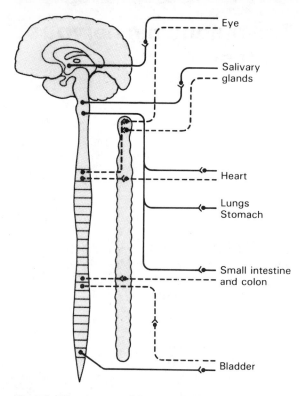

Fig. 3.1 The anatomy of the autonomic nervous system. Sympathetic in broken line, parasympathetic in solid line.

PHYSIOLOGY

Stimulation of a nerve liberates a substance at the nerve ending which activates a receptor in the organ supplied or in another nerve cell. This is known as the *chemical transmission of nerve impulses* and is an important concept because many drugs act by interfering with this process. In the autonomic nervous system transmission occurs in this way in both the sympathetic and parasympathetic divisions but the substances involved differ.

The parasympathetic system (see Fig. 3.2)

Following stimulation of a parasympathetic nerve, a substance called *acetylcholine* is liberated at the nerve ending which acts on a receptor in the organ supplied. To prevent the effect of acetylcholine being too prolonged and powerful there is also present at the nerve ending a substance called *cholinesterase* which rapidly breaks down the acetylcholine and this terminates its effect.

cranial nerves (III, VII, IX and X) and with the sacral nerves.

The relay ganglia of the parasympathetic system are situated peripherally near the organs supplied (Fig. 3.1).

The autonomic system also carries a large number of sensory nerves which supply the various organs. These nerves enter the spinal cord where they may form a spinal reflex arc with the autonomic nerves leaving the cord or they may ascend to the brain where more complex reflexes are built up which may be influenced by impulses arising from the higher levels of the brain. It is a matter of common experience that some visceral sensation may enter consciousness and that events in consciousness may themselves stimulate various visceral effects. The rapid beating of the heart after a fright, being a typical example.

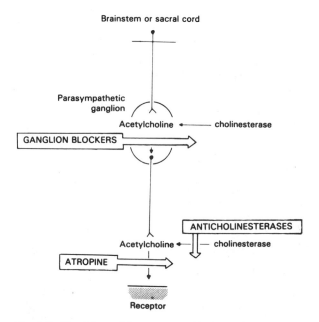

Fig. 3.2 Physiology of the parasympathetic nervous system and its modification by drugs.

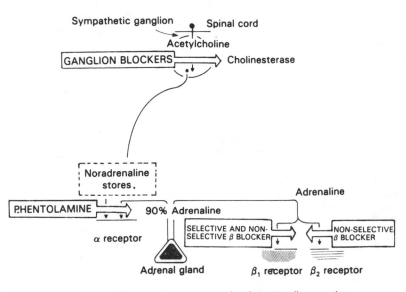

Fig. 3.3 The sympathetic nervous system, showing naturally occurring stimulating agents and drugs which block their action.

The sympathetic system (see Fig. 3.3)

The sympathetic system is rather more complicated because two substances may be liberated and there is more than one type of receptor. The sympathetic nerves release *noradrenaline* from stores at the nerve endings in the peripheral tissues. In addition, the sympathetic system releases *noradrenaline* and *adrenaline* from the medulla of the adrenal glands; these substances enter the blood stream and produce widespread effects. There are several types of sympathetic receptors.

α *receptors* are stimulated by noradrenaline released at sympathetic nerve endings and by adrenaline.

Stimulation produces:

1. Constriction of blood vessels particularly at the skin, causing a rise in blood pressure and reflex slowing of the heart.
2. Dilatation of the pupil.

Stimulation of α receptors is blocked by several drugs (see p. 36).

β_1 *and* β_2 *receptors* (see Figs 3.4 and 3.5) are both stimulated by isoprenaline and adrenaline. In addition noradrenaline acts as a β_1 stimulator on the heart, and the drug salbutamol produces a β_2 response largely on the bronchi. The effects are:

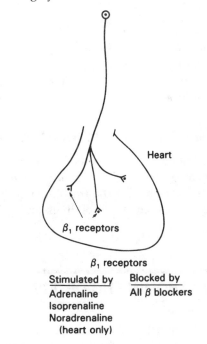

Fig. 3.4 Important β_1 receptors, showing agonists (stimulators) and blocking agents.

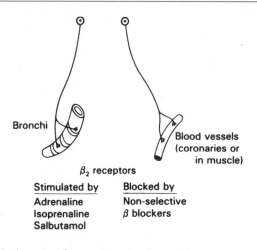

Fig. 3.5 Important β_2 receptors, showing agonists (stimulators) and blocking agents.

a. β_1 responses. Increase in rate and excitability of the heart with increased output of blood.
b. β_2 responses. Dilatation of bronchi and blood vessels.

Stimulation of β receptors can be blocked by drugs known as β *blockers*. Some of these are termed *selective* as they block the stimulation of β_1 receptors only, whereas others are *non-selective* and block the stimulation of both β_1 and β_2 receptors (see p. 35).

Overactivity of the sympathetic nervous system produced by fright or anger causes a mixed picture due to stimulation by noradrenaline and adrenaline of α, β_1 and β_2 receptors (see Table 3.1).

Transmission at autonomic ganglion

Acetylcholine is also liberated at the synapses of both sympathetic and parasympathetic ganglia and is responsible for the transmission of nerve impulses between nerve endings and ganglion cells.

SYMPATHOMIMETIC DRUGS

Sympathomimetic drugs have effects similar to those produced by activity of the sympathetic nervous system.

Table 3.1 The chief effects of sympathetic and parasympathetic activity

	Sympathetic activity	Parasympathetic activity
Heart rate	Increased	Slowed
Blood vessels	Constricted	Dilated
Stomach and intestine	Decreased activity	Increased activity
	Increased secretion	Decreased secretion
Salivary and bronchial glands	Decreased secretion	Increased secretion
Urinary bladder	Body relaxed	Body contracted
	Sphincter contracted	Sphincter relaxed
Bronchial muscle	Relaxed	Contracted
Blood sugar	Raised	
Eye	Pupils dilated	Pupils constricted
		Accommodates for near vision

Adrenaline. Adrenaline is one of the substances produced by sympathetic activity; for medical use it is, however, prepared synthetically. It acts on the sympathetic receptors of the visceral organs. Adrenaline is destroyed by the acid of the stomach and is therefore not effective if taken orally. It is usually given by subcutaneous or intramuscular injection, its effects being produced more rapidly from the latter site. Following injection, its various actions become apparent within a minute. They are:

1. An increase in force and rate of contraction of the heart (β_1 effect), so that the patient may complain of palpitation.
2. A rise in systolic blood pressure due to the increased output of blood by the heart (β_1 effect). The diastolic pressure shows little change as adrenaline produces vasoconstriction only in the skin and in the splanchnic area (mixed α and β_2 effects) and vasodilatation in arteries in muscle (β_2 effect).
3. Adrenaline relaxes smooth muscle, including that of the bronchial tree.
4. Adrenaline raises the blood sugar by mobilizing glucose from the tissues.

Following injection, adrenaline is rapidly broken down in the body by *amine oxidase* and *methyl O transferase*, and its effects only last a few minutes.

Therapeutics. Adrenaline is less used now than in former times. It is still the best immediate treatment for anaphylactic reactions (see p. 265). By causing constriction of blood vessels it relieves oedema and swelling. The usual dose is 0.5 ml of a 1:1000 solution, intramuscularly and it is important not to inject the drug into a vein by mistake as a sudden intravenous injection can precipitate a fatal cardiac arrhythmia.

It is given as an intravenous bolus in a dose of 1 mg (10 ml of a 1:10 000 solution) as a stimulant to the heart in cardiac arrest.

Note: Do not inject into the same intravenous line as sodium bicarbonate.

Noradrenaline. Noradrenaline is closely related to adrenaline and is produced in the body by sympathetic activity. It can also be prepared synthetically. Its most important action is to produce widespread vasoconstriction and thus a rise in both systolic and diastolic blood pressure (α effect). Noradrenaline is rapidly inactivated by the body and, therefore, to produce a continuous effect on the blood pressure, it is given by intravenous infusion.

Therapeutics. Noradrenaline has been used in the treatment of various forms of shock associated with a very low blood pressure. There are two solutions available:

1. *Injection of noradrenaline acid tartrate* contains 4 mg of noradrenaline base in 4 ml and is diluted before infusion.
2. *Special injection of noradrenaline acid tartrate* contains 400 micrograms of noradrenaline base in 4 ml.

Note: 4 mg of noradrenaline base = 8 mg of noradrenaline acid tartrate.

4 mg of noradrenaline base is added to 1 litre of 5% glucose. The initial rate of infusion is 2–3 ml/minute which may be reduced to 0.1–1.0 ml/minute according to response. A patient receiving noradrenaline requires careful nursing and observation with frequent estimations of the blood pressure which may fluctuate widely with small changes in the rate of infusion. Care should be taken to avoid extravasation which can cause necrosis.

Opinion has moved against using noradrenaline to raise blood pressure except in extreme circumstances, for although a satisfying rise in blood pressure can be obtained due to vasoconstriction, this also reduces blood flow in essential organs, particularly the kidney, with troublesome results.

Isoprenaline is related to adrenaline but it stimulates only β_1 and β_2 receptors. It is well absorbed from the buccal mucosa and following inhalation. It relaxes smooth muscle, including that of the bronchial tree and also stimulates the heart but has little or no effect on the blood pressure. It is important to avoid over-dosage as it can cause dangerous cardiac arrhythmias. It is rapidly inactivated after absorption and its effects are short-lived.

Therapeutics. Isoprenaline was formerly used in the treatment of asthma, both by inhalation and orally. Because its action of cardiac stimulation can precipitate fatal arrhythmias it has now been replaced for this purpose by the safer β_2 agonists. It can also be given in cardiac arrest. 4.0 mg is diluted in 500 ml of 5% glucose (8 micrograms/ml), the dose being 2.5–5.0 micrograms/minute. Isoprenaline is also available as 30 mg slow release tablets (*Saventrine*). They are used in certain cardiac arrhythmias.

Adverse effects include palpitation, nausea, headaches and tremors.

Selective β_2 agonists

These stimulate predominantly β_2 receptors so that although they are effective bronchodilators they have little effect on the heart. This is an important improvement over drugs like isoprenaline as the risk of cardiac arrhythmias is removed.

Salbutamol. This is the most widely used β_2 agonist and a powerful bronchodilator. It can be given by various routes but if given orally a

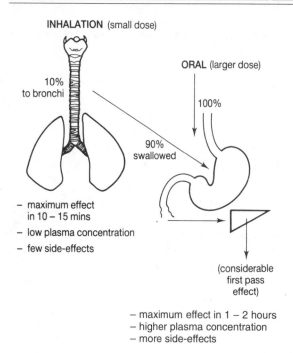

INHALATION (small dose)

10% to bronchi

ORAL (larger dose)

100%

90% swallowed

– maximum effect in 10 – 15 mins
– low plasma concentration
– few side-effects

(considerable first pass effect)

– maximum effect in 1 – 2 hours
– higher plasma concentration
– more side-effects

Fig. 3.6 Comparison of inhalation and oral dosage of salbutamol.

considerable proportion is broken down in the liver (first pass effect). Its action lasts about 4 hours. In large doses it may cause tremor and tachycardia and occasionally night cramps.

Therapeutics. Salbutamol is used to treat bronchospasm due to asthma or bronchitis. It may be taken to relieve an attack or, on a regular basis, to control the spasm. It can be given:

1. Orally in doses of 2–4 mg three or four times daily. Note that a relatively large dose is required because of the large first pass effect and side-effects are frequent.
2. Intravenously in doses of 4 micrograms/kg body weight to treat a severe asthmatic attack. *This is rarely necessary as a nebulizer is very effective. It also requires careful monitoring for cardiac arrhythmias.*
3. By inhalation. Given by this route in the treatment of bronchospasm it is possible to get the maximum effect on the bronchi with minimal effect elsewhere. Even so, only 10% of the dose reaches the bronchial tree, the rest being swallowed (Fig. 3.6).

There are various delivery systems for inhalation (see Fig. 3.7). The dose by pressurized inhaler is 100 micrograms per puff (usually one or two puffs are given); by rotahaler it is 200 or 400 micrograms per capsule and by nebulizer it is 1 ml of respirator solution (5 mg of salbutamol) made up to 4 ml with sterile saline. If inhalations are given on a regular basis they are required 4–6 hourly.

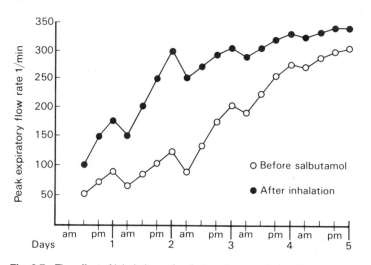

Fig. 3.7 The effect of inhalations of salbutamol on a patient with severe asthma. Note the progressive improvement in respiratory function and the morning dips which are characteristic of asthma.

Table 3.2 Other β₂ agonist bronchodilators

Drug	Dose by aerosol	Special features
Terbutaline	250–500 micrograms (250 micrograms/ puff) 3–4 times daily	Only small first pass effect so useful orally
Fenoterol	180–360 micrograms (180 micrograms/ puff) 3–4 times daily	Slightly longer action than salbutamol (6 hrs) May be associated with fatal or near fatal asthmatic attacks
Rimiterol	200–600 micrograms (200 micrograms/ puff) up to 8 times daily	
Pirbuterol	200–400 micrograms (200 micrograms/ puff) 4 times daily	Short acting Similar to salbutamol

There are other selective β₂ agonists which are very similar to salbutamol shown in Table 3.2.

Salmeterol is a β₂ agonist which is effective over 12 hours. It is used regularly in doses of 50 micrograms twice daily by inhalation. It has also been claimed to have some anti-inflammatory action but this is controversial.

Inhalation delivery systems

Inhalation is a useful and effective way of giving some of the drugs used to treat asthma and other forms of bronchospasm.

1. Pressurized aerosol inhalers (Fig. 3.8) are the most convenient systems for home use. The drug is dissolved or suspended in a propellant and on pressing the plunger a standard amount is released in the form of fine particles measuring 2–5μm. It is essential that the patient is taught the technique of using the inhaler if the treatment is to be effective (Fig. 3.8).

Nursing point

Many patients require repeated instruction in the use of aerosols particularly the young and the elderly. Inhalers containing a placebo are available for teaching.

---

a. Remove the cap from the mouthpiece and shake the inhaler.

b. Breathe out slowly but not fully.

c. Place the mouthpiece in the mouth and close the lips around it.

d. Breathe in slowly and at the same time depress the plunger thus releasing the drug.

e. Hold the breath for at least 10 seconds and longer if possible.

f. If a second inhalation is required, wait for 1 minute.

g. If steroids and β₂ agonists are both prescribed give the β₂ agonist first and wait for 5 minutes.

Spacers. Some patients lack the coordination required to use a pressurized aerosol. A spacer is a reservoir between the aerosol and the mouthpiece. Pressing the plunger releases the drug into the reservoir from whence it may be inhaled.

2. Rotahalers are used for those who find the pressurized aerosols difficult to operate. Capsules containing the drug in powder form are placed in the rotahaler which opens the capsule and delivers the drug to be inhaled. The capsules may become soft and fail to function and some patients find the powder irritant. The *Diskhaler* is a similar arrangement where the powdered drug is carried in blisters on a disc. The apparatus releases the drug which is inhaled.

3. Nebulizers are used in severe asthma and chronic bronchitis and enable a larger dose to reach the bronchi. Air, or sometimes oxygen, is driven through a solution of the drug and the resulting mist is inhaled via a mask. It is important to have the correct particle size and it is best obtained by using an air flow rate of 6–8 litres/ minute. Piped air or oxygen may be used or various mechanical compressors are available which some patients use at home. It is important that these are cleaned regularly to prevent bacterial contamination.

Alternative drugs used in asthma and other types of bronchospasm can be given by inhalation including β₂ agonists, corticosteroids (see below), sodium cromoglycate and ipratropium bromide.

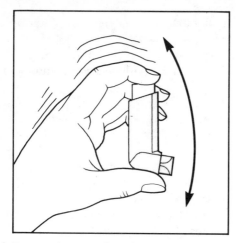

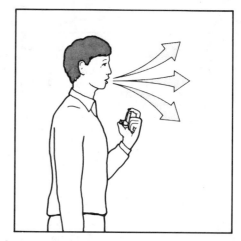

1 Remove the cover from the mouthpiece, and shake the inhaler vigorously.

2 Holding the inhaler as shown above, breathe out gently (but not fully) and then immediately...

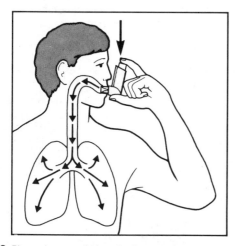

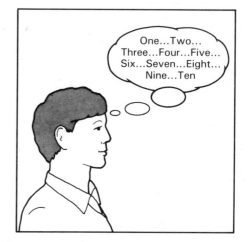

3 Place the mouthpiece in the mouth and close your lips around it. After starting to breathe in slowly and deeply through your mouth, press the inhaler firmly as shown above to release the medication and continue to breathe in.

4 Hold your breath for 10 seconds, or as long as is comfortable, before breathing out slowly.

5 If you are to take a second inhalation you should wait at least one minute before repeating steps 2, 3 and 4.

6 After use replace the cover on the mouthpiece.

Fig. 3.8 How to use an inhaler properly.

4. Delivery systems for children. Asthma is a common disease in childhood affecting about 10% of children. It usually disappears in adolescence. Drug treatment with inhalers may be required but may be difficult to administer.

Less than 1 year — Inhalers cannot be used.

1–2 years — Nebulizer can be used.

2–5 years — Nebulizer and spacers can be used.

5–10 years — As above with the addition of rotahalers.

Over 10 years — As for adults.

THE DRUG TREATMENT OF CHRONIC ASTHMA

Drugs may be given on a *regular basis* to *prevent* an attack or they may be used to *relieve* an attack which has developed. Sufferers will also require advice on their general mode of life and may need considerable psychological support.

There are two processes which narrow the bronchi and are responsible for asthmatic attacks:

1. Spasm of the bronchial muscle
2. Inflammation and oedema of the bronchial mucosa.

Bronchodilators relieve bronchospasm but have little effect on inflammation which responds to corticosteroids.

1. Bronchodilator drugs play an important part in the treatment of asthma.

a. β2 *agonists* are widely prescribed. They are given by inhalation to treat a developing attack or to prevent an attack when it seems likely (e.g. exercise-induced asthma). Their regular use as a preventive is more controversial. They do not control the inflammatory component of asthma and there is some evidence that their regular use can lead ultimately to more severe and sometimes fatal attacks. If regular use of a β2 agonist is required to control asthma an inhaled corticosteroid should be added to the regime.

b. Oral salbutomal tablets are not very efficient but salbutamol controlled release tablets, one at night, have a prolonged action and are useful in preventing attacks of asthma at night.

c. Oral aminophylline in slow release form (e.g. Phyllocontin 1 tablet twice daily) taken regularly can be used to prevent attacks particularly at night. (See p. 146.)

d. Ipratropium bromide is related to atropine and acts as a bronchodilator by virtue of its anticholinergic action. It is given via an inhaler or a nebulizer and any of the drug which is swallowed is not absorbed from the intestine. It thus has a powerful local action on the bronchi but avoids the unwanted side-effects of atropine (see p. 37). It should be used for those patients who have failed to respond to β2 agonists. Its bronchodilator effect begins after about 45 minutes and lasts for 3–4 hours, therefore it is best if taken regularly to *prevent* an asthmatic attack. It may be combined with a β2 agonist or corticosteroids.

2. Corticosteroids are useful in reducing the inflammatory and allergic aspects of asthma and decreasing bronchospasm in severe and persistent asthma. Prednisolone can be taken regularly by mouth to *prevent* attacks, the dose being the lowest required to control the disease. *Beclomethasone* (a steroid well absorbed from mucous surfaces) can be given by inhalation. Three strengths are available, 50, 100 or 200 micrograms per puff. The usual dose is one or two puffs 2–4 times daily; this enables the maximum concentration to be obtained in the bronchi with minimal systemic side-effects. Occasional candida infection of the mouth may occur, presumably due to the lowering of local resistance by the steroid, and occasionally a hoarse voice develops.

3. Sodium cromoglycate prevents asthmatic attacks by stopping the release of substances from mast cells in the bronchi which are responsible for bronchospasm. It is given regularly by pressurized aerosol or rotahaler. The usual dose is four inhalations daily. It is most effective in young asthmatics with an allergic history but is of some use in non-allergic asthma.

Nedocromil is also a mast cell stabilizer and anti-inflammatory agent and is very similar to sodium cromoglycate. It is given as a pressurized aerosol, the starting dose being 4.0 mg twice daily and is used to prevent rather than treat attacks.

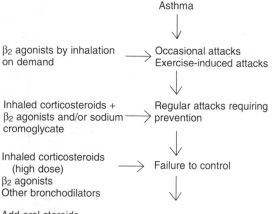

Fig. 3.9 The use of drugs in chronic asthma.

Special points for patient education

It is very important that the patients should learn to manage their own disease as far as possible and for children the parents should be fully involved. This means that they should be taught to:

1. Modify their lifestyle as far as possible to avoid attacks yet lead a normal life.
2. Understand the use of their drugs, whether they are for an acute attack or used prophylactically.
3. Understand the care and maintenance of their home nebulizer if they use one.
4. Learn to monitor their disease by means of a peak flow meter and adjust their treatment accordingly.
5. Recognize the danger signs of deterioration in their asthma and know when to call their doctor.

Nursing points

Do not forget that β blockers can make asthma worse and should be avoided in asthmatics, and that NSAIAs may precipitate an attack.

MANAGEMENT OF STATUS ASTHMATICUS

A prolonged and severe attack of asthma can be very distressing to the patient and may be dangerous. The immediate treatment is:

1. Ensure adequate hydration of the patient if necessary by infusion as this will prevent the sputum becoming sticky.
2. Use bronchodilators:
   - Salbutamol given by nebulizer in doses of 1 ml (5 mg of salbutamol) made up to 4 ml with sterile saline every 4 hours.
   - Aminophylline 250 mg given slowly intravenously (*provided they are not taking oral aminophylline or theophylline*).
3. Hydrocortisone 100 mg i.v. every 3 hours reduces inflammation and relaxes bronchi. Corticosteroids, even if given intravenously, take several hours to be effective.
4. Minimal sedation owing to risk of respiratory depression.
5. Amoxycillin 250 mg three times daily as chest infection frequently complicates the attack.
6. Oxygen as required.
7. Occasionally, patients who respond poorly will require artificial ventilation.

OTHER SYMPATHOMIMETIC AGENTS

Amphetamine and dexamphetamine are similar drugs whose main effect is on the central nervous system. They produce some euphoria, abolish fatigue, increase activity and reduce appetite. They are taken orally. They carry a considerable risk of dependence and their use is now confined to:

1. Narcolepsy starting dose 5.0 mg twice daily.
2. Some hyperactive children on whom, paradoxically, they have a sedative effect.

They should not be used for appetite control.

ADRENERGIC BLOCKING AGENTS

It is possible to block α and β adrenergic receptors.

Table 3.3 Features of some β blockers in common use. *Key*: LA, long acting slow release preparations

Drug	Selectivity	Elimination Hepatic	Renal	Half-life (hours)	Equivalent initial daily dose
Propranolol	$\beta_1 + \beta_2$	+	−	3	80 mg b.d., LA 160 mg daily
Oxprenolol	$\beta_1 + \beta_2$	+	−	2	80 mg b.d., LA 160 mg daily
Sotalol	$\beta_1 + \beta_2$	(+)	+	12	160 mg daily
Timolol	$\beta_1 + \beta_2$	(+)	(+)	5	5 mg b.d.
Nadolol	$\beta_1 + \beta_2$	−	+	16	80 mg daily
Metoprolol	$\beta_1 > \beta_2$	+	−	4	50 mg b.d., LA 200 mg daily
Pindolol	$\beta_1 > \beta_2$	(+)	+	4	5 mg b.d.
Acebutolol	$\beta_1 > \beta_2$	(+)	(+)	6	200 mg b.d.
Atenolol	$\beta_1 > \beta_2$	+	−	12	50 mg daily
Bisoprolol	$\beta_1 > \beta_2$	(+)	(+)	10	10 mg daily
Betaxolol	$\beta_1 > \beta_2$	?	(+)	16	20 mg daily

α adrenergic blockers

α adrenergic blocking agents are used in the treatment of *hypertension*. By removing the vaso-constrictor action of noradrenaline they dilate arterioles and thus lower blood pressure. They are considered on p. 58. They are also used in the diagnosis of *phaeochromocytoma* (a rare tumour of the adrenal gland) and when *phentolamine* is used.

α adrenergic receptors control the smooth muscle round the neck of the bladder. By block-ing these receptors it is possible to relax this muscle and partially relieve *bladder neck obstruc-tion* due to an enlarged prostate. Several α blockers including prazosin can be used when surgical treatment is contraindicated.

β adrenergic blockers

This group of drugs which block the effects of adrenaline and noradrenaline on β adrenergic receptors is widely used. In general, their thera-peutic effects and uses are very similar but individual members of the group show minor differences:

1. Some block predominantly β_1 receptors (i.e. cardiac receptors) and are called *selective* β block-ers, others block both β_1 and β_2 receptors (i.e. cardiac + bronchial + peripheral blood vessel receptors) and are called *non-selective* β blockers.

2. Members of the group differ in their speed and site of elimination and in their duration of action.

General actions of β blockers (Table 3.3)

1. By blocking β_1 receptors in the heart the rate is slowed, the output of blood from the heart is reduced and the work done by the heart is thus decreased. This is particularly marked when there is increased activity of the sympathetic nervous system such as occurs with excitement or exercise. In addition the excitability of heart muscle is reduced.

2. By blocking β_2 receptors β blockers cause bronchospasm particularly in asthmatic patients. This is particularly marked with non-selective β blockers as selective β blockers have less effect on β_2 receptors. This is usually of little consequence in normal subjects but in asthmatic patients may make bronchospasm worse and increase dysp-noea.

3. β blockers lower blood pressure.

4. Some β blockers have metabolic effects and they prevent the rise in blood glucose which normally follows increased sympathetic activity.

5. It is believed that at least some β adrenergic blockers penetrate the central nervous system. Some sedation is quite common in patients re-ceiving β blockers and occasionally this may be severe. In addition, vivid dreams and more rarely hallucinations occur.

6. Many of the symptoms of anxiety such as palpitations, sweating and tremor are mediated via the sympathetic nervous system. These symptoms can often be relieved by β blockers. Whether this is only a peripheral action or

whether in addition there is some other effect on the brain is not known.

Therapeutics. β Blockers are used to treat:

1. Angina of effort (see p. 56) because they reduce the work of the heart especially on effort or excitement.
2. Cardiac arrhythmias because they reduce the excitability of the heart.
3. Hypertension as they lower blood pressure, perhaps by setting the regulation of blood pressure at a lower level.
4. Thyrotoxicosis and anxiety because they reduce the increased sympathetic activity which occurs in these disorders.
5. Essential tremor, a rare familial condition characterized by severe intention tremor.

Adverse effects other than exacerbation of heart failure and of bronchospasm can be troublesome but are not usually serious. Occasionally they cause vivid dreams and hallucinations, and by decreasing cardiac output they reduce the blood flow to the extremities, which may feel unduly cold, and are best avoided in peripheral vascular disease. They mask the usual warning symptoms of hypoglycaemia and can be dangerous in diabetics who are taking insulin (see p. 172). Active people may feel less energetic whilst taking these drugs.

Labetalol is a combined α and β blocker which is used in treating hypertension (see p. 62).

PARASYMPATHOMIMETIC DRUGS

Parasympathomimetic drugs have effects similar to those produced by activity of the parasympathetic nervous system.

Acetylcholine. Acetylcholine is release from the *parasympathetic nerve endings* throughout the body and also from motor nerve endings in *voluntary muscle*. Its effects as a result of parasympathetic release are shown in Table 3.1 and, in addition, it activates voluntary muscle when a motor nerve is stimulated and is essential for all voluntary movements. Its action is very short-lived as it is quickly broken down by cholinesterase so it is not used therapeutically. However, a prolonged effect can be produced either by giving an acetylcholine-like drug which is not broken down or by using a drug which inhibits the action of cholinesterase thus prolonging and intensifying the actions of naturally occurring acetylcholine. This type of drug is called an *anticholinesterase.*

Carbachol is a synthetic substance chemically related to acetylcholine. Its actions resemble those of parasympathetic stimulation. It is not broken down by the body cholinesterases and its actions are therefore much more prolonged than those of acetycholine.

After subcutaneous injection, flushing and sweating appear in about 20 minutes, followed by increased intestinal peristalsis sometimes with colic and contraction of the bladder muscle. These actions last up to an hour. Carbachol may be given by subcutaneous injection or by mouth.

Therapeutics. The most important therapeutic use of carbachol is in the treatment of urinary retention following surgical operation or childbirth. In doses of 250 micrograms subcutaneously it causes contraction of the bladder muscle resulting in the passage of urine.

Adverse effects include colic, diarrhoea and marked fall in blood pressure. They are controlled by atropine.

Bethanechol is similar.

The anticholinesterases

Physostigmine (eserine) prevents the breakdown by cholinesterase of acetycholine produced at nerve endings throughout the body. The actions of acetylcholine are therefore intensified at their two sites of action.

1. The parasympathetic nerve endings
2. The nerve endings in voluntary muscle.

It can be seen, therefore, that the final picture produced by these groups of actions is mixed. The action at the parasympathetic nerve endings usually predominates and the action on nerve endings in voluntary muscle is only seen under special circumstances.

The most important effects of physostigmine are:

The eye. Physostigmine is absorbed through the conjunctiva and following application to the eye causes constriction of the pupil and spasm of accommodation; this appears rapidly and may last more than 24 hours.

Intestinal tract. Physostigmine causes increased intestinal tone and motility.

Physostigmine can be given orally, by subcutaneous injection or locally to the eye. It is largely broken down in the body and its effects last about 2 hours.

Therapeutics:

1. The constricting effect of physostigmine on the pupil is used in the treatment of glaucoma. A 0.25% solution is instilled into the eye as often as is required.
2. Physostigmine has been used in the treatment of myasthenia gravis but has now been replaced by neostigmine.

Neostigmine is a synthetic substance. It is an anticholinesterase with actions very similar to those of physostigmine but with an effect on the neuromuscular junction of voluntary muscle and less on the eye and cardiovascular system. It is rapidly effective following subcutaneous or intramuscular injection and is also absorbed after oral administration, although larger doses are required by this route.

Therapeutics. Used widely in the treatment of disorders in the neuromuscular junction of voluntary muscle (see p. 137). Neostigmine has been used in cases of paralytic ileus and atony of the bladder and the analogue *distigmine* is used in urinary retention.

Pyridostigmine and edrophonium. These are anticholinesterases used in the treatment of myasthenia gravis.

There are a number of other anticholinesterase preparations which are not used therapeutically but which are extensively employed as *insecticides* and are also potential lethal weapons for use in war. As some are absorbed through the intact skin and produce powerful anticholinesterase effects, they have been termed 'nerve gases'.

Adverse effects of anticholinesterases

The adverse effects of the various anticholinesterases are similar. The symptoms include intestinal colic and diarrhoea, sweating and salivation, the pupils are constricted, the pulse rapid and the blood pressure low.

The immediate treatment is atropine 1 mg intravenously.

There are now a number of drugs available which will reactivate cholinesterase by separating it from anticholinesterase. *Pralidoxime* is the best known. The dose is 1 g diluted in 15 ml of water and given slowly intravenously.

DRUGS INHIBITING THE ACTION OF ACETYLCHOLINE

The drugs which inhibit the action of parasympathetic nerve endings belong to the belladonna group or are synthetic substitutes.

All these drugs produce their effect by blocking the action of acetylcholine on the receptors in the organ concerned.

Atropine. Atropine is well absorbed from the intestine after oral administration; it can also be given subcutaneously, intramuscularly or intravenously. Atropine is largely broken down by the liver. Its effects last 2 hours or longer.

The most important action of atropine is to block the action of acetylcholine released by parasympathetic nerve endings. As a result of this action the following are observed.

Gastrointestinal tract. Atropine diminishes motility of the stomach and both small and large intestine with relief of spasm. It decreases salivary secretion and reduces gastric acid secretion.

Heart. Atropine diminishes cardiac vagal tone and thus leads to an increase in pulse rate.

Lungs. By blocking vagal action atropine leads to some relaxing of the bronchial muscle. The secretion of the bronchial glands is diminished.

Involuntary muscle. Other involuntary muscle is also relaxed, notably that of the biliary and renal tracts.

The eye. The parasympathetic nerve supply to the eye is blocked thus leading to dilatation of the pupil and paralysis of accommodation with an inability to see near objects clearly.

Warning. It is important that atropine or similar drugs should not be given to those with a tendency to glaucoma. In this condition the drainage of fluid from the eye is reduced and the pressure rises within the eyeball. Atropine further reduces the flow of fluid from the eye and may precipitate an acute attack of glaucoma (see p. 285).

Therapeutics. Atropine has several therapeutic uses, the more important of which are:

1. *Relief of involuntary muscle spasm.* Most forms of smooth muscle spasm are relieved by atropine, 600 micrograms subcutaneously or intravenously being useful in the relief of intestinal, biliary or renal colic.

2. *Peptic ulcer.* Atropine itself is rarely used at the present time and has been replaced by one of the H₂ blockers which are more effective in reducing acid secretion and have fewer side-effects (see p. 79).

3. *Congenital pyloric stenosis of infants.* The narrowed pylorus which occurs in this condition may be relaxed by atropine. It is more usual to use *atropine methonitrate (Eumydrin)* in doses of 200–400 micrograms half an hour before feeds (one drop of the oral solution contains 200 micrograms).

4. *Eye conditions.* Atropine may be applied locally to the eye as an eye drop to dilate the pupil in a variety of conditions. Homatropine is often used in 2% solution for this purpose as its effects are not so prolonged as those of atropine.

5. *Pre-operative medication.* Atropine is given pre-operatively in doses of 600 micrograms subcutaneously to dry up the salivary and bronchial secretions and to protect the heart from undue vagal depression.

6. *Bronchial spasm.* An atropine derivative *(ipratropium)* is given by inhalation to relieve bronchospasm in asthma (see p. 33).

Adverse effects are dose related. Dry mouth, constipation, difficulty with micturition (in the elderly) and paralysis of ocular accommodation are common. With higher doses restlessness, hallucination and delirium can occur.

Hyoscine (scopolamine). The peripheral actions of hyoscine are the same as those of atropine. Its action on the central nervous system differs, however, in that hyoscine, even in small doses, is a central nervous system depressant leading to drowsiness and sleep.

Therapeutics. Hyoscine is particularly used for its central as well as peripheral effects. It is used pre-operatively in doses of 400 micrograms and as an anti-emetic.

THE SYNTHETIC SUBSTITUTES

These drugs are now rarely used to treat peptic ulcers but are still given to patients suffering from the irritable bowel syndrome and related conditions and occasionally for nocturnal enuresis.

Among those available are:

Dicyclomine	30–60mg daily in divided doses
Mebeverine	135 mg three times daily
Propantheline	15 mg three times daily

Adverse effects are similar to those of atropine.

Oxybutynin 5 mg twice daily is used for similar problems.

THE ERGOT GROUP

Ergot is a fungus which grows on rye. It contains two substances which are of pharmacological importance and which can be used therapeutically; although the actions of these substances are by no means confined to the autonomic system. Ergotamine is considered below and ergometrine under drugs affecting the uterus (p. 183).

Ergotamine. Ergotamine is an α sympathetic stimulant which causes vasoconstriction, particularly of the smaller arteries.

If ergotamine is taken consistently, it will result in impaired blood supply to the extremities and ultimately in gangrene.

Therapeutics. Ergotamine is used in treating migraine, a common type of headache which is believed to be due to increased pulsation with stretching of the walls of the cerebral arteries. The mode of action of ergotamine in relieving migraine is not fully understood. It is certainly not an analgesic drug and it seems most probable that it works by causing some constriction of the cerebral vessels and thus decreases their amplitude of pulsation.

Ergotamine can be given orally. The initial dose is 1–2 mg and it may be repeated hourly to a total of 4 mg in 24 hours or 10 mg in 1 week. It may be prescribed as Cafergot (1 mg per tab)—this also contains caffeine which enhances the effect of ergotamine, or as Migril (2 mg per tab) which consists of caffeine and the anti-emetic cyclizine.

Ergotamine is absorbed into the respiratory mucosa and can be given by inhalation using a Medihaler which is calibrated so that a dose contains 360 micrograms of ergotamine.

It can also be given rectally in the form of suppositories which contain 2 mg of ergotamine. No more than three suppositories should be taken in 1 day or five in 1 week.

Adverse effects include vomiting, diarrhoea and peripheral vasoconstriction which may be serious enough to cause gangrene if an overdose is given. It is contraindicated in coronary artery disease, peripheral vascular disease and pregnancy. Its vasoconstricting action is increased in patients taking β blockers.

Ergotism

Chronic poisoning by ergot may occur in those who eat rye contaminated by the ergot fungus. This has been particularly liable to happen in eastern Europe. The symptoms are gangrene of the extremities and disorders of the central nervous system with drowsiness, convulsions and mental changes.

MIGRAINE

Migraine is a disorder characterized by recurrent attacks of severe headache, often associated with vomiting and various visual disturbances and is due to cerebral vasoconstriction followed by vasodilatation.

Treatment of the acute attack

The acute attack often responds to simple analgesics such as aspirin or paracetamol. The addition of metoclopramide (see p. 89) given early in the attack is useful in preventing vomiting and, by increasing the rate of gastric emptying, it hastens the absorption and effect of the analgesic. It often helps to lie down in a quiet room and some patients find a small dose of diazepam (2.5–5.0 mg) useful for promoting sleep.

If these measures are inadequate, as occurs in about 20% of sufferers, specific drug treatment is required.

Ergotamine, as described above, has long been the drug most often used. Recently, a new one has been introduced.

Sumatriptan stimulates certain 5HT (serotonin) receptors in blood vessel walls and causes vasoconstriction thus relieving the migraine attack. It is given by subcutaneous injection of 6 mg, relieving the headache in most patients within an hour. Its action lasts about 2 hours when the headache may sometimes return. It is also available for oral use, the dose being 100 mg, and it takes 4 hours to relieve symptoms. There is little doubt that sumatriptan is effective against a migraine attack; however, it is much more expensive than ergotamine and will probably be reserved for patients in whom other treatment is ineffective.

Adverse effects include tingling, and tightness in the chest. These are usually mild. It should not be given to patients with ischaemic heart disease as it may cause coronary artery spasm.

Special points for patient education in migraine

1. Patients must be taught which drugs are used to relieve an acute attack and which are used for prevention.

2. It must be stressed that ergotamine should only be taken to relieve attacks and for a limited number of doses, not taken regularly for prevention as this will lead to serious side-effects and may actually cause headaches.

3. Migraine attacks may be precipitated by a variety of external factors, such as certain foods and the 'Pill'. The patient should learn to recognize these and avoid them if possible.

Prevention of migraine attacks

If attacks occur more than weekly in spite of the elimination of 'trigger' factors, prophylactic drug treatment may be needed.

β blockers (e.g. propranolol, 40 mg twice daily) are effective in about half the patients but their contraindications must be remembered.

Pizotifen is concerned with the action of 5HT and reduces the contraction and dilatation of blood vessels. It is widely used to prevent migraine. It may cause drowsiness and the initial dose is 500 micrograms at night. This may be increased up to 3.0 mg daily. It can also cause weight gain.

Antidepressants (dothiepin or amitriptyline) may also be effective, especially if the patient is depressed.

Methysergide blocks the action of 5HT on smooth muscle. It has a number of serious adverse effects and is only used when safer treatments have failed.

Therapeutics. The initial dose is 1–2 mg daily and increased as necessary. Courses of treatment last up to 4 months.

Adverse effects include vomiting and diarrhoea. Prolonged use occasionally causes fibrosis of the peritoneum with renal obstruction.

Clonidine which can also be used to lower blood pressure (see p. 58) reduces the reactivity of blood vessels and can prevent migraine attacks.

Therapeutics. The initial dose is 25 micrograms twice daily and increased as necessary.

FURTHER READING

Barnes P J 1989 A new approach to the treatment of asthma. New England Journal of Medicine 321: 1517

British Thoracic Society 1993 Guidelines for the management of asthma: a summary. British Medical Journal 306: 776

Current problems No 33 1992 Beta-agonist use in asthma.

Editorial 1987 Nebulisers in the treatment of asthma. Drug and Therapeutics Bulletin 25: 101

Editorial 1990 Guidelines for the management of asthma in adults. British Medical Journal 301: 651

Editorial 1991 Salmeterol. Drug and Therapeutics Bulletin 29: 19

Editorial 1992 Sumatriptan, serotonin, migraine and money. Lancet 339: 151

Ellis P 1992 Drugs Update: Antagonising asthma. Nursing Times 88: 37

Lance J W 1992 Treatment of migraine. Lancet 339: 1207

4

Drugs affecting the cardiovascular system

DRUGS ACTING ON THE HEART

There are three major disorders of the heart itself which can be treated by drugs. They are:

1. Cardiac failure
2. Cardiac arrhythmias
3. Cardiac ischaemia.

CARDIAC FAILURE

The heart is a pump receiving blood from the systemic and pulmonary veins and driving it, under pressure, into the pulmonary arteries and the aorta. The volume of blood passing through the heart each minute is known as the *cardiac output*. This is largely determined by four factors:

1. The pressure in the venous system filling the heart and stretching the heart muscle, which is known as the *preload*. In health, a rise in venous pressure causes a rise in cardiac output.
2. The arterial pressure that is the resistance against which the heart must pump, known as the *afterload*.
3. The heart rate—increase in rate leads to an increased output, except in heart failure when an increased rate decreases cardiac efficiency.
4. The contractile efficiency of the heart muscle.

In good health the cardiac output varies considerably depending on the needs of the body, being low at rest and rising with exercise. The healthy heart has a great functional reserve and can cope with demands for increased output which occur from time to time.

In cardiac failure the contractility of the muscle decreases, the neck veins and heart become distended with blood and cannot respond to increased filling pressure (preload) by raising output and instead this results in a fall in output, at first only apparent on exercise but, later, even at rest. It becomes insufficient for the needs of the body and various organs receive an inadequate blood supply. This is particularly important in the kidney where it activates the angiotensin/renin system (see p. 57) causing the kidney to retain salt and water. Oedema of dependent parts and lungs develops, the latter being responsible for marked dyspnoea (shortness of breath) which is a prominent feature of cardiac failure. Angiotensin is also responsible for arterial constriction which increases the work (afterload) of an already labouring heart.

The low cardiac output carries less oxygen to the tissues. The oxygen supply to the heart and brain is kept up at the expense of other organs which are starved of oxygen and this accounts for the fatigue which may be a prominent symptom (Fig. 4.1)

There are many causes of cardiac failure. The heart muscle may be damaged by previous coronary thrombosis or by cardiomyopathy or an increased workload over a long period due to high blood pressure or valve disease ultimately causes it to fail.

Drugs in congestive cardiac failure

Three main groups of drugs are used:

1. Drugs which improve the function of the myocardium so the heart contracts more powerfully and empties more completely thereby raising the cardiac output. This is called a *positive inotropic effect*. The only drug of this type which is used successfully in chronic cardiac failure is digitalis, other drugs of this type are used in cardiac shock (see p. 47).
2. Diuretics which cause the kidney to excrete excess salt and water (see p. 45).
3. ACE inhibitors which act by suppressing the angiotensin/renin mechanism (see p. 46) which is overactive in cardiac failure.

Drugs which improve heart muscle function

Digitalis has been used by physicians for hundreds of years. In 1785 William Withering of Birmingham described its used in dropsy and noted that it appeared to act on the heart.

There are two types of digitalis in common use—*digoxin* which is obtained from the white foxglove and *digitoxin* from the purple foxglove. Both drugs are usually given orally but they can be injected intravenously. They are well absorbed and become attached to the heart muscle where they improve its function. Digoxin is excreted by the kidneys and this is important as accumulation occurs in patients with poor renal function unless a lower dose is used. Digitoxin is broken down by the liver.

	Maximal effect after oral dose	Duration of action
Digoxin	12 hours	2 days
Digitoxin	24 hours	7 days

It will be noted that the action of these drugs lasts for several days. This is not due only to slow elimination but because, once bound to heart muscle, their action is prolonged.

Digoxin is the type of digitalis most commonly used in the United Kingdom though digitoxin is usually used in the USA.

The effects seen in the failing heart are:

1. Increased force of contraction of the ventricular muscle. This action is due to an increase in calcium ions in the heart muscle cells. In large doses this may be associated with increased excitability of the ventricle.
2. Slowing of the heart rate, partially due to increased activity of the vagus nerve and partly to a direct action on the sinu-atrial node.
3. Depression of conduction in the AV node and the bundle of His (see Fig. 4.3). This action does not affect the heart in sinus rhythm, but in atrial fibrillation it decreases the number of impulses reaching the ventricles from the fibrillating atria, and thus decreases the rate of ventricular contraction.

The most important of these three actions is slowing of the ventricular rate particularly in

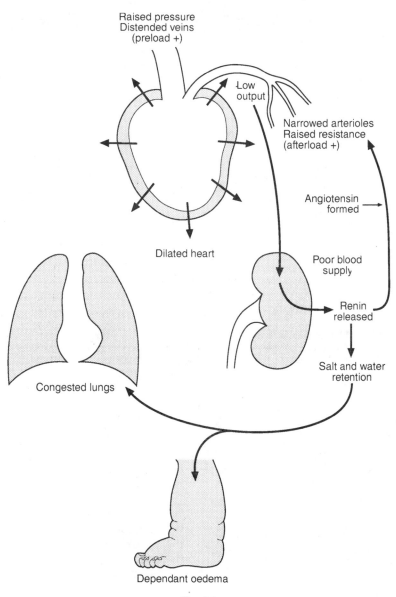

Fig. 4.1

atrial fibrillation where the slower and more regular contractions allow the heart to function more efficiently and raise cardiac output. The *positive inotropic effect* is less important and if the heart is in sinus rhythm the benefits are less obvious.

Therapeutics. Treatment is started with a full dose of the drug until a satisfactory response is obtained as judged by the general condition of the patient, a ventricular rate of 60–80 per minute, a diuresis followed by reduction of oedema. This usually starts about 6 hours after dosing (see Fig. 4.2).

If the patient has atrial fibrillation the apex rate is the best guide because the pulse rate at the wrist may appear to be slower as weak beats may not be felt.

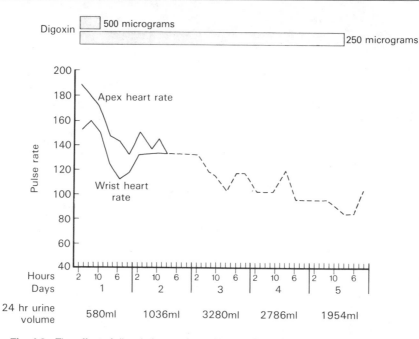

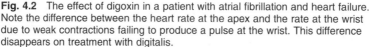

Fig. 4.2 The effect of digoxin in a patient with atrial fibrillation and heart failure. Note the difference between the heart rate at the apex and the rate at the wrist due to weak contractions failing to produce a pulse at the wrist. This difference disappears on treatment with digitalis.

The initial dose for an adult should be 500 micrograms of digoxin orally, followed by 250 micrograms three times daily for a day or two until a full therapeutic response is achieved. Thereafter the maintenance dose to replace the day-to-day loss will usually lie between 125–500 micrograms daily. Elderly patients and those with impaired renal function require smaller doses to avoid accumulation of the drug and in these cases 62.5 micrograms daily or less may be sufficient.

The introduction of powerful and fast-acting diuretics has reduced the need for rapid digitalization but 500 micrograms of digoxin can be given *slowly* intravenously. It is important to ensure that the patient is not already receiving digitalis or overdose may occur.

Plasma levels of digoxin can now be measured, the correct therapeutic range being between 0.9–2 micrograms/litre. There is, however, considerable interperson variation and the estimation of plasma levels is more useful to confirm non-compliance or overdose than in

the control of treatment where clinical observation is usually adequate.

Digitalis may also be used in certain *cardiac arrhythmias*, even if they are unassociated with heart failure.

Atrial fibrillation. By suppressing conduction between the atria and ventricles digitalis controls the ventricular rate in atrial fibrillation whether there is associated cardiac failure or not. It does not however, abolish the fibrillation.

Atrial flutter. Digitalis may change the arrhythmia into atrial fibrillation. If the drug is then stopped, normal sinus rhythm may be restored.

Supraventricular paroxysmal tachycardia. By slowing conduction digitalis breaks the abnormal circus movement responsible for the arrhythmia and allows the heart to return to normal rhythm.

Digitalis must *not* be used in ventricular paroxysmal tachycardia, because it may lead to ventricular fibrillation and death.

Comparative potency of digitalis preparations. 125 micrograms digoxin = 100 micrograms digitoxin.

Adverse effects. There is only a small difference between the therapeutic dose of digitalis and the toxic dose so dosage should be carefully regulated. Elderly patients, those with renal impairment and with hypothyroidism are more liable to suffer adverse effects. *The nurse should keep a watch for toxicity* and should know the common manifestations of overdose. They are:

1. Undue slowing of the heart due to excessive effect on the conducting system or the sinu-atrial node. A pulse rate below 60 indicates that the drug should be omitted for a day or two.
2. Coupled beats. These are due to ventricular extrasystoles following normal beats. They are felt at the wrist as a double pulsation followed by a pause. The extrasystoles result from increased excitability of the ventricles and are an indication to omit the drug. Continued overdosage may lead to ventricular paroxysmal tachycardia or even ventricular fibrillation which is rapidly fatal.
3. Sometimes a combination of complete heart block with a ventricular rate of about 100 is seen. This disorder is difficult to diagnose without an electrocardiogram.
4. Nausea and later vomiting. This is due to stimulation of the vomiting centre in the medulla by digitalis. However, as heart failure itself may produce vomiting, it is not a very reliable symptom of overdosage.
5. Rarely, coloured vision may be found in overdosage.
6. In elderly patients digitalis may cause confusion.

It is also important to remember that *lowering the level of potassium in the blood increases the toxicity of digitalis*. This may occur with certain diuretics (p. 192) and their administration may result in the appearance of signs of digitalis overdosage in a patient who has been satisfactorily treated for a long time.

Interactions:

1. The action of digoxin is increased by verapamil, diltiazem and amiodarone and the dose should be halved if these drugs are introduced.
2. Any drug which lowers plasma potassium (i.e. diuretics) potentiates the toxicity of digoxin.

Nursing point

Mistakes with digitalis dosage are not uncommon. Three strengths of digoxin tablet are currently available—62.5, 125 and 250 micrograms. The paediatric elixir contains 50 micrograms/ml. To avoid confusion, the dose should be written in micrograms not mg.

Diuretics

These are considered in detail on page 189. Both thiazide and loop diuretics are used in cardiac failure. By increasing the excretion of salt and water they help to get rid of oedema and pulmonary congestion and by reducing blood volume they relieve distension of the heart. However, the reduced blood volume tends to activate renin release by the kidney and this may partially reverse their beneficial effects by stimulating the kidney to retain fluid and, by vasoconstriction, to increase the work of the heart. Nevertheless, the benefits usually outweigh the disadvantages and they are the most widely used drugs for the relief of chronic cardiac failure.

Both thiazide and loop diuretics increase potassium loss via the kidney. If small doses are used this is unlikely to require correction but:

a. If large doses of diuretic are used
b. If dietary potassium is deficient (e.g. in the poor or elderly)
c. If concurrent digitalis is given

potassium deficiency increases digitalis toxicity. Supplementary potassium or a potassium sparing diuretic should be added to the regime (see p. 192). In all cases the plasma potassium concentration should be monitored and kept above 3.2 mmol/litre.

Angiotensin converting enzyme (ACE) inhibitors

This group of drugs which is also used to treat

hypertension has emerged as an important addition to the management of chronic heart failure. By blocking the renin/angiotensin mechanism (see p. 57) they reduce the retention of salt and water by the kidneys and, in addition, by dilating arterioles they lower the resistance to blood flow from the heart (afterload), reduce cardiac work and raise cardiac output.

Nursing point

When patients with heart failure are given an ACE inhibitor they may experience a marked fall in blood pressure, especially if they are already taking a diuretic. This is due to the combination of vasodilatation and reduced circulating blood volume resulting from diuretic treatment. These patients should be under observation with regular measurements of blood pressure after the first dose. With captopril hypotension only lasts a few hours, but with enalapril its onset may be delayed up to 8 hours and last up to 36 hours. The initial dose should be low, e.g. captopril 12.5 mg or enalapril 2.5 mg.

The treatment of cardiac failure

The three main objectives in treating cardiac failure are to increase the efficiency and output of the heart so that there is sufficient blood and oxygen supply to the various organs, to reduce congestion and oedema and to try where possible to remove or diminish the factor or factors which caused the heart to fail.

Patients with cardiac failure are nursed in a sitting position so that the accumulated oedema fluid drains away from the lungs and abdominal viscera to the legs and does not therefore embarrass respiration. Although the legs may be slightly elevated on a stool when the patient is sitting out of bed they should not be raised above the horizontal as this may shift fluid to the abdomen and lungs. Constipation may be a problem requiring modification of diet and sometimes, a purgative or suppository.

These patients usually require easily digested and light foods. Retention of salt is as important as retention of water by the kidneys in producing oedema. Modern diuretics will usually enable the kidneys to excrete salt and a low salt diet is rarely required. Opinions vary as to the correct fluid

intake but it is not usually necessary to restrict it. However, in severe heart failure or when sodium deficiency has developed as a result of prolonged and intensive diuretic therapy, intake should be cut to 1500 ml daily and the regime arranged to minimize the patient's discomfort.

In mild or moderate heart failure treatment is usually started with *diuretics*, either thiazides for minimal failure or loop diuretics for more severe failure. They are given once daily by mouth. Patients should be weighed regularly at the same time of day and in the same clothes to assess the efficacy of treatment. This may be sufficient treatment and can be carried on at home under the family doctor.

There is a tendency to introduce *ACE inhibitors* into the therapeutic regime early in treatment. They should certainly be used if the response to diuretics is not satisfactory or if cardiac failure is severe but many physicians think there is a place for their use even in moderate failure, and there is evidence that they not only control symptoms but also prolong life.

Digitalis was formerly used extensively in heart failure both to stimulate contraction of the heart and to slow the pulse rate thus raising the cardiac output. It is now realized that the effect on the contraction is short lived and less important than it was once considered to be, so its main use in heart failure is to slow the pulse rate, particularly in atrial fibrillation.

Various ancillary drugs may be used in the treatment of cardiac failure. A hypnotic drug may be required if the patient cannot sleep. In the very restless and ill patient, morphine is extremely useful, particularly in acute failure of the left ventricle, but it must be used with care in patients who are cyanosed as depression of respiration may occur. If cyanosis is a marked feature, *oxygen* is given at full concentration unless the patient has concurrent chronic respiratory disease, in which case the concentration should be controlled.

Patients in bed with cardiac failure are liable to develop venous thrombosis and it is common practice to give prophylactic treatment with *heparin* 5000 units subcutaneously twice daily.

It is not so easy to remove the cause of the cardiac failure, but in recent years some of the precipitating factors can be treated. High blood pressure can be reduced by drugs, and advances in cardiac surgery have enabled many defects of the valves of the heart to be relieved.

Nursing point

β Blockers and calcium antagonists may make cardiac failure worse and should be avoided if possible in this condition, NSAIAs reduce the effect of diuretics and can cause fluid retention with oedema.

Special points in patient education

Unless the underlying cause can be removed, most patients with chronic heart failure will require some medication for the rest of their lives. It should be explained to them that the main objectives of treatment are to give them a reasonable exercise tolerance and to keep them free of oedema. The importance of taking their drugs regularly should be stressed. They should be told of the main adverse effects particularly those producing symptoms (e.g. nausea in digitalis overdose). All patients with chronic heart failure should be seen regularly either as outpatients or by their family doctor.

Acute failure of the left ventricle which commonly occurs in patients with a high blood pressure or following a cardiac infarct leads to rapidly developing oedema of the lungs with distress and shortness of breath. It is best treated with a rapidly acting *diuretic* (frusemide 10–40 mg i.v.), *morphine* 10 mg i.v. or diamorphine 5 mg i.v. which sedates the patient and also by dilating veins reduces congestion of the lungs. If necessary, they may be combined with *prochlorperazine* 12.5 mg deep i.m. to control vomiting.

If the above treatment is not effective vasodilators are used. These decrease the peripheral resistance (afterload) and allow the heart to work more efficiently. *Sodium nitroprusside* is given intravenously (p. 61) and the dose adjusted to produce the optimum cardiac output. This type of treatment should be carried out in an intensive care unit as careful monitoring is essential.

Drugs in shock

In a state of shock the output of blood from the heart is acutely reduced, the blood pressure is low and circulation to the organs of the body is inadequate. Clinically, the patient is pale, sweating and confused, the pulse is rapid, the blood pressure low and the limbs cold; kidney failure may supervene. This state may occur for two main reasons:

1. Sudden reduction of blood volume, usually due to bleeding which is treated by replacing the lost fluid by infusion.
2. Reduced pumping action of the heart (pump failure) following damage (e.g. after a myocardial infarct).

Sometimes both reasons are combined as in septicaemia, when bacterial toxins damage the heart, dilate the blood vessels and cause leakage of fluid from the circulation.

If the main fault is pump failure, drugs can be given to increase the force of contraction of the heart muscle (**positive inotropic effect**) and thus improve cardiac output and circulation and raise the blood pressure.

Digitalis is not effective in these circumstances and may precipitate a dangerous cardiac arrhythmia. The most commonly used drugs are dopamine and dobutamine. This type of treatment requires careful monitoring, usually in an intensive care ward.

Dopamine is a naturally occurring substance which is changed to noradrenaline in the body. However, it has actions of its own and is used to treat shock which may follow cardiac infarction or major cardiac surgery.

It is a β_1 stimulant and also increases the release of noradrenaline in the heart, thus causing the heart muscle to contract more powerfully. In addition, dopamine stimulates receptors in the renal blood vessels causing them to dilate and increase both renal blood flow and urinary output. This action is useful as shock often causes a decline in renal function.

Dopamine is given by continuous intravenous infusion. In doses of 2–5 micrograms/kg/minute it affects mainly the kidneys and is used to improve their function, often combined with a diuretic.

In doses of 5–20 micrograms/kg/minute it is used for its action on the heart and its renal effect disappears.

Higher doses should not be used as the intense vasoconstriction which develops may cause gangrene of the extremities.

Interactions. Patients on MAOIs should be given one-tenth of the usual dose of dopamine.

Dobutamine is similar to dopamine but has no effect on the kidneys. It is, however, less likely to cause cardiac arrhythmias. The dose is 5–10 micrograms/kg/minute by continuous infusion.

Dopamine and dobutamine may be combined, a low dose of dopamine being used for its effects on the kidneys and dobutamine for its cardiac action.

Both dopamine and dobutamine should be infused via a central vein to minimize peripheral vasoconstriction.

Other cardiac stimulants

Efforts are continually being made to find a drug which will stimulate heart muscle to raise the cardiac output. Several have been introduced including *xamoterol* but as yet there is no really effective newcomer.

CARDIAC ARRHYTHMIAS

In the normal heart the initial stimulus of contraction starts in the sinu-atrial node (the pacemaker of the heart) situated at the junction of the superior vena cava and the right atrium. The rate of discharge from the node is under control of the vagus and sympathetic nerves. Vagal activity slows the heart rate and sympathetic activity increases it. The wave of contraction spreads over both atria forcing blood into the ventricles. The stimulus then pauses for a fraction of a second at the *atrioventricular (AV) node* before passing down the *bundle of His* and spreading through the muscles of both ventricles, which contract and drive blood into the pulmonary artery and the

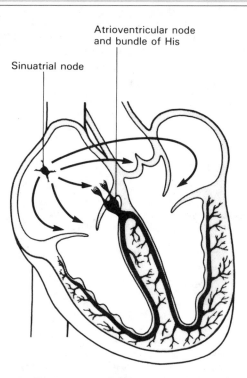

Fig. 4.3 The heart, showing the sinu-atrial node and conducting system (atrioventricular node and bundle of His).

aorta (Fig. 4.3). The heart then relaxes, refills with venous blood and awaits the next stimulus for contraction. Under certain circumstances this cycle may be disturbed.

Disorders of cardiac rhythm can be divided into those due to overexcitability of the heart which are by far the most common, and those due to conduction defects in the bundle of His.

Arrhythmias due to overexcitability

Extrasystoles (ectopic beats). These are caused by an excitable focus either in the atria or ventricles which stimulates the heart to contract while relaxed and awaiting the next normal stimulus. This normal stimulus then falls on a heart in the unresponsive or refractory phase which immediately follows a contraction and there is a pause before normal rhythm is resumed. Extrasystoles are very common in healthy people and are usually of little significance. They may be related to excessive smoking or to the consumption of tea, coffee or alcohol. They rarely require treatment.

Paroxysmal tachycardia may arise from the ventricle (*ventricular*) or from the atria or atrioventricular node (*supraventricular*). In *ventricular tachycardia* an excitable focus in the ventricle stimulates the ventricle to contract regularly at about 160–180 times a minute. It frequently occurs in diseased hearts, for instance after a cardiac infarct.

Supraventricular tachycardias are believed to have a rather different mechanism. They are usually due to a rapid circus movement within the AV node which fires off ventricular contractions via the bundle of His at about 160/minute. This is known as a *re-entrant phenomenon*. If the circus movement is supressed, the heart returns to normal rhythm.

Attacks of paroxysmal tachycardia may last for anything from a few seconds to hours or even days. They may occur in quite healthy people or they may complicate heart disease.

Atrial flutter. Sometimes the atria may contract at an even higher speed, usually about 240–300/minute. This is called atrial flutter. Under these circumstances the ventricles are unable to 'keep up' with the atria and therefore respond to every other or perhaps every third atrial contraction, a condition known as 2:1 or 3:1 heart block.

Atrial (auricular) fibrillation. In atrial fibrillation each individual bundle of muscle fibres in the atria contracts individually at a rate of about 450 contractions/minute. This results in complete disorganization of atrial contraction, and furthermore the ventricles are bombarded, via the bundle of His, with rapid and irregular stimuli and are unable either to fill properly with blood or to contract satisfactorily. Although atrial fibrillation rarely occurs in healthy hearts, it is usually found in heart disease, often in thyrotoxicosis or rheumatic mitral stenosis.

Arrhythmias due to conduction defects

Heart block. Sometimes the bundle of His may fail to transmit the impulse from the atria to the ventricles. This condition is known as heart block. If there is no association between atria and ventricles, the block is said to be *complete* and, if only a proportion of impulses get down the bundle, the block is said to be *partial*.

Cardiac arrhythmias are not necessarily associated with cardiac failure, but certain arrhythmias, commonly atrial fibrillation, may, by throwing an extra strain on the heart, either precipitate or augment cardiac failure.

Drugs used to treat arrhythmias

Cardiac arrhythmias can be terminated and normal rhythm restored by drugs. If, however, the heart is functioning poorly it is safer to stop the arrhythmia by DC cardioversion or, if it is a conduction defect, to use electrical pacing.

Arrhythmias due to overexcitability

When the arrhythmia is due to an excitable focus in the heart muscle (usually in the ventricle), drugs which reduce excitability are appropriate and include:

- Lignocaine
- Mexiletine.

When the arrhythmia is due to a circus movement, as in supraventricular tachycardias, drugs which slow conduction in the AV node and/or the bundle of His are used. They include:

- Verapamil
- β Blockers
- Adenosine
- Digitalis.

In addition, three drugs which have both actions and can therefore be used in both types of arrhythmia are:

- Disopyramide
- Amiodarone
- Flecainide.

Lignocaine suppresses the excitability of the ventricular muscle with only moderate depression of the heart's action. It is not likely therefore

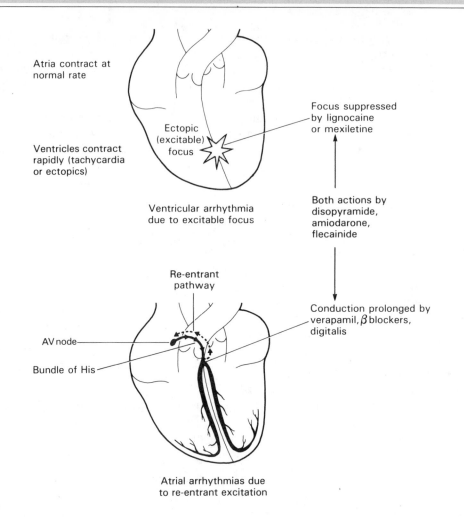

Atria contract at normal rate

Ventricles contract rapidly (tachycardia or ectopics)

Ectopic (excitable) focus

Focus suppressed by lignocaine or mexiletine

Ventricular arrhythmia due to excitable focus

Both actions by disopyramide, amiodarone, flecainide

Re-entrant pathway

AV node

Bundle of His

Conduction prolonged by verapamil, β blockers, digitalis

Atrial arrhythmias due to re-entrant excitation

Fig. 4.4 The mechanisms of paroxysmal tachycardias.

to cause cardiac arrest or a fall in blood pressure except in overdose.

Therapeutics. Lignocaine is particularly used to treat arrhythmias due to ventricular excitability a hich are liable to occur in the first few days after a cardiac infarct. It must be given intravenously because if it is given by mouth it is very rapidly broken down by the liver after absorption from the intestine (*first pass effect*). Unfortunately its action only lasts about 20 minutes. The initial dose is 50–100 mg injected over 2 minutes, and this may be followed by an intravenous infusion of a solution containing 4.0 mg of lignocaine in 1.0 ml of 5% dextrose solution (0.4%) at the rate

of 1–4 mg of lignocaine/minute. In patients with cardiac failure or shock the breakdown of lignocaine by the liver is much slower, and dangerous accumulation can occur with continuous infusion. In these circumstances the infusion rate should not exceed 1 mg/minute. The therapeutic blood level is 2–5 micrograms/ml.

Contraindications and adverse effects. Lignocaine should be avoided in shocked patients when it may further depress cardiac function. It should not be given if the conducting system of the heart is damaged as may happen after cardiac infarction.

The most common adverse effects are caused

by stimulation of the central nervous system with restlessness, tremor and possibly fits. It can also cause a fall in blood pressure and bradycardia, particularly if heart function is already compromised.

Interactions. A low plasma potassium level reduces the effectiveness of lignocaine and the plasma potassium concentration should be kept above 4 mmol/litre.

Mexiletine is similar in its action to lignocaine. It suppresses cardiac arrhythmias and it is particularly valuable because it is effective when given orally.

Therapeutics. The oral dose is 400 mg followed after 2 hours by 200 mg 8 hourly. Intravenously, the initial bolus is 100–250 mg slowly followed by an infusion of 250 mg over 1 hour and then 250 mg over 2 hours.

Adverse effects include nausea and dizziness and are rather frequent.

Verapamil (see p. 60). Verapamil blocks the flow of calcium ions into the muscle cells of the heart. This reduces the force of contraction of the heart muscle and slows conduction in the atrioventricular node, and is thus particularly useful in supraventricular tachycardia as it breaks the circus wave of stimulation. Because of its depressing effect on cardiac muscle contraction *it should not be used if a β blocker has been given in the preceding 24 hours* as the combination can seriously reduce cardiac efficiency and may cause cardiac arrest. For the same reason it should not be used in cardiac failure.

The oral dose is 80 mg 8 hourly or it can be given by infusion, the dose being 5–10 mg over 1 hour, maximum 100 mg in 24 hours or as an i.v. bolus of 5–10 mg given over 2 minutes.

β blockers. The general pharmacology of this group of drugs is considered on page 35. By preventing the stimulation of adrenergic receptors by adrenaline, these drugs decrease the excitability of the heart and thus stop arrhythmias due to an excitable focus or to a supraventricular circus movement as in tachycardia.

It must be remembered that in reducing adrenergic drive to the heart and depressing the heart muscle, these drugs may exacerbate or precipitate heart failure in those whose hearts are under stress from some disease.

Therapeutics. β blockers can be used in arrhythmias due to overexcitability of the heart.

Dosage:

- Propranolol 20–40 mg three times daily, orally
- Atenolol 50–100 mg once daily.

They are usually given to prevent ventricular or supraventricular tachycardia or ectopic beats.

Sotalol is believed to have an additional action which is useful in ventricular arrhythmias.

Interactions. β blockers may also exacerbate the depressing effect on heart muscle of such drugs as verapamil.

Adenosine suppresses conduction through the AV node and is used to terminate supraventricular arrhythmias. It is given intravenously, the usual dose being 6 mg. Its action begins very rapidly and only lasts a very short time, but this is usually sufficient to restore sinus rhythm.

Adverse effects are flushing, chest pain and dyspnoea coming on immediately after injection and lasting up to 30 seconds.

Digitalis. In addition to its use in heart failure, digitalis is sometimes useful in supraventricular arrhythmias where by slowing conduction it may abolish the arrhythmia or control the ventricular rate.

Disopyramide. This drug decreases excitability and slows conduction so it can be used for both supraventricular and ventricular tachycardias. It can be given either orally, the initial dose being 100 mg three times daily, or intravenously at a dose of 2mg/kg slowly over no less than 5 minutes. Disopyramide is excreted via the kidneys and reduced dosage is necessary if renal function is impaired.

Adverse effects include dry mouth, worsening

of glaucoma and difficulty with micturition, all due to an anticholinergic action. It may also cause nausea, vomiting and diarrhoea.

Amiodarone. This most interesting drug is effective in both ventricular and supraventricular arrhythmias. It acts by prolonging the refractory period of heart muscle: this is the short period after each contraction of the heart when the muscle will not respond to any stimulus. Its other important property is that, unlike most anti-arrhythmic drugs, it has little depressing effect on cardiac function. The initial oral dose is 200 mg three times daily and this is reduced after a week to a satisfactory maintenance dose, usually 100 mg daily. This unusual dosage scheme is required because it is very readily bound by the tissues and only when these binding sites have been saturated does it produce its effect on the heart. This also means that it is slowly eliminated and its actions continue for some time after dosage has stopped. Amiodarone can be used intravenously but it must be given over at least 20 minutes and preferably longer via a *central venous line* otherwise it may cause a considerable fall in blood pressure.

Adverse effects are rather common and to some extent limit its use. They include:

1. Photosensitivity rash and bluish-grey pigmentation of exposed areas.
2. It contains a high concentration of iodine and may cause both hypothyroidism and thyrotoxicosis. Thyroid function tests (TSH and T4) should be performed every 6 months in those on long-term treatment.
3. Pulmonary fibrosis requires chest X-rays every 6 months.
4. Deposits in the cornea of the eye occasionally cause visual haloes.
5. Rarely liver damage and neuropathy.
6. Rapid i.v. injection causes marked hypotension.

Interactions. It potentiates the actions of warfarin and digitalis.

Flecainide reduces excitability and slows conduction in the AV node and bundle of His, so it can be used for both ventricular and supraventricular arrhythmias.

Therapeutics. Flecainide can be given by slow intravenous injection (over 10 minutes) in a dose of 2mg/kg (half dose in the elderly) to terminate arrhythmias. Given orally, in doses of 100–200 mg daily and reduced after 3 days to the minimum effective dose, it is useful in preventing ventricular arrhythmias.

Although flecainide is an effective drug it can induce dangerous arrhythmias in patients who have poorly functioning or damaged ventricular muscle, particularly following myocardial infarction, and should be avoided in this group.

Adverse effects. Dizziness is not uncommon. It has some depressant effect on heart muscle and should be used with care, if at all, in patients with conduction defects on a pacemaker. Rarely, it actually provokes, rather than diminishes, ventricular arrhythmias.

Propafenone is effective in suppressing both ventricular and supraventricular arrhythmias and those complicating the Wolff–Parkinson–White syndrome. It can be given orally in doses of 450–900 mg daily in divided doses and has also been used intravenously. Its efficacy appears similar to that of lignocaine and flecainide. The dose may need to be individualized as there is considerable interindividual difference in the blood levels for a given dose due to variation in drug metabolism. Its place in therapeutics can only be determined by further experience.

Direct current cardioversion

A direct current shock is applied to the heart via electrodes placed on the chest. This shock obliterates the ectopic focus or circus movement which causes the arrhythmia and allows normal rhythm to be resumed. This form of treatment has been widely and successfully used in treating atrial fibrillation and about 70% of these patients can be converted to sinus rhythm. Unfortunately, in spite of maintenance treatment with anti-arrhythmic drugs many patients relapse within a few months. It is also useful in other arrhythmias.

Electrolytes and arrhythmias

A low plasma potassium concentration (hypokalaemia) increases the risk of developing an arrhythmia and makes the arrhythmia more difficult to terminate. This is particularly liable to occur after an infarct or in patients taking diuretics. Following an infarct the plasma potassium level should be kept above 4.0 mmol/litre.

Magnesium deficiency also predisposes to arrhythmias and in some units magnesium sulphate is infused immediately after a myocardial infarct to reduce cardiac excitability.

Treatment of individual arrhythmias

In *atrial fibrillation* the pulse rate is usually controlled by digitalis, particularly if present for a long time, and if associated with heart failure. Occasionally the addition of verapamil is required to increase efficacy. If the fibrillation is of recent onset and its underlying cause has been removed, as in treated thyrotoxicosis or after a successful mitral valvotomy, an attempt can be made to restore sinus rhythm by DC shock. Relapse may be prevented by small doses of a β blocker and digoxin or, more rarely, by amiodarone.

Atrial flutter. Digitalis may restore normal rhythm. It may however produce atrial fibrillation which can then be treated as above.

Ventricular tachycardia or extrasystoles. Intravenous lignocaine damps down the excitable focus and usually stops this type of tachycardia. DC shock is also very effective and may be preferred if the facilities are available, particularly if the heart is showing signs of strain. Disopyramide or amiodarone given orally are used to prevent extrasystoles although often no treatment is necessary.

Supraventricular tachycardia. Acute attacks are terminated by depressing conduction through the AV node and thus breaking the circuit. This may be achieved by the patient performing the Valsalva manoeuvre (expiring against the closed glottis) which causes reflex vagal stimulation and slows AV conduction. A similar effect can be produced by pressure over *one* carotid sinus.

The most effective drug is verapamil in a dose of 5–10 mg i.v., a further 5 mg may be given i.v. after 10 minutes if the first dose is unsuccessful. Amiodarone given *slowly* intravenously may be effective and can be tried if verapamil fails.

An alternative approach is to give adenosine which may terminate the attack. It is perhaps safer because its action is very short lived and is now preferred by some experts.

β blockers are used by some but due to their negative inotropic effect (depression of the heart muscle) *they must not be combined with verapamil.*

If drug treatment fails DC shock may be used.

> **Nursing point**
>
> The Valsalva manoeuvre or carotid massage should be carried out with the patient lying flat when it is more effective and he is less liable to faint.

The Wolfe–Parkinson–White (WPW) syndrome

The WPW syndrome is an interesting congenital abnormality occurring in about 0.2% of the population. It is due to an extra (accessory) conducting system between the atria and the ventricles. In itself it causes no trouble but is associated with supraventricular arrhythmias due to re-entry (i.e. down one bundle and up the other) and atrial fibrillation which are occasionally dangerous.

In treating these arrhythmias it must be remembered that the accessory bundle may not respond to drugs in the same way as the normal conducting system. In particular, digoxin and verapamil enhance rather than depress conduction through the accessory bundle and are therefore contraindicated. Depending on circumstances amiodarone, disopyramide or flecainide are used.

Arrhythmias due to conduction defects

Conduction defects can sometimes be relieved by

sympathomimetic drugs (p. 29). Isoprenaline is most commonly used and is most easily given as *Saventrine*, a slow release preparation. However, in most patients with conduction defects, rhythm will have to be maintained by a *pacemaker*.

Bradycardia, particularly when it occurs following a coronary thrombosis, may be due to failure of the cardiac pacemaker (SA node). Atropine 0.6 mg i.v. is useful to restore normal function of the pacemaker.

Nursing points

Much of the treatment of cardiac arrhythmias takes place in hospital with continuous monitoring, often in an intensive care unit. Careful observation is required and changes in rhythm must be noted as they may indicate the need to stop a drug or change treatment.

Remember that no mechanical system is perfect and the nurse should check all mechanical aids, particularly infusion pumps administering drugs, at regular intervals.

DRUGS USED IN ANGINA OF EFFORT

With increasing age the walls of the coronary arteries become thickened and the lumen partially obstructed by a process known as atheroma. If this is severe it interferes with the blood supply to the heart muscle. The coronary blood flow is usually adequate when the patient is at rest, but with effort the demands of the heart muscle for oxygen increase and cannot be met by the narrowed coronary arteries. This results in chest pain which characteristically comes on with effort and is relieved by rest. The coronary arteries can also be narrowed by spasm. The cause of the spasm is not known but it too can give rise to chest pain. Drugs are available which relieve the symptoms of angina but they do not reverse the underlying atheroma.

Sometimes a thrombus forms on a patch of atheroma causing obstruction of the artery and cutting off the blood supply to an area of heart muscle. This is considered on page 70.

The nitrates

This group of drugs acts directly on all the plain muscle of the body causing it to relax. This action is particularly marked on the muscle in the walls of arteries and veins and is due to the release of *nitric oxide* which acts as a vasodilator. Nitrates relieve the pain of angina:

a. By dilating the coronary vessels so that blood flow to ischaemic areas of heart muscle is improved
b. By venodilatation which decreases the return of blood to the heart and thus reduces heart work.

There are a number of drugs in the nitrate group; some having a powerful but short-lived action, others acting less powerfully but over a longer period (Table 4.1; Fig 4.5).

Those in common use are:

Glyceryl trinitrate. Glyceryl trinitrate is an oily liquid which is used in making an

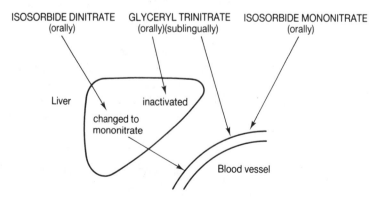

Fig. 4.5 The absorption and metabolism of some commonly used nitrates.

explosive. It is prepared as tablets by mixing with an absorbent base. It is taken orally and sucked, the drug being absorbed from the mucous membrane of the mouth. If swallowed whole, it is not effective because the drug is rapidly destroyed by the liver. Its effects start within a minute and last for 15–20 minutes. It causes a marked general vasodilatation with a fall in blood pressure. The tablets lose potency and should not be kept for more than 2 months, and they should be stored in a closed container and not exposed to light or cotton wool.

A very useful alternative is to give glyceryl trinitrate via a *metered aerosol*. Each dose contains 400 micrograms, which is sprayed under the tongue and the mouth is then closed.

Glyceryl trinitrate is also absorbed through the skin and impregnated patches are available for application. They release the drug slowly over 24 hours thus producing a prolonged effect. They have not proved particularly useful as it is difficult to control dosage and tolerance of the drug's action may develop.

Glyceryl trinitrate can be given by intravenous infusion. This approach is reserved for patients with severe chest pain usually following a cardiac infarct when it may relieve the pain and also improve any complicating heart failure. It is best given in saline or 5% dextrose by a syringe pump and the initial dose is 20 micrograms/minute. PVC containers (Viaflex and Steriflex) must not be used.

Isosorbide dinitrate is similar to glyceryl trinitrate. It is broken down in the liver to isosorbide mononitrate which is the active agent. It is available in several forms:

Chewable tablets	— active within a minute or two.
Oral tables	— active in about 20 minutes and last 4–6 hours.
Oral modified release tablets	— active in about 20 minutes and last about 12 hours.

The dose varies between 5–60 mg and is adjusted to suit the needs of the patient.

Isosorbide mononitrate is the active breakdown product of the above and is now available for clinical use. The dose is 20–40 mg orally, usually twice daily as its action is quite prolonged.

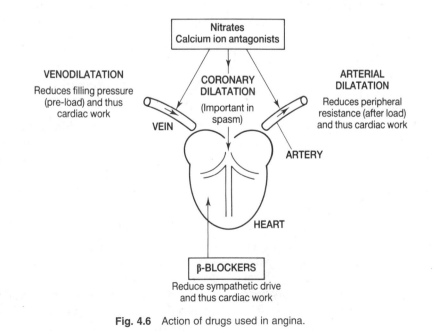

Fig. 4.6 Action of drugs used in angina.

Therapeutics. The main use of nitrates is in the treatment of angina of effort. The nitrates, by dilating the coronary arteries, increase blood supply to the myocardium and at the same time, by lowering the blood pressure, and venodilatation, they decrease the work of the heart (Fig. 4.6). Nitrates can be used in several ways to treat angina. They may be taken intermittently to relieve the pain in an attack, or better, taken *before* performing some action which the patient knows from experience will cause pain. Glyceryl trinitrate is the best drug for this purpose.

One tablet (300 or 500 micrograms) is sucked and the dose may be repeated as frequently as it is required. Some patients taking nitrates complain of throbbing headaches due to dilatation of the cerebral vessels, and may occasionally faint from the fall in blood pressure. In patients who are getting repeated attacks, a long-acting nitrate such as sustained release isosorbide dinitrate or isosorbide mononitrate can be given *regularly* to prevent attacks or diminish their severity.

In patients with severe and continuous anginal pain nitrates can be given by intravenous infusion either as glyceryl trinitrate or isosorbide dinitrate. They may also be effective in severe heart failure. When nitrates are given in this way the patient requires very careful monitoring and the facilities of an intensive care unit are desirable.

Adverse effects. In addition to flushing, headaches, and palpitations these drugs may cause a fall in blood pressure which can be particularly troublesome with long-acting preparations when the patient may feel faint. Rarely, large doses cause methaemoglobinaemia leading to a cyanotic appearance.

Tolerance to the action of nitrates occurs with continuous or frequent dosage but sensitivity is rapidly restored if the drug is stopped for a few hours. Intravenous infusions should not be given for more than 36 hours without a break. The last dose of sustained-release or long-acting preparations should be taken with the evening meal unless nocturnal angina is a problem. Glyceryl trinitrate is unlikely to produce tolerance as it is so short acting.

Table 4.1 Duration of action of nitrates

	Onset of effect	Duration of effect
Glyceryl trinitrate		
(sucked or chewed)	2 minutes	30 minutes
(patch)	1–2 hours	up to 24 hours
Isosorbide mononitrate		
(swallowed)	20 minutes	10 hours
Isosorbide dinitrate		
(chewed)	2 minutes	2 hours
(swallowed)	10 minutes	5 hours

β blockers (see p. 36)

β blockers have proved very useful in treating angina of effort. The rise in heart rate and heart work which occurs on exercise is partially brought about by the activity of the sympathetic nervous system. By blocking this stimulating effect the β blockers protect the heart from overactivity and prevent the development of anginal pain.

Therapeutics. Most β blockers have been used successfully in treating angina of effort and there is no evidence that any one drug is to be preferred. The usual method of giving these drugs is to start with a small dose and increase it until a satisfactory control of symptoms is obtained. The drug is given *regularly to prevent pain* rather than to treat attacks.

Nifedipine, verapamil and diltiazem (see p. 59)

These drugs decrease cardiac work by dilating the peripheral blood vessels and this lowers resistance to blood flow. In addition, they dilate the coronary blood vessels, therefore they are useful in treating angina, particularly if it is believed that coronary spasm is playing a part in producing the symptom.

Therapeutics. They are taken regularly to prevent angina. Nifedipine is given in doses of 10 mg three times daily before meals and increased as necessary. Verapamil in doses of 80–120 mg three times daily and diltiazem in doses of 60 mg three times daily.

Adverse effects (see p. 60).

Special points for patient education

Patients with angina can learn to avoid or treat their attacks.

1. If possible, they should avoid situations known to precipitate attacks, e.g. undue exertion, heavy meals.
2. They should differentiate between drugs which are used intermittently to treat an attack or taken immediately before exertion to prevent one, and those which are taken regularly as a prophylactic measure.
3. They should be aware of the main adverse effects they may encounter and it is helpful if the first dose glyceryl trinitrate is taken under supervision so that patients may become familiar with the side-effects.
4. Patients may ask if the drugs will become less effective with continued use. This is unlikely with glyceryl trinitrate, but not for the longer-acting nitrates (see above). Tolerance does not occur with β blockers or calcium antagonists.
5. Patients should be told to call their doctor if an attack is prolonged and fails to respond to glyceryl trinitrate.

DRUGS USED TO LOWER BLOOD PRESSURE

The blood pressure depends on:

1. The peripheral vascular resistance
2. The output of blood from the heart
3. The volume of blood within the circulation.

By decreasing one or more of these factors it is possible to lower the blood pressure.

The peripheral vascular resistance depends on the bore of the smaller arteries (arterioles). The walls of these arteries contain circular muscle fibres which are controlled by the sympathetic nervous system (p. 27). Stimulation of this system releases *noradrenaline* which causes these muscles to contract and leads to narrowing of the arterioles and a rise in blood pressure.

Angiotensin (see below) also causes constriction of blood vessels and a rise in blood pressure.

The cardiac output depends on several factors, but one important control is again the sympathetic nervous system which, by releasing

adrenaline, causes a rise in pulse rate and output of blood.

The volume of blood within the circulation is ultimately controlled by the kidneys. There are receptors which 'sense' changes in the blood volume and if it falls the kidney secretes a substance called *renin* which, via a complex series of changes, causes retention of salt and water by the kidneys (Fig. 4.7).

HYPERTENSION

In certain people the blood pressure is consistently raised above normal limits probably as a result of arteriolar constriction—the condition is known as *hypertension*. In the majority of patients the cause is not known although there are probably inherited and environmental factors and the condition is then called *essential hypertension*. Much more rarely it is secondary to kidney or endocrine disorders. The actual elevation of blood pressure, unless severe, rarely produces symptoms but it damages the heart, blood vessels and kidneys which leads to coronary thrombosis, heart failure, strokes and less often to renal failure.

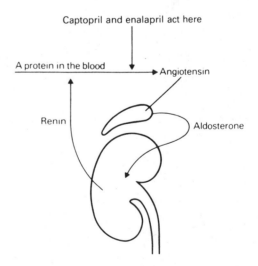

Fig. 4.7 Renin released from the kidney acts on a protein in the blood to form angiotensin. Angiotensin constricts blood vessels and raises BP. Angiotensin also releases aldosterone from the adrenal gland which causes salt and water retention by the kidney. Net result = a rise in blood pressure.

It is logical therefore to prevent these complications by lowering the blood pressure and this can be achieved by drugs which: (a) Lower peripheral resistance (b) Lower cardiac output (c) Decrease blood volume, or a combination of these effects.

DRUGS WHICH LOWER PERIPHERAL RESISTANCE BY DECREASING SYMPATHETIC ACTIVITY

As stated above the peripheral vascular resistance is maintained by the sympathetic nervous system. It follows therefore that a drug which blocks the action of the sympathetic system will decrease peripheral resistance and lower blood pressure.

Sympathetic blocking drugs (see Fig. 4.8)

Prazosin, doxazosin and terazosin block the vasoconstrictor sympathetic nerve supply to the small arteries (α receptors) and the resulting vasodilatation causes a fall in blood pressure. With these drugs there is no compensatory rise in pulse rate or cardiac output. The fall in blood pressure is inclined to the postural (greater on standing than lying). Prazosin is short-acting and dosage is required two or three times daily, doxazosin and terazosin have a longer action so once a day dosage is adequate.

Therapeutics. The initial dose can sometimes cause a profound fall in blood pressure with fainting so it is advisable that this dose is given before retiring and should be low. Subsequent doses do not appear to provoke this problem and can be increased until a satisfactory blood pressure is achieved.

Prazosin	500 micrograms initially then 1.0 mg three times daily up to 20 mg daily.
Doxazosin	1.0 mg daily increased to 4.0 mg daily.
Terazosin	1.0 mg daily increased up to 10 mg daily.

Drugs with several sites of action
(see Fig. 4.8)

Methyldopa. This drug lowers blood pressure by an action on the brain which results in decreased activity of the sympathetic system. In addition, it is converted by the body to methylnoradrenaline which then blocks the action of noradrenaline on blood vessels and thus lowers the blood pressure.

Therapeutics. Methyldopa was formerly used widely in the treatment of hypertension. It is effective and easy to use because the fall in blood pressure is not precipitous. However, it has a number of adverse effects which patients sometimes find unacceptable and its use has declined considerably.

The initial dose is 250 mg orally three times daily and this can be increased to 1.5 g daily. Further increases in dosage do not seem to be more effective.

Adverse effects are rather common. Drowsiness and depression often occur early in treatment but may pass off after a few weeks, more rarely fluid retention producing oedema can be troublesome but is controlled by a diuretic. Haemolytic anaemia and drug fever have also been reported. It is still, however, used by some when hypertension complicates pregnancy, but does not have any particular advantage in this situation.

Clonidine has both a central action on the brain and a peripheral action on the arteries. It produces a moderate fall in blood pressure which is little altered by posture. The initial dose is 50 micrograms three times a day, and increased as required.

Adverse effects, particularly tiredness and depression, have led to a decline in its use. *It is important not to stop treatment with clonidine suddenly as this may be followed by a 'rebound' rise in blood pressure which can be dangerous.*

DRUGS WHICH ACT DIRECTLY OR INDIRECTLY ON THE ARTERIOLE
(Fig. 4.8)

Hydralazine. Hydralazine lowers the blood pressure by relaxing the blood vessels. It acts

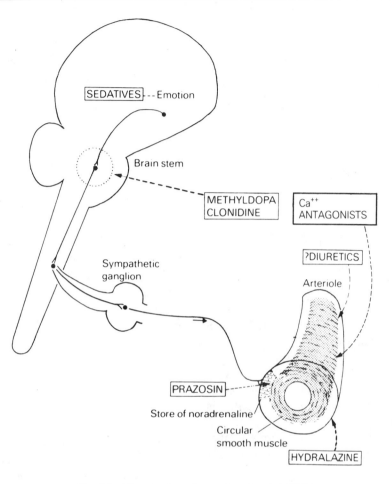

Fig. 4.8   Site of action of some hypotensive drugs.

directly on the muscle and not via the sympathetic nervous system. Unfortunately it also causes a rise in pulse rate and cardiac output which to some degree cancels its hypotensive action. This problem can now be overcome by combing hydralazine with a β blocker which will prevent the rise in pulse rate and cardiac output and thus increase the fall in blood pressure. Initial dose is 25 mg twice daily.

Adverse effects include headache and rashes, and arthritis similar to SLE can be troublesome with high dosage.

Calcium antagonists. This group of drugs blocks the entry of calcium ions into the muscle cells in the arterial walls resulting in relaxation of the muscle and dilatation of the arteries. They are used to lower blood pressure in hypertension and to dilate coronary arteries in angina (see p. 56). In addition verapamil slows conduction in the AV node and is used in treating cardiac arrhythmias (see p. 51).

Therapeutics. Although their actions and uses are similar they differ in detail. They are all given orally and broken down by the liver.

Short-acting used for hypertension or angina:

Nifedipine   5–20 mg three times daily. Retard and slow-release preparations are available needing only one or two doses daily.

Nicardipine   20–30 mg three times daily.
Isradipine   1.25–5.0 mg twice daily.
Diltiazem   60 mg three times daily.

Long-acting used for hypertension or angina:

Amlodipine   5–10 mg once daily.

Used for hypertension, angina and cardiac arrhythmias:

Verapamil   80–480 mg three times daily orally.
5–10mg slowly i.v.

At present there is no clearly preferred drug for hypertension although the longer-acting preparations are more convenient.

Adverse effects. Headache, flushing and ankle oedema, due to vasodilatation can occur with all these drugs but are more common with nifedipine and nicardipine.

Constipation, only with verapamil.

Depression of heart. Marked with verapamil and to a lesser extent with others. Verapamil should not be given intravenously to patients receiving β blockers.

Great care is necessary if calcium channel blockers are given to patients with heart failure as this may be made worse.

Interactions. The action of nifedipine and nicardipine is increased by cimetidine.

The blood levels (and therefore the action) of carbamazepine, theophylline and digoxin are increased by these drugs.

Angiotensin converting enzyme (ACE) inhibitors. ACE inhibitors interfere with the formation of angiotensin II and thus block the renin/aldosterone system (see p. 57). This reduces the vasoconstricting action of angiotensin and the sodium retaining properties of aldosterone and causes a fall in blood pressure. They are used in treating hypertension and cardiac failure (see p. 45). They also reduce proteinuria in diabetic patients with kidney disease and slow the decline in renal function.

Several of these drugs are now available, having similar actions and uses.

Therapeutic use. Captopril was the first to be introduced and is still widely used. It is rapidly absorbed when given orally, its action starts after half an hour and lasts up to 8 hours. The initial dose is 12.5 mg (6.25 mg for the elderly) twice daily before meals and this may be increased, if necessary, to 50 mg twice daily.

Enalapril is a pro-drug and is itself inactive but is converted into an active metabolite in the liver. It therefore takes longer to act (3 hours) but its effects are prolonged (24 hours). The initial dose is 5.0 mg once daily and increased to 40 mg daily if necessary.

Other ACE inhibitors are:

Drug	Pro-drug	Dosage frequency	Special Points
Fosinopril	+	Daily	Hepatic and renal excretion
Lisinopril	–	Daily	
Perindopril	+	Daily	
Quinapril	+	Daily or b.d.	
Ramipril	+	Daily	

A marked fall in blood pressure occurs occasionally after starting to take an ACE inhibitor especially if the patient is already taking a diuretic. For this reason the initial dose should be low and taken before retiring; patients should be warned of the possibility of a sharp fall in blood pressure if they get up in the night.

ACE inhibitors should not be used in pregnancy and the dose kept as low as possible in renal impairment.

Before starting treatment, electrolytes and renal function should be measured.

Adverse effects and interactions:

1. A few patients, particularly the elderly and those with impaired renal function, develop renal failure so the plasma creatinine should be measured every 6 months.
2. Dry cough.
3. Fatigue, headaches, diarrhoea.
4. Rashes, change in taste (captopril).
5. Captopril may produce proteinuria and neutropenia though rarely with the lower doses now used.
6. Hyperkalaemia in patients with renal disease or who are taking potassium-sparing diuretics or supplementary potassium.

7. Declining renal function if combined with NSAIAs.

Sodium nitroprusside must be given intravenously and is therefore only suitable for treating a hypertensive crisis and some patients with acute heart failure. It is given by infusion in a dose of 0.5–8 micrograms/kg/minute. It is usual to start at the lower end of the dose range and increase it until the blood pressure is satisfactorily controlled. This will require close observation and is usually carried out in an intensive care unit.

There are four important practical points in its use:

1. It should be dissolved in 5% dextrose (nothing else is suitable).
2. The infusion must be protected from the light and discarded after 4 hours.
3. It should also be discarded if the colour changes from pale orange to dark brown or blue.
4. Infusion should not be continued for more than 72 hours.

Adverse effects. Headaches, dizziness, palpitations and chest pain.

Minoxidil is a powerful vasodilator and thus causes a fall in blood pressure. Its use is confined to patients who are resistant to more usual treatment (see below).

Therapeutic use. When minoxidil is given it should be combined with:

1. A diuretic, otherwise it will cause salt and water retention.
2. A β blocker, or it will cause the heart rate to rise.

The usual initial dose is 5 mg daily which may be increased as required.

Adverse effects. Increasing hairiness is a strange but common and upsetting complication.

In addition to salt and water retention, pericardial effusions sometimes develop.

DRUGS WHICH LOWER CARDIAC OUTPUT

β blockers. β blockers will lower the blood pressure to a satisfactory level in about 40% of hypertensive patients, but the hypotensive effect may be delayed for several weeks after starting treatment. It is not known exactly how these drugs produce this effect. By interfering with the sympathetic nervous system they certainly prevent the rise in cardiac output and blood pressure which occurs with excitement or effort. It may be that this damping down of the circulation ultimately causes a permanent fall in blood pressure. In certain circumstances β blockers decrease renin release by the kidney which would tend to lower the blood pressure (see p. 57) and some of them (particularly propranolol) have some central sedative action.

The effect of some β blockers is predominantly on the heart (β_1 receptors) and they are called *'selective'* β blockers; others affect also the bronchi and possibly the peripheral circulation (β_2 receptors) and are known as *'non-selective'* β blockers.

Therapeutics. There is no evidence that any particular β blocker is more effective in lowering blood pressure, but if the patient is prone to obstructive airways disease a selective β blocker is preferred. Among those used are:

Selective β *blockers*	*Non-selective* β *blockers*
Metoprolol 100–200 mg daily	Propranolol 80–320 mg daily
Atenolol 50–100 mg daily	Oxprenolol 160–480 mg daily
	Nadolol 80–160 mg daily
	Timolol 15–45 mg daily
	Pindolol 15–30 mg daily

Atenolol, pindolol and nadolol can be given once daily. The others are usually given two or three times daily although such frequent dosage may not be necessary to control blood pressure. There are also slow release preparations available of propranolol, oxprenolol and metoprolol.

Serious adverse effects are not common. Patients with bronchospasm from asthma or chronic bronchitis may get worse on β blockers which should be *avoided in asthmatics* and used with care in bronchitis for which a selective β blocker is indicated (see above). They may also exacerbate heart failure and should not be used in this condition.

Diabetic patients taking insulin are at some risk as β blockers mask the symptoms of hypoglycaemia and this should be explained to them.

Apart from these three dangerous effects β blockers have other side-effects which, although not dangerous, may interfere with the quality of life—an important consideration if treatment is to be continued over long periods. Some patients complain of lacking energy and aggression and feel tired and depressed. Others may complain of vivid dreams and occasionally of hallucinations.

Owing to the fall in cardiac output, the peripheral circulation decreases and this results in cold hands and feet and can be a serious problem in patients with peripheral vascular disease in whom β blockers should be avoided.

Occasionally, the resting pulse rate is considerably reduced by β blockers. Provided it does not fall below 50/minute this is not usually a matter of concern. Lower rates require a change to oxprenolol or pindolol which allow a rather higher pulse rate at rest.

Interactions:

1. Myocardial function is reduced if combined with intravenous verapamil.
2. β blockers increase the peripheral vasoconstricting action of ergotamine (see p. 39).
3. The action of some β blockers is increased by cimetidine.

Labetalol combines β blocking activity with some α blocking effect. The result is that the cardiac output is decreased and at the same time there is some peripheral vasodilatation. This leads to a fall in blood pressure.

Therapeutic use. The initial dose is 100 mg twice daily and this may be increased gradually until satisfactory control is achieved. Dosage requirements are variable and this makes treatment difficult. It can also be given i.v. in doses of 50 mg over 2 minutes to control a hypertensive crisis.

Adverse effects. Labetalol should be used with care in patients with heart failure as it may make it worse, and avoided in asthmatic patients. Other side-effects include stuffy nose, lethargy and vivid dreams and tingling of the scalp.

Celiprolol combines a selective β_1 blocking action on the heart with a β_2 action on the blood vessels causing vasodilatation. Theoretically this dual action should be advantageous in lowering blood pressure; however, clinical trials suggest that its efficacy is similar to that of other β blockers.

DRUGS WHICH DECREASE BLOOD VOLUME

Diuretics. Diuretics cause a small fall in blood pressure. This may be partly due to the fall in the blood volume and partly to a direct effect on the arteriole wall making it less sensitive to substances causing vasoconstriction.

The thiazide diuretics are most suitable for this purpose. A small dose is sufficient as a larger one causes very little further fall in blood pressure but increases the incidence of adverse effects. These include impotence in 20% of males; long-term treatment can induce a diabetic-like state and diabetics may be more difficult to control. Uric acid retention can precipitate attacks of gout. Potassium depletion is rare with low doses of thiazides but the plasma potassium should be checked after 4 weeks of treatment.

Diuretics may be used as the sole treatment or combined with other hypotensive agents such as β blockers. The combination of diuretics with ACE inhibitors can cause a profound fall in blood pressure so care is required if these two drugs are given together.

Indapamide is similar to the thiazides and offers no particular advantage.

THE TREATMENT OF HYPERTENSION

When a raised blood pressure is detected, it is important to exclude underlying renal or endocrine causes, although essential hypertension is responsible in 90% of cases. Hypertension, by itself, rarely causes any symptoms and the object of treatment is to prevent the development of complications e.g. stroke, coronary thrombosis, cardiac and renal failure. Many hypertensive patients live for years without these complications and this means that the drugs used in treatment should be safe and free from adverse effects. Unfortunately, no hypotensive drug entirely fulfils these criteria. It is generally accepted that severe hypertension carries a poor prognosis and adequate treatment considerably reduces morbidity and mortality. It is in patients with milder degrees of hypertension that a decision to embark on drug treatment is more difficult.

In healthy subjects with no evidence of cardiac, vascular or renal complications it is justifiable to observe the patient with regular measurement of blood pressure for 6 months because, in some people, it may return to normal levels, particularly when they become used to visiting the doctor. At this stage, non-drug measures may be considered (see under Special points for patient education, p. 64). If, however, the diastolic pressure remains persistently above 90 mmHg (95 mmHg in the elderly) and particularly if there are additional risk factors (hyperlipidaemia, bad family history) it is usual to start treatment with a single drug and if this fails a combination should be given. The aim is to reduce the blood pressure below 160/90 and a similar figure is acceptable in the elderly.

There have been many trials of hypotensive drugs in this group of patients and the results can be roughly summarized as follows:

1. There was some reduction in overall mortality—probably about 20%.
2. The incidence of stroke was halved but there was less reduction of coronary thrombosis.
3. In elderly patients the incidence of stroke was reduced by about 40% and there was some reduction in the occurrence of coronary thrombosis.

A variety of agents is now available and the best drug or combination of drugs for treatment is still being investigated. The usual approach is to start with β blocker in the younger or middle-aged patient.

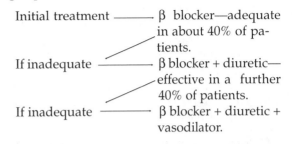

In elderly patients it may be better to start treatment with a diuretic.

There is increasing concern about the quality of life of patients receiving treatment for hypertension as these regimes may be associated with various adverse effects which, although usually minor, can be troublesome. ACE inhibitors, though not without risk, do not make life a burden and may well have a place in initial therapy. α blockers and calcium channel blockers may also be used and there are numerous possible combinations where the effects are at least additive. It is usually possible to plan a regime which is therapeutically effective without interfering with the patient's lifestyle.

A few patients require admission to hospital so that they can be fully investigated and when treatment is started, frequent observation of blood pressure can be made. In milder hypertension, with no complicating disease, treatment can be started and carried through on an outpatient basis. When adequate control is obtained, further supervision is required by the family doctor or hospital outpatients' department.

Occasionally it may be necessary to reduce a *very high blood pressure rapidly*. Sodium nitroprusside (see p. 61) is the drug of choice for initial treatment. Great care must be taken when lowering a very high blood pressure as a precipitate fall may cause renal failure or cerebral damage due to sudden reduction of the blood supply to the kidney and brain. The early stages of this treatment should be carried out in an intensive care unit if possible and the blood pressure monitored at frequent intervals. The aim of treatment should be to reduce the diastolic blood pressure to around 100 mmHg. Thereafter treatment for hypertension should be carried out in the normal way (see above).

If facilities for intensive monitoring are not available and if the clinical situation is less acute, some physicians use oral nifedipine 10 mg or oral captopril. The problem here is that the fall in blood pressure is less predictable and less easily controlled and there is a risk of dangerous hypotension.

Hypertension in pregnancy presents a special problem as occasionally it may progress to pre-eclampsia and eclampsia with serious risk to both mother and child. Mild transient elevation of blood pressure occurring towards the end of pregnancy rarely needs drug treatment. More severe hypertension, particularly if the patient was hypertensive before the start of her pregnancy, may require drugs to lower the blood pressure. Methyldopa has been found satisfactory for many years. β blockers are also used but may retard fetal growth. In severe hypertension hydralazine orally or intravenously is effective. Diuretics and ACE inhibitors should be avoided.

Measuring the blood pressure

It is often the nurse's duty to measure the blood pressure. The technique is beyond the scope of this book but there are some important points to remember when treating hypertension.

1. The blood pressure should usually be recorded with the patient both *lying and standing* as some hypotensive agents cause a much greater fall in blood pressure when the patient is standing than when he is lying down. In certain cases it should also be recorded after exercise.
2. Some patients are nervous when visiting the doctor. Quiet reassurance and a rest period of 5 minutes is necessary before measuring the blood pressure. Sometimes it is helpful to teach intelligent patients to take their own blood pressure so a home record can be obtained which will give a better idea of day-to-day fluctuations. Because smoking may alter the blood pressure temporarily, patients should be asked to avoid it for 30

Special points for patient education

1. Some patients do not realize that once drug treatment is started it will probably continue for the rest of their lives, although it may be altered or attenuated with advancing years.
2. There are several non-drug ways of lowering blood pressure. Adding no salt to food or cooking will reduce blood pressure and enhance the effect of drugs but some patients find that this spoils the joy of eating. Various forms of relaxation, meditation and stress reduction produce a small but useful fall in blood pressure in many subjects.
3. It is very important that 'risk' factors which increase their liability to the complications of hypertension be avoided, so the following advice should be given:

   a. Stop smoking.
   b. Reduce weight if obese and correct blood lipids if abnormal (see p. 72).
   c. Reduce alcohol consumption if excessive (this actually lowers blood pressure).

4. Patients should be warned of the main adverse effects of the drugs prescribed for them.
5. It is impossible for patients to know and understand all the possible interactions but if given a new drug they should remind the prescriber that they are already receiving medication.
6. Some patients can be taught to take their own blood pressure and thus obtain a more accurate assessment of day-to-day levels.

Nursing point

Nurses are often involved in treating hypertension. They may work in special outpatient clinics or it may be part of their duties as general practice nurses and they will often be responsible for taking blood pressures and arranging attendances, etc. They should be familiar with the drugs being used, particularly their adverse effects so that they can advise the patient and if necessary, together with the doctor, change the treatment.

---

minutes before having their blood pressure measured.

3. A well-applied cuff and a good stethoscope are necessary for accurate readings.
4. Measurements of blood pressure tend to show 'observer bias'. This may happen in trials of new drugs and it is necessary in these circumstances to use a special sphygmomanometer in which the blood pressure is recorded 'blind' so that the recording is not known by the observer.

DRUGS USED IN THE TREATMENT OF PERIPHERAL VASCULAR DISEASE

For many years various drugs, which in normal individuals dilate arteries, were used in vascular disease in the hope that they would increase the blood supply to the ischaemic limb. Unfortunately, vascular disease usually affects the large arteries and these diseased arteries were unresponsive to vasodilators which are now recognized as being useless in this condition.

They are however useful in Raynaud's disease which is due to spasm in the small arteries of the hands and feet brought on by cold.

Therapeutics. Nifedipine (see p. 59) used as for hypertension is the most useful drug. Other measures include keeping warm in cold weather. Do not forget that β blockers and ergotamine make peripheral vascular disease worse.

FURTHER READING

Breckenridge A 1988 ACE inhibitors. British Medical Journal 296: 618

Cobbe S M, Rankin A C 1988 Drug treatment of cardiac arrhythmias. Prescribers Journal 28: 48

Collins R et al 1990 Blood pressure, stroke and coronary artery disease. Lancet 335: 827

Cool S M 1982 'Mr Jones has pump failure'. Nursing lst series 33: 1435

Dahlof B et al 1991 Morbidity and mortality in the Swedish trial in old patients with hypertension. Lancet 338: 1281

Editorial 1988 Aspirin all round? British Medical Journal 296: 307

Editorial 1988 The place of angiotensin—converting enzymes inhibition in the treatment of cardiovascular disease. New England Journal of Medicine 319: 1541

Editorial 1988 Modern treatment of heart failure. British Medical Journal 297: 83

Editorial 1989 Treating mild hypertension. British Medical Journal 298: 694

Editorial 1990 Do drugs help intermittent claudication? Drug and Therapeutics Bulletin 28: 1

Editorial 1991 Hypertensive emergencies. Lancet 338: 229

Editorial 1991 ACE inhibitors a cornerstone in the treatment of heart failure. New England Journal of Medicine 325: 351

Editorial 1992 Managing heart failure. Drug and Therapeutics Bulletin 30: 61

Feely J, Pringle T, McLean D 1988 Thrombolytic agents and the new calcium antagonists. British Medical Journal 296: 705

Fogarty A 1986 et al Finding the facts on glyceryl trinitrate tablets. Nursing Times 82(35): 37

Kitchen I 1984 Congestive cardiac failure and cardiogenic shock. Nursing 2nd series 25: 743

Nitrates and heart disease 1984 Drug and Therapeutics Bulletin 22: 120

Sever P et al (1993) Management guidelines in essential hypertension. British Medical Journal 306: 983

Swales J D 1990 First line treatment of hypertension. Editorial, British Medical Journal 301: 1172

Vallance P, Moncarda S 1994 Nitric oxide—from mediator to medicine. Journal of the Royal College of Physicians, London 28: 209

5

Anticoagulants and thrombolytic agents

THROMBOSIS

When the wall of a blood vessel is damaged or severed the blood coagulates and thus arrests bleeding. The mechanism is complicated and depends on the activation of various factors in the blood. A simplified version is:

> Prothrombin + Thromboplastin + Calcium + other factors → Thrombin
> Thrombin + Fibrinogen → Fibrin.

Fibrin is deposited in the damaged areas and blocks the source of bleeding. This action is assisted by platelets which plug small defects in the vessel wall. This is the normal process.

Coagulation or thrombosis may sometimes occur in blood vessels which have not been injured and in these circumstances blockage of the vessel concerned may have serious consequences. There are two types of thrombosis:

1. Venous thrombosis (phlebothrombosis)
2. Arterial thrombosis.

Although both may result in obstruction to a blood vessel they occur under different circumstances, have different mechanisms and differ in their treatment.

VENOUS THROMBOSIS (PHLEBOTHROMBOSIS)

This usually occurs in the deep veins of the legs. It is due to stagnation of blood in the veins when a patient is lying still after an operation (particularly if the pelvis or hip is involved), associated with pregnancy or during a severe illness. The risk is increased in the obese, in patients with malignancy or who have a history of previous thrombosis. *Oral contraceptives* containing oestrogen are also a risk factor and should be stopped 6 weeks before a major operation or any surgery involving the pelvis or hip. The danger of this type of thrombosis is that part of the clot may break off, forming an *embolus* which is swept back via the heart to the lungs where it blocks a branch of the pulmonary artery, an event which can be fatal.

In atrial fibrillation a thrombus may develop in the left atrium because of impaired blood flow and fragments can become detached resulting in emboli to the brain and elsewhere. Anticoagulants, which interfere with clotting (coagulation) of blood can be used either to prevent the formation of thrombi or to treat established venous thrombosis.

ANTICOAGULANTS

These drugs by interfering with clotting are used to prevent and treat venous thrombosis.

Heparin

Heparin is a complex substance. It is not absorbed by mouth and is usually given by intravenous or sometimes by subcutaneous or intramuscular injection. Heparin is an anticoagulant. Its actions on the clotting mechanism are multiple and complicated, but the end result is a prolongation of clotting time. The anticoagulant effect of heparin is seen within a minute or two of injection, but passes off within a few hours.

Therapeutics. Heparin is often used at the beginning of anticoagulant treatment because its effects are so rapid. It may be given by continuous intravenous infusion or by intermittent subcutaneous or intravenous injection.

Infusion is best given via a syringe pump at the rate of 25 000–30 000 units in 24 hours following an initial bolus of 5000 units. If a pump is not available the heparin can be added to 1 litre of saline or 5% dextrose and given as an infusion.

Whichever method is used the infusion rate must be carefully controlled.

The rate of infusion is monitored by measuring the *kaolin cephalin time or partial thromboplastin time* 6 hours after starting infusion and then at least once daily and these should be kept between $1\frac{1}{2}$ and $2\frac{1}{2}$ times the control value. If intermittent injections are given the dose is about 10 000 units 6 hourly and estimations of clotting time are not usually required.

When used to *prevent* thrombosis, heparin is given in doses of 5000 units in 0.2 ml subcutaneously twice daily. It is injected into the subcutaneous tissue of the abdominal wall via a fine needle (gauge 25 length 16 mm). An inch of skin should be picked up at the site of injection and the needle inserted perpendicularly to its full length. Local pressure is applied for 5 minutes after injection to prevent excessive bruising.

Adverse effects. The only common adverse effect from heparin is bleeding due to overdose. As with all anticoagulants this often first appears as haematuria, but may occur from any site. The treatment is to stop the heparin.

Protamine sulphate which reverses the action of heparin can be given intravenously in a dose of 1 mg for every 100 units of heparin. Protamine sulphate may cause a fall in blood pressure. If blood loss is excessive it should be replaced by transfusion.

Low molecular weight heparins. These drugs are similar in their action to heparin but the anticoagulant effect lasts much longer so that one daily subcutaneous injection is adequate in preventing thrombosis. After hip operations they are possibly a little more effective than conventional heparin but the incidence of bleeding complications is similar. They are considerably more expensive.

Twice daily subcutaneous injections have also been used in treating deep vein thrombosis and appear to be as effective and as safe as continuous intravenous infusion.

Available at present are *deltaparin* and *enoxaparin*. Others will probably be introduced and their place in anticoagulant treatment will become better defined.

The coumarin group

There are two substances in this group which are commonly used in anticoagulant therapy, **warfarin** and **phenindione**. Their mode of action is similar and they will therefore be considered together.

They are effective by mouth and prevent the conversion of vitamin K to various clotting factors. Their exact site of action is not settled, but there is evidence that the liver is concerned and patients with liver disease are certainly more sensitive to these drugs than is usual.

Therapeutics. This group of drugs is given orally. It is very important that strict accuracy is observed in the timing of doses. The effectiveness of the drug in interfering with coagulation is measured by *prothrombin time* estimations.

Contraindications include active peptic ulcer, severe liver disease and renal failure.

Warfarin. The initial dose of warfarin for an adult is 9 mg daily for 3 days. Various factors such as old age, poor nutrition, liver disease, heart failure, previous surgery and concurrent drugs will increase the patient's sensitivity to warfarin and require smaller dosage.

The prothrombin time should be measured before starting treatment. As warfarin is rather slow to take effect it need not be repeated for 3 days, thereafter it must be measured daily. The ratio:

$$\frac{\text{Patient's prothrombin time}}{\text{Normal prothrombin time}}$$

is known as the *International Normalized Ratio* (INR) and the dose is adjusted to keep this between 2.0 and 3.0 which gives effective anticoagulation with minimal risk of bleeding. The daily dose for most patients lies between 3–6 mg. The initial stages of anticoagulation are carried out in hospital but thereafter they are controlled on an outpatient basis and only monthly measurements of prothrombin time may be required.

Phenindione. The initial 24-hour dose of phenindione is about 200 mg in divided doses. The maximum effect is within 24–36 hours.

Adverse effects. Overdosage is the most important side-effect of the coumarin group of drugs and may lead to haemorrhage from any site. It is worth remembering, however, that phenindione sometimes colours the urine a pinkish-red. It is best treated by withdrawal of the drug. If necessary the effect of the anticoagulant can be reversed rapidly by an infusion of fresh frozen plasma. Alternatively, phytomenadione (vitamin K)1–2 mg i.v. can be given but takes about 12 hours to become effective. Larger doses of phytomenadione interfere with further anticoagulation for some days. Rarely transfusion with fresh blood is required if blood loss has been excessive.

In addition skin rashes, drug fever and jaundice can occur rarely with phenindione.

Use in pregnancy. Warfarin crosses the placenta and may cause fetal abnormalities if given in the first 3 months of pregnancy. If anticoagulation is required during pregnancy, either heparin can be used throughout or heparin used up to 16 weeks, warfarin from 16–36 weeks and heparin until delivery. Prefilled syringes of heparin calcium containing 5000 units are available for self-injection by pregnant women at home.

Interactions of oral anticoagulants with other drugs are important because even a small increase or decrease in their effectiveness may render them dangerous or useless. Warfarin activity is increased by antibiotics, aspirin, alcohol, cimetidine, dipyridamole and phenytoin and decreased by barbiturates. This list is by no means complete and if possible, the use of other drugs

---

Special points for patient education

1. The dose of anticoagulants is critical—the correct dose must be taken at the correct time.

2. Overdosage is dangerous—any evidence of bruising or bleeding must be reported immediately. In hospital the urine should be tested daily for blood.

3. As far as possible patients should not alter their lifestyle, but even one night of heavy drinking may alter the efficacy of oral anticoagulants.

4. There are many interactions with other drugs. These (even those obtained over the counter) should not be taken without medical advice.

5. All patients on oral anticoagulants should carry a card and attend regularly for estimations of prothrombin time.

with anticoagulants should be avoided. If the drug regime has to be changed the prothrombin time must be monitored carefully.

PREVENTION OF VENOUS THROMBOSIS

Patients *immobilized in bed* as a result of surgery, severe illness or trauma are at risk of venous thrombosis and pulmonary embolism. Overall about 20% of untreated postoperative patients develop a thrombosis and about 1% have a fatal pulmonary embolus. These risks can be considerably reduced by giving 5000 IU of heparin subcutaneously, twice daily or low molecular weight heparin once daily (see above) over the operative and postoperative period. With correct dosage it is possible to achieve thrombus prevention without undue bleeding at operation.

The risk of thrombosis continues for several weeks and although it is usual to stop heparin on discharge from hospital, the possibility of continuing prophylaxis as an outpatient should be considered. The use of full-length anti-embolism stockings further reduces the risk.

Patients with *prosthetic heart valves* require full anticoagulation with warfarin to prevent thrombosis on the valve.

In patients with *established atrial fibrillation* long-term anticoagulation with warfarin is effective in preventing emboli, and aspirin, taken regularly, confers some benefit.

THE TREATMENT OF VENOUS THROMBOSIS

Patients in whom immediate anticoagulant treatment is required should be started on heparin after a baseline *kaolin cephalin clotting time* (KCCT) and prothrombin time have been obtained. It is usually given by intravenous infusion, preferably by a syringe pump, an initial bolus of 5000 units followed by an infusion of 25 000–30 000 units over 24 hours. The KCCT should be repeated after 6 hours and then daily, and the dose adjusted to keep it at about twice the normal time. Some authorities consider twice daily subcutaneous injection to be equally effective. At the same time

the patient is started on oral warfarin, the dose being adjusted to produce the required prothrombin time which, initially, is measured daily. When this is achieved the heparin is stopped.

If there is less urgency, treatment should be started with warfarin.

The duration of treatment depends on circumstances but should be continued (usually on an outpatient basis) for at least 1 month and in some patients (e.g. with recurrent episodes) up to a year or longer.

ARTERIAL THROMBOSIS

This arises in a rather different way from venous thrombosis. With increasing age the lining (endothelium) of the arterial wall may become damaged by the flow and eddying of blood, stress and strains due to raised blood pressure, high levels of circulating cholesterol and possibly other factors such as irritants from tobacco smoke. This leads to patchy accumulation of cholesterol-containing lipoproteins and macrophage cells under the arterial endothelium together with the deposition of platelets. Ultimately, the patch may break down leaving a rough area (atheromatous plaque) on which a thrombus may form and block the artery. Sometimes, clumps of deposited platelets or a fragment may break off and obstruct a small, more peripheral artery, particularly in the brain.

It can be seen therefore that the possible therapeutic approaches are:

1. Dissolve the thrombus with thrombolytic drugs and thus remove the block to the artery.
2. Prevent the deposition of platelets on the atheromatous plaque by reducing 'platelet stickiness'.
3. Prevent damage to the lining of the artery by reducing stress (e.g. blood pressure), by lowering blood cholesterol levels and by stopping smoking.

FIBRINOLYTIC AGENTS (Fig. 5.1)

Streptokinase. Streptokinase is a streptococcal exotoxin. It reacts with a plasma globulin plasmi-

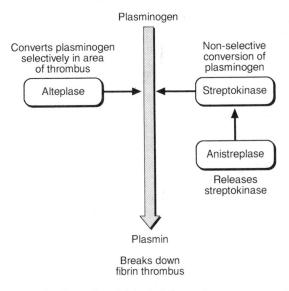

Plasminogen

Converts plasminogen selectively in area of thrombus

Non-selective conversion of plasminogen

Alteplase

Streptokinase

Anistreplase

Releases streptokinase

Plasmin

Breaks down fibrin thrombus

Fig. 5.1 The action of thrombolytic agents.

nogen, liberating plasmin which breaks down fibrin. Following a thrombosis intravenous streptokinase thus breaks down fibrin within the clot forming soluble fibrin degradation products (FDP). Circulating plasmin, however, is rapidly neutralized by antiplasmins.

Therapeutic use. Streptokinase has been used for many years to treat venous thrombosis. It appeared to have no advantage over the anticoagulants described above and was more difficult to use as it was necessary to neutralize circulating antistreptokinase from previous streptococcal infections before plasminogen was activated.

At present its most important use is in lysing the thrombus in coronary thrombosis. For this purpose 1.5 million units of streptokinase are infused over 1 hour. This may be preceded by chlorpheniramine 10 mg and hydrocortisone 100 mg to reduce allergic reactions. If this is combined with 150 mg of oral aspirin which should be chewed before swallowing, the immediate mortality following coronary thrombosis is more than halved. However, treatment must be started within 24 hours of the onset of symptoms.

Adverse effects. The main risk with streptokinase is bleeding and this is particularly liable to

occur at sites of recent trauma or invasive vascular procedures which must be avoided if possible.

Allergies are common and include fever, bronchospasm and rashes.

It should not be used if the patient has had previous streptokinase within the last 12 months.

Hypotension can occur and the blood pressure should be monitored.

Other plasminogen activators are:

Alteplase (tissue plasminogen activator) directly converts plasminogen to plasmin and its action is largely confined to the site of the thrombus. It is not neutralized by circulating streptococcal antibodies, therefore it can be used in patients who have had streptokinase or a streptococcal infection. It is, however, considerably dearer than streptokinase. The dose is 100 mg i.v. given in divided doses over 3 hours. Alteplase should be followed by heparin to prevent re-occlusion.

Anistreplase is a plasminogen–streptokinase complex which liberates streptokinase and can be given as a single intravenous injection of 30 units, over 5 minutes. It is also expensive.

On the present evidence streptokinase appears to be at least as effective for patients requiring thrombolytic therapy as the alternative plasminogen activators and is a lot cheaper. Alteplase should be used in those with circulating streptococcal antibodies.

Nursing points

When giving thrombolytic drugs:

1. Avoid intramuscular injections.
2. Avoid subclavian catheters for central venous lines.
3. Use indwelling venous or arterial catheters for access.
4. Look out for bleeding.
5. There are several contraindications to the use of thrombolytic agents. Check that they have been considered and excluded.

DRUGS AND PLATELET CLUMPING

Arterial thrombosis such as occurs in coronary thrombosis and strokes is partly due to an aggregation of platelets which ultimately forms small plugs in blood vessels. Certain drugs have been shown to reduce platelet 'stickiness' so that aggregation is less likely to occur. These drugs are undergoing extensive trials to see whether it is possible to prevent thrombotic disease. Among those which may be useful are *aspirin* (see p. 105), *dipyridamole* and *sulphinpyrazone* (see p. 111).

Aspirin, by inhibiting prostaglandin synthesis in platelets, reduces their stickiness and thus their tendency to form clumps which lead to thrombosis. Unfortunately it also inhibits prostacyclin synthesis in the walls of the blood vessels and this may increase the liability to thrombosis.

There have been several large trials on the role of aspirin in preventing and treating thrombotic disease. The results have often been contradictory, possibly because the aspirin dosage has varied between trials, and so far the best dose to have maximal effect on platelet stickiness and minimal effect on prostacyclin production has not been determined. At the time of writing 150 mg daily or on alternate days seems to be the best compromise.

It appears that the role of aspirin so far determined is:

1. Acute coronary thrombosis—combined with streptokinase (see above).
2. Prevention of coronary thrombosis—probably some preventive effect.
3. Transient cerebral ischaemic attacks—some reduction in attacks and in development of strokes.

Dipyridamole, like aspirin, prevents platelet clumping. It is not very effective when given alone but may be combined with aspirin or warfarin. The dose is 300–600 mg daily.

Fish oil. Eskimos have a low incidence of coronary thrombosis and this appears to be related to their large consumption of fish. The fatty acids in fish differ from those of meat and reduce the production in the body of prostaglandins (which promote thrombosis and inflammation) and increase that of prostacyclin (which is anti-inflammatory). The role of fish oil in preventing thrombotic disease and also rheumatoid arthritis

and psoriasis is being studied and the results are encouraging.

THE HYPERLIPIDAEMIAS

The hyperlipidaemias are a group of disorders of metabolism in which there are increased amounts of various lipoproteins in the blood. Lipoproteins are substances which are composed of fats and proteins and are produced by the liver. The concentration of blood lipoproteins is determined partly by the dietary intake of fats and partly by metabolic processes within the body. It is therefore possible to lower the lipoprotein levels either by decreasing the intake or absorption of fats or by changing the metabolism.

The most important lipid in lipoproteins is cholesterol and there is strong evidence that a high level of cholesterol in the blood is associated with an increased risk of atheroma and coronary thrombosis.

Approximate relationship between blood cholesterol levels and coronary thrombosis:

Blood cholesterol level in mmol/litre	Coronary deaths/1000
4.5	5
6.0	8
7.0	12

It seems reasonable therefore to lower the blood cholesterol concentration and thereby reduce the risk of coronary artery disease. Whether in fact, this object is achieved in practice is still open to debate and study.

There are several ways of lowering plasma cholesterol levels:

1. **Diet and weight reduction.** A decrease in the total fat intake and the proportion of saturated (animal) fat to unsaturated (fish and vegetable) fat will reduce plasma cholesterol; however, unless the diet is fairly strict the reduction will be small and have a minimal effect on the risk of coronary disease.
2. **Drugs.**
   a. Agents which *combine with bile acids and cholesterol* in the gut thus preventing their absorption and increasing faecal excretion.

Although they decrease the blood cholesterol they are unpleasant to take and can cause dyspepsia and flatulence.

- Cholestyramine A, 8–16 g daily.
- Colestipol, 5–30 g. daily.

b. *Fibrates* alter the metabolism of lipoproteins so lower blood cholesterol and have been shown to reduce the risk of coronary disease. They are given orally:

- Bezafibrate Mono, 400 mg daily.
- Gemfibrozil, 900–1200 mg daily in divided doses.

They can cause headaches, fatigue, rashes and dyspepsia.

c. *Statins* block the synthesis of cholesterol in the liver and thus lower the blood level.

- Simvastin, 10–40 mg at night.
- Pravastatin, 10–40 mg at night.

They are given at night because cholesterol synthesis is greatest at this time.

Adverse effects. Liver disturbances can occur, and liver function tests should be carried out every 2 months for the first year of treatment.

Rarely, severe muscle pains.

Management of hyperlipidaemias

Subjects with mild hyperlipidaemia (plasma cholesterol 5.2–6.5 mmol/litre) are advised about diet and lifestyle to minimize the risk of getting atheromatous disease. This is a very large group embracing up to 40% of the adult population of the UK. The problem is really one of public health rather than therapeutics. For those with higher levels of cholesterol and/or complex abnormalities of lipoproteins specialist care is needed as the patient may require drug treatment in addition to advice about prevention.

Nursing point

Hyperlipidaemia may be due not only to an inherited disposition and dietary indiscretion but to i.e. myxoedema diabetes, nephrotic syndrome and alcohol abuse.

FURTHER READING

Barry M, Orme M 1991 Anticoagulants: benefits and complications. Prescriber 19th August: 15

Editorial 1988 Thrombolytic therapy for acute myocardial infarction: Round 2. Lancet 1: 565

Editorial 1991 Orthopaedic surgery on the leg and thromboembolism. British Medical Journal 303: 531

Editorial 1992 Preventing and treating deep vein thrombosis. Drug and Therapeutics Bulletin 33: 129

Editorial 1992 How to anticoagulate. Drug and Therapeutics Bulletin 30: 77

ISIS 3 1992 A comparison of thrombolytic régimes. Lancet 339: 753

Manson J E 1992 Primary prevention of myocardial infarction. New England Journal of Medicine 326: 1406

Nurmohamed M et at 1992 Low molecular weight heparin versus standard heparin. Lancet 340: 152

O'Connor P et al 1990 Lipid lowering drugs. British Medical Journal 300: 667

Ornish D et al 1990 Can lifestyle change reverse coronary disease? Lancet 336: 129

Patrono C 1994 Aspirin as an antiplatelet drug. New England Journal of Medicine 330: 1287

Steering Committee of Physicians Health Study Research Group 1989 Final report on aspirin. New England Journal of Medicine 321: 129

6

Drugs affecting the alimentary tract

THE MOUTH

DISORDERS OF SALIVATION

A proper flow of saliva is necessary to keep the mouth fresh and free from infection. Salivary flow will be diminished in fever and dehydration and also by certain drugs, notably those of the belladonna group and the tricyclic antidepressants. Severe oral infection may supervene if salivary flow is markedly decreased and was a frequent complication in very ill patients in former times when dehydration was not adequately corrected and measures to ensure oral hygiene not practised. Patients receiving cytotoxic drugs are especially at risk as their resistance to infection is lowered and some cytotoxics cause ulceration of the mouth.

Prevention of oral infection

1. Before major surgery or any other procedure with a special risk of oral infection, the mouth should be inspected and infected gums or teeth should be treated. The help of the dentist or dental hygienist may be needed.
2. Dehydration must be avoided.
3. Mouthwashes play a useful part in preventing infection and making the patient more comfortable.

Mouthwash solution tablets contain thymol, a mild antiseptic, and are adequate for most patients. One tablet is dissolved in half a glass of warm water and used three or four times daily.

For patients at special risk various regimes can be used.

Chlorhexidine gluconate, a more powerful antiseptic, is used in a 0.2% solution (Corsodyl). The mouth is rinsed out two to three times daily with 10 ml for about 1 minute. The tongue and teeth may be stained brown but this can be largely avoided by brushing the teeth *before* use. Chlorhexidine 1% dental gel is useful for children and the handicapped. Mouthwash solution can be used 2 hourly in between.

If dry mouth is a special problem, *hypromellose* (an artificial saliva) up to 5 ml can be used instead of mouthwash solution. The maximum daily dose is 20 ml. The regime is expensive and should not be used routinely.

In the unconscious patient the mouth should be cleaned regularly. *Sodium bicarbonate* $\frac{1}{4}$ teaspoonful in 50 ml is particularly valuable in clearing mucus.

Hydrogen peroxide is used in some hospitals to remove debris from ulcers, etc. A 20 volume solution (6%) is diluted, one part in three parts warm water and used two or three times daily.

In seriously ill patients the care of the mouth is a particularly important aspect of nursing care. Hospitals used different regimes and nurses will have to draw their own conclusions as to the most effective.

Nursing point

In oral infection, prevention is better than cure and recognition that it is a potential problem is important as it can cause considerable discomfort.

Oral infections

In spite of care some patients will develop infections in the mouth, particularly those on cytotoxics or at special risk. The main infections are:

Candida. This is common and is best treated by *nystatin*, an antifungal antibiotic (see p. 210). It can be given as tablets (500 000 units of nystatin) four times daily, which are dissolved in the mouth and should be continued for 48 hours after the infection has resolved. Some patients find the taste objectionable and the tablets are hard and form sharp edges. Pastilles (100 000 units of nystatin) or the suspension may be more acceptable. An alternative is to use *amphotericin*, another antifungal antibiotic, as lozenges, four to eight times daily.

In young children *miconazole* gel smeared round the mouth is easier but expensive.

Dentures must be removed during treatment and should be soaked in 1% *sodium hypochlorite* solution overnight and rinsed before being replaced.

Oral herpes simplex. *Acyclovir* suspension 200 mg five times daily for 5 days is used.

Herpes labialis (cold sores) must be treated when symptoms (local burning) just develop. There is no ideal remedy. Acyclovir 5% cream, corticosteroid cream or ice cubes applied locally have all been tried with some success.

Nonspecific stomatitis with/without ulceration. Dehydration, if present, should be corrected.

Chlorhexidine mouthwashes as above. *Hydrogen peroxide* can be used to cleanse ulcers.

Benzydamine mouthwash, which acts as a local anaesthetic, is extremely effective in relieving the discomfort of oral ulceration. The mouth should be rinsed out every 2–3 hours with the undiluted solution.

Choline salicylate (Bonjela) is a mild local anaesthetic in gel form which may be applied before meals and at night.

Aphthous ulceration. These small, painful, recurrent oral ulcers are common in healthy people. The cause is unknown and treatment only partly effective. *Hydrocortisone pellets* (2.5 mg) dissolved in the mouth four times daily or tetracycline mouthwashes are used.

Infections of the pharynx and tonsils are very common and are usually viral. Most of them require no specific treatment as recovery is rapid. Many people use gargles although there is little evidence that they do any good. *Thymol glycerine*, a mild antiseptic, is popular and does no harm. *Soluble aspirin* is also used as a gargle. It is doubtful whether it has any effective local action but when swallowed will rapidly produce its systemic analgesic and anti-inflammatory effect.

Serious throat infections require the use of the appropriate antibiotic given systemically and there is little indication for the local use of antibiotics in these circumstances.

THE OESOPHAGUS

Inflammation may occur at the lower end of the oesophagus; it is usually due to regurgitation of acid from the stomach and can be relieved by antacids. Preparations are available which combine an antacid with a local anaesthetic and these are particularly valuable in relieving the pain of swallowing.

Gaviscon and Gastrocote are combinations of an antacid with alginates which float on the gastric contents. If reflux occurs they protect the mucosa of the lower oesophagus.

Mucaine contains the antacids aluminium hydroxide and magnesium hydroxide with oxethazaine, a local anaesthetic which, it is claimed, relieves the pain arising from the inflamed oesophagus.

H₂ blockers can be combined with antacids but are less effective than in peptic ulcer.

Omeprazole (see p. 79) which abolishes gastric acid secretion almost entirely, is more effective and is used in severe cases of reflux oesophagitis.

Drugs that stimulate oesophageal motility and thus keep the oesophagus empty are also useful. **Metoclopramide** (see p. 89) is the first choice but adverse effects may preclude its use. Alternatives are **domperidone** or **cisapride** which are free from central adverse effects but are considerably more expensive. Finally, nondrug measures such as weight loss in the obese, elevation of the bedhead and stopping smoking are advised.

THE STOMACH

The stomach is a hollow organ receiving food from the oesophagus and passing it on, after a variable interval, to the intestines. It is concerned with the mechanical breaking down of the food to render it more easily digested and more easily absorbed. Its muscular walls are capable of powerful waves of peristalsis which mix and macerate the food. The mucosa lining the stomach secretes hydrochloric acid and pepsin which together initiate the digestion of proteins.

ANTACIDS

Antacids were once widely used in the treatment of peptic ulcers and other forms of dyspepsia. They act by reducing the acidity in the stomach and they also reduce pepsin activity. They are very effective at temporarily relieving the pain from an ulcer, but unless used intensively, do not accelerate healing. They are also used in various minor gastric upsets; whether they do any good in these circumstances is open to doubt but they are useful placebos. Magnesium or aluminium salts are the most popular. Magnesium is available as magnesium oxide, hydroxide or trisilicate.

Magnesium trisilicate is a white, gritty powder usually prescribed as the mixture which contains sodium bicarbonate and magnesium carbonate as well. Taken in the usual dose of 10 ml it is effective for about 40 minutes. If, however, it is taken 1 hour after food it assists the neutralizing effect of food and its action may be considerably longer. Magnesium salts are very poorly absorbed from the gut and cause diarrhoea.

Aluminium hydroxide is a white powder, insoluble in water and usually given as a mixture or a tablet which is sucked to prolong its effect. In addition to reducing gastric acidity, aluminium salts inactivate gastric pepsin. This antacid is slightly astringent and can cause constipation. The usual dose is 10 ml or one tablet.

Frequency of dosage of antacids is important.

They are usually given 1 hour after meals throughout the day and on retiring. This produces a moderate reduction in acidity and keeps symptoms at bay; however, to accelerate healing larger than usual doses must be given more often.

Antacid mixtures. There are many available (20 in the 1992 BNF). They contain a variety of antacids sometimes combined with substances which protect the mucosa, anticholinergics or local anaesthetics. Generally they have little advantage except in special circumstances (see Gaviscon and Mucaine above) and are usually more expensive.

Antacids in renal failure and other disorders

Although the amount of magnesium or aluminum absorbed is very small and harmless in patients with normal renal function, accumulation can occur in renal failure.

Some antacids contain quite large amounts of sodium and cause fluid retention and oedema in patients with cardiac, renal or hepatic failure; also in pregnancy and in infants under 6 months.

Interactions. Antacids may interfere with the absorption of digoxin, tetracycline, iron salts, indomethacin and isoniazid.

THE TREATMENT OF PEPTIC ULCERS

Peptic ulcers may be either in the stomach (gastric) or the duodenum (duodenal). Although their causal factors may differ the treatment for both types of ulcer is similar. Whether or not hydrochloric acid secreted by the stomach *initiates* peptic ulcers is a matter for debate. It seems unlikely to be of major importance in gastric ulcers as most patients have no evidence of increased acid production. In duodenal ulcers, however, about half the patients produce more acid than normal subjects, and it may be that in this type of ulcer excess acid production is more important. Patients who do not secrete acid do not have peptic ulcers.

The relationship between bacterial infection with *Helicobacter pylori* and peptic ulceration is important. This organism may be found in the stomach of subjects without evidence of gastric or duodenal disease; however, it is more frequently isolated from those with gastritis or peptic ulcer. Further, eradication of the organism with antibiotics decreases the number of ulcer patients who relapse after treatment.

It is clear that once an ulcer has developed, *acid is largely responsible for pain*, which is the leading symptom, and reduction of acid leads to relief of pain and probably to healing.

The two possible methods of reducing gastric acidity are:

1. To neutralize the acid within the stomach with *antacids* (see above) and with *frequent feeds.*
2. To reduce the secretion of acid by the stomach.

Acid secretion is a complex process. It seems probable that there are two ways in which it can be provoked (Fig. 6.1):

a. Stimulation of the vagus nerve leads to the release of *acetylcholine* and thus to increased secretion of acid. In the intact individual this is brought about by the thought, sight or smell of appetizing food. Adequate acid and pepsin are thereby produced to start the digestion of food when it arrives in the stomach. In patients with ulcers, the acid causes the typical pain, particularly if the hoped-for food is delayed.

b. Distension of the stomach (for instance by food) causes the production of the hormone *gastrin* and this in turn stimulates the stomach to produce acid.

It appears that the common factor in acid production by both these mechanisms is the release in the stomach wall of *histamine*, from cells called histaminocytes, which then causes increased acid secretion. The effect of histamine on the stomach is said to be mediated by H_2 *receptors;* in addition it has effects at other sites including the bronchial muscle and on blood vessels, which are said to be mediated by H_1 *receptors.*

Gastric acid secretion can therefore be blocked in two ways:

1. Histamine receptor (H2) blockers—cimetidine, famotidine, ranitidine and nizatidine. These drugs block the action of histamine on receptors in the stomach wall and thus reduce the excretion of acid by about 70%.

Therapeutics. They are given orally.

Cimetidine — 800 mg at night (or 400 mg twice daily) for 6 weeks and then 400 mg at night if necessary.

Ranitidine — 300 mg at night (or 150 mg twice daily) for 6 weeks, then 150 mg at night if necessary.

Famotidine — 40 mg at night for 6 weeks and then 20 mg at night if necessary.

Nizatidine — 300 mg at night for 6 weeks, then 150 mg at night if necessary.

This reduces acid secretion over most of the night and day. Ulcer symptoms usually disappear within a week and some 85% of duodenal ulcers heal in a month, gastric ulcers may take rather longer. Unfortunately, about half the patients will develop a recurrence of symptoms after treatment is stopped. If this occurs, long-term maintenance treatment (ranitidine 150 mg nocte or cimetidine 400 mg nocte) may be required.

In the small number of patients who fail to respond to H₂ blockers, omeprazole or De-Nol (see below) can be tried. An alternative approach for patients who respond poorly to H₂ blockers is to eradicate *Helicobacter pylori* infection or resort to surgery (see Fig. 6.2).

H₂ blockers can also be used in reflux oesophagitis (see above) or to prevent the development of ulcers in patients under severe stress. Injections of cimetidine and ranitidine are available.

There is little to choose between these drugs; cimetidine and ranitidine have been in use the longest. Adverse effects are a little more troublesome with cimetidine.

Adverse effects are rare with cimetidine but include gynaecomastia, impotence due to interfering with the action of normally occurring androgens and confusional states in the elderly. Cimetidine *interacts* with various drugs by interfering with their metabolism in the liver. Drugs whose action may be prolonged are:

Phenytoin	Morphine
Warfarin	Methadone
Theophylline	Labetalol
Propranolol	Diazepam
Metoprolol	

These effects have not been reported with the other H₂ blockers.

2. Omeprazole is not an H₂ blocker but it directly prevents the excretion of hydrogen ions (and thus, acid) by the stomach. It inhibits acid secretion more powerfully than the H₂ blockers. It is used in patients with peptic ulcer who have failed to respond to H₂ blockers, in reflux oesophagitis and in the rare Zollinger–Ellison syndrome in which there is gross oversecretion of acid. The usual dose is 20 mg daily.

Adverse effects include headache, nausea, diarrhoea and rashes.

Eradication of *Helicobacter pylori*

The ideal method has yet to be decided. Usually a combination of an antibiotic (tetracycline or ampicillin) with metronidazole and De-Nol is used for a period of from 1–2 weeks. An alternative is omeprazole combined with an antibiotic.

Other drugs

In addition to reducing acid, ulcer healing can be encouraged by drugs which protect the ulcer and increase the resistance of the gastric and duodenal lining to acid.

Bismuth chelate (De-Nol) is a bismuth-containing compound. It is believed to relieve the symptoms of peptic ulcer by causing coagulation at the base of the ulcer and thus protecting it and promoting healing. It also has some action against *Helicobacter pylori*. The dose is 5 ml in 15 ml of water half an hour before meals and before retiring.

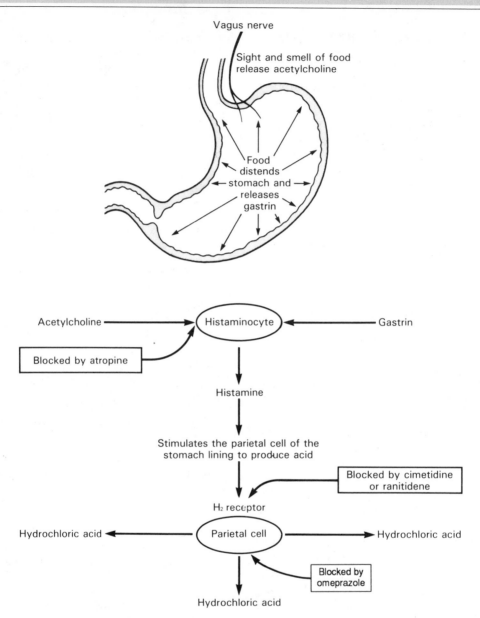

Fig. 6.1 The mechanisms involved in the secretion of acid into the stomach and the effect and site of action of H₂ blockers.

This solution has an unpleasant taste and some patients prefer tablets which are crushed in the mouth and washed down with water. The stools may appear black and it should *not* be combined with antacids.

Sucralfate is a compound of aluminium and sucrose which coats the base of an ulcer, protect-

ing it from pepsin and allowing healing to take place. The dose is one tablet four times daily before meals and at bedtime.

Prostaglandins. It is believed that prostaglandins (p. 183) exert some protective effect on the gastric mucosa and this may be one reason why drugs which inhibit prostaglandin production (e.g. NSAIAs) can cause peptic ulcers. *Misoprostol* has been shown to reduce the risk of gastric ulcer in patients at special risk (e.g. the elderly, those with history of ulcer) who are taking NSAIAs. Misoprostol can cause diarrhoea.

CARMINATIVES

Carminatives are substances which when taken by mouth produce a feeling of warmth in the stomach. They cause relaxation of the cardiac sphincter and allow the 'belching up' of wind and may thus relieve gastric distension. Examples in common use are the oils of ginger and peppermint.

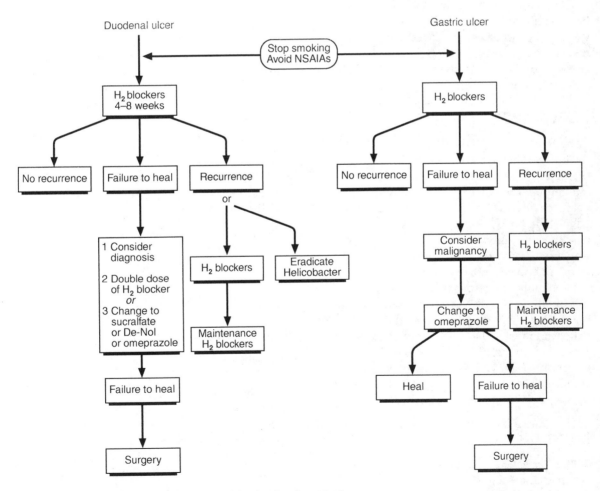

Fig. 6.2 Flow diagram of the management of duodenal and gastric ulcer.

THE INTESTINES

After food has been partially digested in the stomach it passes into the small intestine where digestion of protein, carbohydrates and fat is completed and absorption occurs.

The passage of food through the small intestine takes about 12–24 hours and the residue then enters the colon where further absorption, largely of water, takes place and the intestinal contents become semi-solid. The filling of the rectum produces the characteristic sensation of the 'call to stool' and the bowels are then emptied by a complicated mechanism partially voluntary and partially involuntary.

The passage of food through the intestines is brought about by peristalsis, which consists of a wave of contraction preceded by a wave of relaxation. Parasympathetic stimulation increases peristaltic activity and sympathetic stimulation decreases it.

PURGATIVES

Purgatives may be defined as drugs which loosen the bowel. They are widely used and a great deal of their use is unnecessary and may even be dangerous. The bowel habit of individuals varies very considerably and many people require to have their bowels open less frequently than is usually considered 'normal'. There is nothing to be gained by these people trying to attain a more frequent bowel action by means of purgatives.

Even more dangerous is the indiscriminate use of purgatives for all types of abdominal pain. In many acute abdominal diseases the use of such drugs aggravates the condition, a classical example being the rupture of an acutely inflamed appendix following a purgative. Purgatives should, thus, never be given to patients with undiagnosed abdominal pain.

There are a large number of purgatives which may be classified:

1. *Bulk purgatives.* High residue foods; bran; ispaghula (Isogel).
2. *Stool softeners.* Docusate sodium.
3. *Osmotic purges.* Magnesium sulphate.
4. *Irritant purges.* Anthracenes; phenolphthalein; bisacodyl.

The bulk purges increase the contents of the bowel and thus stimulate peristalsis. The emollient purges aid the passage of faecal material by their lubricating action. The irritant purges increase peristalsis and thus the intestinal contents pass more rapidly through the bowel and remain more fluid.

Bulk purges

High residue foods contain a high proportion of cellulose which is not digested or absorbed and thus increases the bulk of the intestinal contents. Common examples are green vegetables, fruit and wholemeal bread. **Bran**, which is a by-product of milling, contains about 30% of fibre made up of celluloses, pectins and lignins, substances which are not absorbed from the intestine and which swell as they take up water and thus increase the bulk of the faeces. The initial dose is 1 tablespoonful daily and is increased at weekly intervals until a satisfactory result is achieved. The main side-effect is wind.

Methylcellulose is available in a number of preparations either as granules or tablets. It is an effective bulk purge.

Ispaghula husk is of plant origin and swells on contact with water thus acting as a bulk purge. It is available as Isogel and Regulan and other preparations.

Combine both with plenty of water.

Stool softeners

Liquid paraffin may cause leaking via the anal sphincter; lipoid pneumonia (if inhaled) may occur in the very young and very old, and it may interfere with absorption of vitamins A, D, and K. It should not therefore be used on a regular basis. It is best given as the liquid paraffin and magnesium hydroxide mixture, 5–20 ml, which is less likely to cause these difficulties.

Docusate sodium is available as tablets or

syrup. The dose is 50–200 mg daily in divided doses. It acts by softening the stools and this may be sufficient to relieve constipation particularly if a painful condition such as piles or anal fissure is interfering with bowel evacuation. It may be combined with a stimulant laxative.

It can also be used as a micro-enema in the management of faecal impaction when 90 or 120 mg of docurate in solution are injected into the rectum.

Osmotic purges

Saline purges. The most commonly used saline purge is **magnesium sulphate** (Epsom salts). It is poorly absorbed from the intestinal tract. This leads to a rise in osmotic pressure within the bowel and prevents the absorption of water so that the intestinal contents remain more fluid and more bulky.

A saline purge should be given on an empty stomach (before breakfast being a good time) so that it passes rapidly through the stomach and into the intestine. If it is held up in the stomach, it may not be effective. It is given dissolved in water and the concentration should not exceed 8 g of magnesium sulphate to 120 ml of water as a more concentrated dose may cause closure of the pyloric sphincter and delay the drug leaving the stomach. The drugs are usually effective within 1–2 hours.

Therapeutics. Magnesium sulphate 8 g in 150 ml of water before breakfast.

Fruit salts usually contain some sodium bicarbonate and tartaric acid. When these are mixed with water, sodium tartrate is formed with the liberation of carbon dioxide. The sodium tartrate acts as a mild purge.

Lactulose is a sugar which is broken down by bacteria in the large bowel with the production of various acids. These act as osmotic purgatives rendering the bowel contents more fluid, and as mild irritants, both of which produce a laxative effect. It is a liquid, given in doses of 15–20 ml twice daily. It takes several days to act and may cause a certain amount of flatulence and disten-

tion. For these reasons it is not a particularly good purgative but is sometimes used in the long-term treatment of the constipated elderly and for those receiving opiates for intractable pain when constipation may be a problem. It also has a limited use in patients with severe liver disease to reduce the absorption of toxic substances from the bowel.

Irritant purges

The anthracene group of purges all contain the anthraquinone, *emodin*, which is the chief active constituent of the group, the varying properties of the anthracene purges depending on the ease with which this active constituent is released. After liberation in the intestine, emodin is absorbed into the blood stream and acts on the large intestine causing increased peristalsis. All members of this group of drugs therefore take about 8–12 hours to act and are best given at bedtime. They may occasionally cause griping and should be avoided in pregnancy.

The commonly used anthracene purges are:

Senna is the most powerful of the anthracene purges. It is usually prescribed as **Senokot**. This is a proprietary preparation which contains the purified principles called sennoside A and sennoside B. It is highly satisfactory and can be used either as granules or tablets. The dose is 2–4 tablets or 1–2 teaspoonfuls of granules.

Bisacodyl is a preparation which stimulates activity of the colon when it comes in contact with the wall of the bowel. It can be used either orally in doses of 1–3 tablets (5–15 mg) or as a suppository.

Co-danthramer is mixture of a stool softener and a stimulant purge (danthron). Unfortunately, it has been shown to produce tumours in animals with high and prolonged dosage although there is no evidence that this occurs in man. Its use is therefore restricted to the elderly with obstinate constipation or those whose constipation is due to opioid analgesics (e.g. the terminally ill).

Laxative abuse. Some patients become dependent on laxatives because they believe that these drugs wash away poisons from the body. If carried to extremes this can lead to serious electrolyte depletion and damage the bowel.

THE TREATMENT OF CONSTIPATION

Before making a diagnosis of constipation it is important to realize that there is considerable natural variation in the frequency with which people open their bowels. The majority vary between twice daily and once every other day. Constipation has two main causes:

1. Delayed passage of faeces through the colon. This in turn may be due to:
   a. Local lesions of the bowel
   b. Disorders which interfere with bowel muscle function such as hypercalcaemia or myxoedema
   c. Old age
   d. Depression
   e. Weakness of the abdominal muscle
   f. Low bulk diet
   g. Various drugs including opioids, antidepressants and verapamil.
2. Neglect of the call to stool. This may occur for social reasons or may be due to illness, surgery or some painful lesion of the anus such as a fissure. As a result the rectum becomes used to distension of its walls by faeces and loses its ability to contract and empty.

In the ill patient who has been constipated for a few days 2–4 Senokot tablets at night followed by a glycerine suppository next day is often sufficient. In the elderly faecal impaction may not respond to the above measures. It may be treated with retention enemas of docusate sodium followed by rectal washouts. If this fails or rapid evacuation is required manual removal may be necessary.

In chronic constipation the object of treatment is to re-educate the intestines so that a normal bowel habit is restored. This can be achieved by increasing the bulk of the faeces either by a high fibre content in the diet, i.e. bran or similar substances or by the use of bulk purgatives such as methylcellulose. A reasonably high fluid intake is also helpful. This should be combined with regular habits and may require the use of some purgative such as Senokot at night until a normal rhythm is regained.

Laxatives are also used before investigation of the intestinal tract.

> **Nursing point**
>
> In hospital it is essential to establish the normal bowel habit for a particular patient and plan care in relation to this, ensuring privacy and the use of proper facilities whenever possible. Re-education with regard to diet with high fibre content is also important.

Enemas and suppositories

The wall of the rectum contains nerve receptors which respond to pressure to produce the normal call to stool but may also be stimulated by various substances which can be introduced into the rectum as suppositories or micro-enemas to initiate the evacuation of the bowel. Larger volume enemas distend the rectum and lower bowel causing contraction and also have some washout effect.

Suppositories. Glycerol suppositories, one inserted moistened with water, are quite satisfactory. Other suppositories are available but, in general, offer no advantage.

Enemas. These may be used to soften the stool and include arachis oil or docusate sodium. To promote evacuation a phosphate enema, 128 ml run into the rectum, is useful for example, before sigmoidoscopy. An alternative is to use a micro-enema such as Micolette, 5 ml is given rectally and it acts as a colon stimulant.

Laxatives are also used to prepare the bowel before colonic surgery or colonoscopy. Various regimes are used but essentially a low residue

> **Nursing point**
>
> Care is necessary in preparing sodium picosulphate from powder as heat is generated. The powder is mixed with 2 tablespoonfuls of water and left for 5 minutes then diluted to 150 ml.

diet is taken for a few days and two sachets of sodium picosulphate are given on the eve of the procedure. Sodium picosulphate is a bowel stimulant which induces a thorough emptying of the bowel. Other similar preparations are available.

Enemas can also be used to treat conditions of the bowel. In ulcerative colitis steroids (either prednisolone or hydrocortisone) can be introduced into the rectum and retained if possible for at least 1 hour. A certain amount of steroid is absorbed into the circulation and so both local and general therapeutic effects result.

INTESTINAL SEDATIVES

The peristaltic activity of the intestines may be diminished by several groups of drugs.

1. The *belladonna group* (p. 37) decrease gut tone by blocking the action of the parasympathetic nervous system. They are particularly useful in colon spasm. *Mebeverine* has a similar action but fewer side-effects.
2. The *opium group* (p. 94) actually increase gut tone but reduce peristalsis. They are useful in various forms of diarrhoea. The most widely used is *codeine phosphate* in doses of 10–60 mg 4 hourly.
3. *Co-phenotrope* is a combination of atropine and diphenoxylate hydrochloride. The latter drug is related to the narcotic analgesics (see p. 95). It is widely used in controlling diarrhoea but it must be remembered that it is dangerous in overdose, particularly in children, as it can cause depression of respiration.

Loperamide decreases large bowel motility. Toxicity is low and the usual adult dose is 4 mg initially followed by 2 mg three times daily.

It is important to remember that diarrhoea may cause *dehydration* and *electrolyte depletion*, particularly in children, and replacements may be required.

In severe depletion, intravenous replacement may be required but for the majority of patients the oral route is quite satisfactory and preparations containing sodium, potassium, glucose and water in the optimum concentrations are available.

PANCREATIC SUPPLEMENTS

As a result of pancreatic disease (usually cystic fibrosis or chronic pancreatitis) the pancreatic enzymes may be deficient leading to failure to digest fat and protein, malabsorption and loose fatty stools (steatorrhoea). The missing enzymes may be given orally but they are broken down by the acid in the stomach and thus rendered ineffective. This may be circumvented by combining the enzyme with an H_2 blocker to reduce gastric acidity or by using preparations which are coated to protect them against acid.

Available preparations include:

Pancrex, which is supplied as a powder, capsules or tablets and is given before meals (or feeds). The capsules should be broken and mixed with water or milk.

Creon capsules containing coated pellets which may be swallowed whole or opened and the pellets mixed with food. They must not, however, be chewed as they will lose their protective coating. The dose is very variable and is best judged by observing the nature of the stool.

GALLSTONES

Gallstones are a common finding although they do not always cause symptoms. They are usually removed surgically either by open operation or by endoscopy. There are, however, drugs which dissolve cholesterol-rich gallstones and they are used to treat selected patients.

Chenodeoxycholic acid and ursodeoxycholic acid. Most gallstones are largely composed of cholesterol. These two drugs, which are bile salts, reduce the concentration of cholesterol in the bile and make it more soluble so that cholesterol containing stones are slowly dissolved.

Therapeutic use. Only small stones are suitable for this therapy. The two drugs are often given together orally as a single dose at bedtime and it may take from 6–18 months for the stones to disappear. Relapse is liable to occur when the treatment is stopped. Because of the relatively few patients suitable for this method of treatment and the lengthy supervision required, it has not become popular.

FURTHER READING

Allbright A 1984 Oral care of cancer chemotherapy patients. Nursing times 80(21): 40

Avery M E, Snyder J D 1990 Oral therapy for acute diarrhoea. New England Journal of Medicine 323: 891

Bateman D N, Smith J M 1988 A policy for laxatives. British Medical Journal 297: 1420

Booth B, Booth S 1986 Aperients can be deceptive. Nursing Times 82(8): 38

Bouchier I A D 1990 Gall stones. British Medical Journal 300: 592

Editorial 1988 New H2 blockers: Does more choice help? Drug and Therapeutics Bulletin 26(17): 65

Hopkins S 1992 Drugs update: undermining ulcers. Nursing times 88(16): 62

Langman M J S 1991 Omeprazole. British Medical Journal 303: 481

Patterson W L 1991 *Helicobacter pylori* and peptic ulcer. New England Journal of Medicine 324: 1043

Emetics, anti-emetics and cough remedies

EMETICS

Vomiting is a complex series of actions involving the stomach, oesophagus, and pharynx with the voluntary muscles of the chest and abdomen and resulting in the ejection of food from the stomach. These actions are coordinated by a vomiting centre in the medulla. This centre can be stimulated directly from the labyrinth of the ear in such conditions as seasickness or vertigo, by gastric irritants or even by mental activity (i.e. sick with fright). It can also be stimulated via the chemoreceptor trigger zone (CTZ) which lies close to the vomiting centre in the brain stem and which is stimulated by a number of circulating substances including certain drugs (see Fig. 7.1). Finally, there are receptors which are stimulated by 5-hydroxytryptamine (5HT) found in both the peripheral and central connections of the vagus nerve close to the CTZ. Circulating cytotoxic drugs (particularly cisplatin) release 5HT and activate these receptors and, ultimately, the vomiting centre. Before the act of vomiting occurs, stimulation of the vomiting centre produces a sensation known as nausea, which is often associated with increased secretion by the salivary and bronchial glands.

Emetics or drugs which provoke vomiting are rarely used in medical practice except in poisoning. They may be divided into two types, reflex emetics and central emetics.

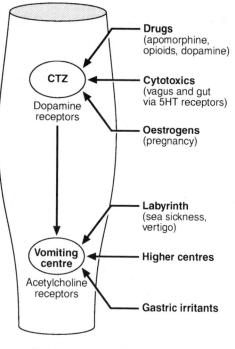

Brain stem

Fig. 7.1 Drugs and other factors stimulating the CTZ and vomiting centre.

REFLEX EMETICS

This group of drugs produces vomiting by irritating the stomach. The only one in common use is **ipecacuanha** which is dispensed as *Ipecacuanha emetic mixture* (paediatric) and the dose is:

Young children	10 ml
Older children	15 ml
Adults	30 ml

It should be followed by 200 ml of water and vomiting should occur in 15–30 minutes. It may be used as a first-aid treatment for overdose provided that:

1. The patient is fully conscious
2. Overdose is not of corrosive substances or petroleum products when inhalation could be fatal.

Ipecacuanha can be used up to 4 hours after ingestion of poison and longer for some, such as tricylic antidepressants and salicylates when gas-tric emptying is delayed. It is not so effective as a stomach washout but is particularly useful in children when the upset of lavage should be avoided if possible and in removing such objects as berries which cannot be washed out of the stomach.

CENTRAL EMETICS

It is possible to stimulate the CTZ directly and the most useful drug having this action is **apomorphine**. This drug is closely related to morphine but has none of its analgesic effect. It has, however, a very powerful stimulating effect on the vomiting centre and also produces some cerebral depression. It was formerly used as an emetic but because of its depressing action it should not be used in treating patients who have taken an overdose.

ANTI-EMETICS

It is believed that acetylcholine, dopamine and 5-hydroxytryptamine (5HT) act as intermediate transmitters in the CTZ and vomiting centre. By blocking the action of these substances it is possible to prevent or diminish vomiting (Table 7.1).

Acetylcholine antagonists

Hyoscine was widely used in the Second World War to prevent troops crossing the sea from becoming seasick. The usual dose for this purpose is 400 micrograms orally. It is also available as a transdermal preparation, a patch being applied behind the ear for maximal absorption, 6 hours before starting a journey. Blurring of vision, due to paralysis of ocular accommodation, can occur.

Antihistamines

Most of the antihistamine group of drugs have some acetylcholine blocking action and are useful anti-emetics. Among the most useful are **cyclizine** in doses of 50 mg three times daily and **meclozine** which is long acting, a dose of 50 mg lasting from 12–24 hours. **Dimenhydrate** is also

Table 7.1 The management of vomiting. There are several causes of vomiting and specific drugs are effective for different types

Types of vomiting	Effective drug	Comment
Vomiting of pregnancy	Promethazine sometimes combined with pyridoxine	Dietary management if possible Keep drugs to a minimum in early pregnancy owing to risk of fetal deformity Promethazine appears safe
Motion sickness	Hysoscine	Dry mouth. Blurred vision. Some sedation. Short journey
	Cinnarizine	Preferred for longer journey
Vertigo	Prochlorperazine Cinnarizine Betahistine	
Opiates	Prochlorperazine Metoclopramide Chlorpromazine Haloperidol	Less sedating Long acting
Cytotoxics	Prochlorperazine Domperidone Metoclopramide Ondansetron Cannabinoids Benzodiazepines	Sedative Not sedative High doses required Being investigated Particularly if anxiety is a factor
Migraine	Dexamethasone Metoclopramide	

effective in doses of 50 mg twice daily but it is rather inclined to cause drowsiness.

Dopamine antagonists

Several of the phenothiazine drugs (see p. 120) are powerful anti-emetics due to blocking the effects of dopamine on the CTZ. Among those used are:

Chlorpromazine 25 mg three times daily, orally, or 25–50 mg by injection.

Prochlorperazine 5 mg three times daily, orally, or 12.5 mg by injection.

Domperidone is less sedative than chlorpromazine and less liable to produce dystonic reactions than metoclopramide (see below) because its action on the nervous system is confined to the CTZ. It also enhances gastric emptying. Unfortunately, only about 15% of the oral dose reaches the circulation and a parenteral preparation is not available. It can be used to suppress vomiting with long-term opioid therapy and with the mildly emetic cytotoxic drugs. The dose is 10–20 mg 4–8 hourly orally or 60 mg as a suppository.

Metoclopramide increases gastric tone and dilates the duodenum. This causes the stomach to empty more quickly. In addition it has some central action on the vomiting centre. It is quite an effective anti-emetic in doses of 10 mg three times daily by mouth or 10 mg by intramuscular injection. It is used in postoperative and opioid-induced vomiting and in migraine. In very large doses it also blocks 5HT receptors and is used to prevent vomiting due to cytotoxic drugs.

Adverse effects. These are rare but, even with normal doses, patients may develop spasm of the facial and neck muscles. This is more common in young people. They pass off within a few hours of stopping the drug and can be controlled by diazepam. Prolonged use has been reported as causing tardive dyskinesia (see p. 121).

Cinnarizine is an anti-emetic which has found particular favour among yachtsmen and others at risk from seasickness but it can also be used in other types of vomiting. The dose is 30 mg 3 hours before sailing and then 15 mg 8 hourly. Sedation is not usually a problem.

5HT antagonists

Ondansetron and granisetron probably block the 5HT receptors associated with the central connections of the vagus nerve in the brain stem in close proximity to the CTZ. They are used to prevent vomiting in patients receiving the highly emetic cytotoxic drugs such as cisplatin, which release 5HT. The usual dose of Ondansetron is 8 mg orally 2 hours before treatment, but with the more emetic drugs, 8 mg i.v. before treatment, followed by 8 mg orally every 12 hours.

Others

Cannabinoids are derivatives of cannabis indica (marihuana); they have an anti-emetic action and have been used with some success in controlling vomiting in patients receiving cytotoxic drugs. They also produce some sedation and occasionally confusion.

Betahistine. This drug differs from other anti-emetics in that its use is confined to Ménière's disease in which vertigo and vomiting are due to a disturbance in the labyrinth of the inner ear. It is believed to lower pressure in the inner ear and thus relieve symptoms. The dose is 16 mg two or three times daily.

Dexamethasone has proved useful as an anti-emetic during cancer chemotherapy (see p. 251).

Benzodiazepines may be used in combination with other anti-emetics. It seems probable that they have no specific anti-emetic effect but are useful in relieving anxiety.

Nursing points

As a general rule anti-emetics are best if given at least half an hour before the emetic stimulus. Prevention is easier than cure.

COUGH REMEDIES

EXPECTORANTS AND COUGH MIXTURES

The cough is a reflex. The stimulus may arise from inflammation or foreign material in the pharynx, larynx, trachea or bronchial tree. It may also be provoked by stimuli arising in the pleura. It is, therefore, advantageous to aid the removal of foreign material from the respiratory passages and this may be achieved by increasing the secretion of the bronchial glands and thus 'loosening' the sputum.

The bronchial glands are supplied by the vagus nerve and when nausea or vomiting occurs there is widespread vagal activity and a considerable increase in bronchial and salivary secretion. Ex-pectorants are drugs which loosen the sputum and thus aid its ejection from the bronchial tree. They are nearly all emetics if given in large enough doses and the theory behind their use is that in smaller doses the emetic action is not provoked but the reflex stimulation of the bronchial glands remains.

There is no evidence that in the doses commonly prescribed expectorants have any useful action and in general their use should be discouraged. There are many excitingly coloured medicines with a powerful and sometimes unpleasant taste which can have a placebo effect and will no doubt continue to be used. Among the ingredients which may be found in such cough mixtures are ammonium chloride, ipecacuanha, guaiphenesin and squill, and many can be bought 'over the counter'.

Certain compound preparations used for treating coughs do contain active drugs but any benefit which follows their use is not due to an expectorant action.

Benylin preparations contain menthol, diphenhydramine hydrochloride and other substances in syrup. The benefit from this mixture is from the sedative effect of the diphenhydramine (antihistamine) and the soothing action of the syrup. It is useful to give a night's sleep to those with a troublesome cough. The dose is 5–10 ml 4–6 hourly and is especially useful at bedtime.

Actifed (syrup or tablets) contains pseudo-ephedrine (vasoconstriction clears the nasal passages) and triprolidine (antihistamine).

Dimotapp (long acting) contains phenylephrine and phenylpropanolamine (vasoconstriction clears the nasal passages) and brompheniramine (antihistamine).

There are many other mixtures of similar type and efficiency. They are useful in the cold + cough situation but it must be remembered that those containing vasoconstrictors *must not be used by patients taking monoamine oxidase inhibitors* (see p. 128).

As a result of government action the antihistamine-decongestant preparations are no longer prescribable under the NHS but are available on private prescription and many of them can be bought 'over the counter'. The only way to obtain the drugs on the NHS is for the main ingredients to be prescribed separately.

INHALATIONS AND MUCOLYTIC AGENTS

In the past various drugs were inhaled, particularly in the treatment of chronic lung infections, although with the advent of antibiotics this treatment has been largely superseded. Steam itself is, however, a very good expectorant as it liquefies the sputum and thus enables it to be coughed up.

Benzoin tincture. This is one of the balsams which contains resins and volatile oils. When it is added to hot water, the volatile oil is given off and may be inhaled; it exerts a mildly soothing effect on the bronchial mucous membrane and is frequently used in acute bronchitis. *Menthol and eucalyptus* inhalation can be used in a similar way and produces a considerable outpouring from the bronchial glands and a transient vasoconstriction of the respiratory mucous membrane with clearing of the air passages.

Great care must be taken when young or elderly patients are inhaling these drugs that they do not spill the hot water over themselves or severe burns may occur.

Nursing point
Avoiding dehydration, giving hot drinks and efficient physiotherapy are more effective than medicines in 'clearing the chest'.

COUGH SUPPRESSANTS

Under certain circumstances it is advantageous to suppress a cough which is tiring the patient and serving no useful purpose. However, undue suppression of a cough can lead to sputum retention and cough suppressants should be used with care.

Demulcents

Coughs arising from irritation of the upper respiratory tract are helped by demulcents. **Simple linctus** which is essentially flavoured syrup in doses of 5.0 ml three to four times daily is satisfactory but should be avoided in diabetics as it contains sugar.

For many years the only really effective cough depressing drugs were those derived from the opium groups, which included **morphine, heroine** and **codeine**. These drugs were included in many cough mixtures and, by virtue of this action on the cough centre, were valuable antitussives.

The most popular of this group was codeine, which was included in **linctus codeine** (BPC). This linctus, although widely used, has been found to be not very effective by many physicians unless given in doses rather above those usually recommended, in which case it was often constipating.

Dose. Linctus codeine (BPC) 5–10 ml.

Pholcodine. This is closely related to codeine and depresses the cough centre. Weight for weight experimental results suggest it is rather more active than codeine, although side-effects are probably similar. Its action lasts 4–6 hours. It is included in various mixtures including linctus pholcodine (BPC).

Dose. Linctus pholcodine (BPC) 10 ml.

Antihistamines

These have some antitussive effect, partly perhaps by a local antihistamine action, but more by their sedative effect on the nervous system.

FURTHER READING

Barnes J, Barnes N 1991 Effective management of nausea and vomiting. Prescriber Issue 34: 29

Editorial 1991 Ondansetron vs dexamethasone for chemotherapy-induced emesis. Lancet 338: 478

8

Analgesics

THE PERCEPTION OF PAIN (Fig. 8.1)

The central nervous system is constantly receiving nerve impulses arising in the body from the skin and internal organs. Under certain circumstances the brain interprets these as pain. There are a number of theories to explain how this occurs and the most popular today is the *'gate' (input control)* theory. This states that high-intensity stimulation activates a network of fine nerves at the periphery which terminate centrally in the posterior horn of the spinal cord. Here nerve impulses are relayed via the spinothalamic tract to the thalamus where they are felt as pain. There is then a further relay system to the cerebral cortex where discrimination and interpretation occur. The passage of nerve impulses through the relay 'gate' in the posterior horn is modified by:

a. Other impulses arising from the periphery. Low intensity impulses damp down transmission and high intensity impulses facilitate it.
b. Nerve fibres arising in the brain and descending in the spinal cord terminate in the posterior horn and damp down transmission through the gate and thus decrease the sensation of pain.

It is common experience that distraction can make pain either better or worse. Patients who have been in pain often benefit when visitors arrive or cope better with their pain when they have something interesting to do, for example, a good book to read or the radio. This does

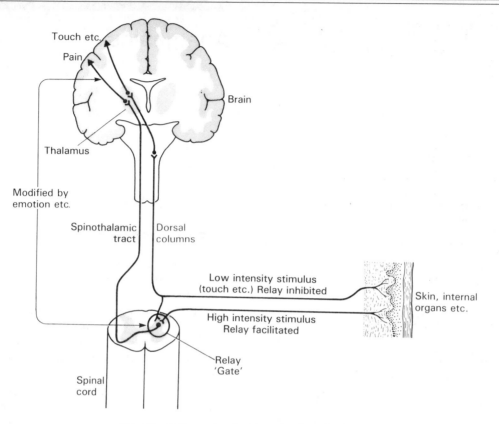

Fig. 8.1 Pathways involved in perception of pain.

not mean that the pain has not been genuine, but that it can be modified by environmental factors.

Analgesics are drugs which relieve pain. They are of great importance in the practice of medicine, as pain is a common and distressing feature of many diseases. It must be remembered, however, that pain has its uses, both as a warning of the presence of disease and also, by its nature, it may help in localization and diagnosis of the underlying cause.

Drugs which relieve pain may act at various sites along the pain pathways.

1. They may act on the brain and spinal cord and reduce the appreciation of pain. This is the site of action of opioid analgesics.
2. They may suppress conduction in nerves car-

rying impulses from the painful area. This is where local anaesthetics act.

3. They may reduce inflammation and other causes of pain in the painful area. This is the site of action of the nonsteroidal anti-inflammatory agents (NSAIAs).

Opioids*

Natural: opium; codeine.

Synthetic: diamorphine; methadone; levorphanol; pethidine; phenazocine; dextromoramide; dipipanone; dihydrocodeine.

Nearly all the opioids are potentially **drugs of dependence** and this subject is discussed on page 273.

---

*The term opioid is applied to any substance which has an opium-like action. These drugs are also called *narcotics*.

Minor analgesics

These include nonsteroidal anti-inflammatory agents (NSAIAs).

THE OPIOIDS

The mode of action of opioid analgesics

There are special receptors in the nervous system particularly in the midbrain and posterior horn of the spinal cord. When these receptors are stimulated transmission of nerve impulses related to pain are inhibited and the appreciation of pain is suppressed. These receptors are stimulated by substances which occur naturally in the brain, called β endorphin and met-encephalin. It seems likely that they are part of a system in the brain which controls pain appreciation and may be involved in such phenomena as acupuncture.

Opioid drugs also react with these receptors and thus relieve pain. This interaction can occur in three ways (see Fig. 8.2):

1. The receptor is stimulated—this happens with many opioids, e.g. morphine, diamorphine, pethidine—this is called an *agonist* effect.
2. The receptor is partially stimulated and partially blocked—this occurs with buprenorphine and is called a *partial agonist* effect (see p. 99).
3. The receptor is blocked—this occurs with naloxone and is called an *antagonist* effect (see p. 100).

There are several types of opioid receptor in the nervous system but the most important are called μ receptors and are responsible for the analgesia, euphoria, respiratory depression and constipation seen with most opioid analgesics.

Endorphins appear to be released during physical exercise and may be responsible for the feeling of well-being that participation in sports so often engenders.

Opium

Opium is obtained from the unripe capsule of a poppy which grows throughout Asia Minor and the East. Crude opium is a brownish gum-like material and contains a number of substances; the most important are morphine, codeine and papaverine.

Morphine is the most powerful of these alkaloids and the actions of morphine and opium are similar and may be considered together.

Morphine

Morphine hydrochloride is a white powder soluble in water. It is administered by mouth or by subcutaneous or intravenous injection. After absorption morphine is combined in the liver to form several substances, one of which (morphine-6-glucuronide) has powerful analgesic properties of its own. These substances are then excreted by the kidney. When given by *injection* it produces analgesia rapidly. When given *orally* as a *single* dose its effect is greatly reduced as about 75% of the dose is broken down by the liver before reaching the circulation. However, with *repeated* oral dosage it is very effective. This may be because morphine-6-glucuronide is slowly excreted and with repeated doses accumulates sufficiently to help to produce satisfactory analgesia. The analgesic effect of morphine usually lasts about 4 hours after injection but depends to some extent on the severity of the pain, the sensitivity of the patient to the drug, and the dose. Morphine will also cross the placental barrier and affect the fetus, a point of importance in obstetrics. Repeated doses of morphine may induce a state of tolerance to the drug so that increasing doses may be required to produce a therapeutic effect. It is a *powerful drug of dependence*. The most important actions of morphine are on the central nervous system. They may be divided into depressing and stimulating effects.

Depressing effects:

1. Morphine depresses the appreciation of pain by the brain and thus acts as a powerful analgesic. It relieves all types of pain. If the pain is felt at all, it seems to have lost is unpleasant nature.
2. It is a euphoric and allays anxiety.
3. It depresses respiration.
4. It depresses the cough centre and thus damps down the cough reflex.

5. It is a mild hypnotic and may produce drowsiness and sleep.

Stimulating effects:

1. Morphine stimulates the CTZ in the brain stem (see p. 87) causing nausea and vomiting in about 30% of patients particularly if they are mobile.
2. The pupils of the eye are constricted due to an effect on the nucleus of the third nerve.
3. Morphine stimulates the vagus nerve. This action is particularly liable to be troublesome when morphine is used for the pain of coronary thrombosis as it may cause undue slowing of the pulse and lowering of the blood pressure.

Other actions. Morphine decreases the peristaltic activity of the bowel and at the same time increases the tone leading to constipation. It causes spasm of the sphincters, including the sphincter of Oddi at the lower end of the bile duct, and thus produces a rise in pressure in the biliary system. It also interferes with bladder function which may cause urinary retention after operation.

Therapeutics. Morphine is still one of the best analgesics for severe pain of a temporary nature such as occurs in surgical emergencies, in the postoperative period, following injury or after a coronary thrombosis, for not only does it relieve the pain but it also relieves the anxieties and miseries of the patient. It is very useful in controlling severe pain in terminal cancer (see p. 102) if given regularly. It is commonly used as a premedication, given half an hour before operation on account of its analgesic, euphoric and tranquillizing effects.

Morphine is also useful in treating the dyspnoea of heart failure, particularly acute failure of the left ventricle with pulmonary oedema. Its mode of action under these circumstances is not clear, though it probably acts by its widespread sedative effect on the central nervous system and also by dilating veins and relieving congestion of the lungs.

The dosage in severe pain or in acute left ventricular failure depends on many circumstances, including the age, weight and general health of the patient, but morphine 10–15 mg subcutaneously is the usual dose for an adult. Morphine can also be given intravenously, the dose being 4–10 mg. The analgesic effect starts within 20 minutes of subcutaneous injection and 10 minutes of intravenous injection.

Morphine in small doses can also be given by continuous subcutaneous infusion. This allows the dose to be modified as required and can be very useful in severe and fluctuating pain. However, this method needs careful titration of the dose in relation to the therapeutic effect and fixed dose regimes are not very successful (see p. 101).

It can be given orally for long-term control of pain as *Slow-Release tablets* which are only needed twice daily or as an *aqueous solution* containing either 2.0, 6.0 or 20 mg/ml or an *immediate release tablet* which must be given 4-hourly.

If vomiting is troublesome, morphine can be combined with the anti-emetic *prochlorperazine* 12.5 mg i.m. or in long-term oral treatment *haloperidol* 500 micrograms—3.0 mg orally twice daily may be preferred. Anti-emetics are usually only required for a few days.

Morphine, in rather smaller doses, is also included in some cough mixtures by virtue of its depressing action on the cough centre. It is used in mixtures usually containing bismuth or kaolin, in the treatment of diarrhoea.

Adverse effects are considered below.

Signs of overdosage. A patient who has received an overdose of morphine is drowsy or unconscious. The skin is cyanosed and sweating. The respirations are depressed and the pupils are pin-point. The fatal dose is variable but death usually occurs after a dose of 200 mg unless tolerance has been induced by repeated dosage.

Papaveretum (Omnopon) is a mixture of morphine and other opioids. Its actions are essentially those of morphine: 10 mg of papaveretum ≡ 6.25 mg of morphine.

Diamorphine (heroin)

Diamorphine is obtained by modification of morphine. When given by injection it enters the

Table 8.1 Adverse effect of morphine, diamorphine and other powerful opioids (Based on the Lewisham and North Southwark Formulary)

Adverse effect	Approximate frequency (%)	Dose related	Tolerance	Comments
Constipation	100	No	No	Prophylactic laxative (e.g. Senokot required)
Nausea	30	No	Yes (5–7 days)	Prophylactic anti-emetic if needed Give oral or i.m. prochlorperazine or oral haloperidol
Sedation	30	Yes	Yes (3–4 days)	Usually mild. Wears off in 48 h
Confusion, nightmares hallucinations (particularly at night)	1	Probably	No	Try reducing dose then consider haloperidol 2–4 mg at night

nervous system more rapidly than morphine so that its action starts a little sooner than that of morphine. Thereafter it is quickly converted to morphine in the body. When given orally diamorphine is all converted to morphine in the liver before it enters the systemic circulation; therefore their actions are similar except that the effects of diamorphine are seen a little earlier after injection. It is more soluble than morphine and this is useful when large doses are required by injection.

Although diamorphine is more popular than morphine among addicts, it is difficult to see a scientific reason for this and it may be for social or mythological reasons.

Therapeutics. Diamorphine can be used instead of morphine. The dose is 5–10 mg by subcuta- neous or intramuscular injection. For more rapid action it can be given intravenously in doses of 2.5–5.0 mg, and for the long-term control of pain, diamorphine elixir given orally should be used in doses sufficient to keep the patient free from pain. Its analgesic action lasts about 4 hours. If vomiting is troublesome it can be combined with *prochlorperazine* 12.5 mg intramuscularly.

Adverse effects of morphine and diamorphine are shown in Table 8.1. Other adverse effects of opioids are:

1. Bradycardia.
2. Urinary retention.
3. Dry mouth.
4. Allergy.

5. Dependence can develop rapidly when narcotics are used in a social context but they very rarely present a problem when used therapeutically either in an acute painful situation or in terminal disease. However, their use in chronic painful, but non-fatal disorders, is asking for trouble.

Interactions. Opioids increase the effect of other central depressants as also do monoamine oxidase inhibitors which are particularly dangerous with pethidine.

Certain patients are very sensitive to powerful opioids and a normal dose may produce signs of overdose. The most important of this group are patients whose respiratory centre is under stress, i.e. those with chronic bronchitis and emphysema, and patients *during* an asthmatic attack. Patients with liver damage or impaired renal function suffer an exaggerated and prolonged response. Finally, the very old and the very young are especially sensitive and they should only be given a small dose until their sensitivity to the drug is known.

Table 8.2 Equivalent doses of morphine and diamorphine if given regularly.

Morphine orally 10 mg	≡	Morphine subcutaneously 7.5 mg
Morphine orally 10 mg	≡	Diamorphine subcutaneously 5 mg
Morphine orally 10 mg	≡	Diamorphine orally 10 mg

Table 8.3 Some other opioid analgesics and equivalent doses

Drug	Dose	Equivalent analgesic effect	Special features
Dextromoramide	5–20 mg orally or by injection	15 mg ≡ 15 mg oral diamorphine	Short acting (3 h) Effective orally
Dipipanone	10–20 mg orally	10 mg ≡ 3 mg oral diamorphine	Given as Diconal (dipipanone 10 mg + cyclizine 30 mg per tablet). Rather sedative
Papaveretum (Omnopon)	10–20 mg orally or by injection	10 mg ≡ 3 mg diamorphine by injection	Contains alkaloids of opium. Action similar to morphine
Phenazocine	5 mg orally or sublingually	5 mg ≡ 10 mg oral diamorphine	Can be given sublingually if there are swallowing problems
Oxycodone	30 mg rectally	20 mg ≡ 10 mg diamorphine	Given as suppository analgesic effect lasts 8 hours (i.e. useful overnight)

Equivalent doses of opioids are only approximate. Much will depend on the circumstances in which the drug is given, previous drug history and individual responses.

Methadone

Methadone is a synthetic analgesic. Its analgesic action is as powerful as that of morphine, but it has little of morphine's euphoric and tranquillizing effect. Like morphine, it also has a depressing effect on the cough centre, but the effect on the respiratory centre is not so marked. It is a drug of dependence. It is rapidly and well absorbed after oral administration or subcutaneous injection and is less liable to produce vomiting than morphine. It is, however, liable to accumulate with repeated dosing.

Therapeutics. Methadone may be used as a substitute for morphine in the treatment of pain, and in small doses is useful as a cough sedative.

It is also used as a substitute for morphine or diamorphine in the treatment of drug dependence. The usual dose is 5–10 mg orally or by injection.

Pethidine

Pethidine is a synthetic substance, which is related chemically to atropine.

It is well absorbed after oral or subcutaneous administration. It is less powerful than morphine, but has less effect in therapeutic doses on the cough or respiratory centre. It causes some spasm of plain muscle of the bile ducts. It is not constipating. It does not cause constrictions of the pupil

and is therefore used in head injuries where observation of the pupil size may be important. Dependence can develop.

Therapeutics. Pethidine is used in the treatment of moderately severe pains, particularly those arising from viscera. It is especially useful in the relief of pain occurring in the later stages of labour, as it is short acting and less likely to depress the respiratory centre of the baby. The usual dose is 50–100 mg orally or by subcutaneous injection. Its action lasts 2–3 hours.

Codeine

Codeine is obtained from opium. It is given orally. It is a mild analgesic having only about one-seventh of the power of morphine. Its most useful action is its depressing effect on the cough centre and it is about half as powerful as morphine in this respect. Like morphine, it also decreases peristalsis of the intestine.

Dependence on codeine is rare but may occur.

Therapeutics. Codeine is widely used in various cough mixtures for its sedative effect on the cough centre. These mixtures usually also contain syrup, whose emollient action is useful in relieving coughs arising from the pharynx. The dose to suppress a cough is 15–30 mg.

It will control diarrhoea, in doses of 15–60 mg 6 hourly. It is combined with aspirin or paracetamol as a mild analgesic (see p. 107) in doses of 8–60 mg.

Dihydrocodeine is similar to codeine and is used as a mild analgesic. It causes constipation and occasionally dizziness and nausea. The dose is 30 mg orally or 50 mg by intramuscular injection.

Dextropropoxyphene is similar to methadone but is a much weaker analgesic. The usual dose is 30–60 mg orally and it is combined with paracetamol as the compound tablet **Co-Prox-amol** (Distalgesic) which is useful in treating pains which do not respond to aspirin or paracetamol alone. It is slightly addictive and like many drugs in this group it can cause vomiting. *Overdose* can be dangerous not only because the paracetamol in Distalgesic can cause liver damage but because dextropropoxyphene can cause respiratory depression and collapse.

PARTIAL AGONISTS

Opioid partial agonists (see p. 95) differ from opioid agonists such as morphine in some of their effects. They are powerful analgesics but are less addictive, less likely to depress respiration and are less euphoric.

Buprenorphine. This analgesic, although only a partial agonist, is as powerful as morphine. It can be given by injection or sublingually but is not effective orally as it is broken down in the liver (large first pass effect). Its analgesic action lasts longer than that of morphine (6–8 hours) and it is less likely to depress respiration. The risk of dependence is low but it can occur.

Buprenorphine shows a 'ceiling effect' so that increasing the dose above 5.0 mg daily will not improve its efficacy. Although it competes with powerful opioids such as morphine for receptor sites in the brain, in the therapeutic dose range buprenorphine does not reduce the analgesic action of other opioids when they are combined.

Therapeutics. Buprenorphine is used to treat moderate and severe pain. It can be given by injection in doses of 300–600 micrograms for postoperative pain but it is rather slow to take effect. It is also given sublingually in doses of 200–400 micrograms 6–8 hourly for various forms of chronic pain.

Adverse effects. Buprenorphine sometimes causes troublesome vomiting which requires the drug to be stopped. Respiratory depression, although not so marked as with morphine, is only partly reversed by naloxone.

Meptazinol is similar. When given by injection it has a short action (2–3 hours) and is used in obstetrics where its rapid elimination by both

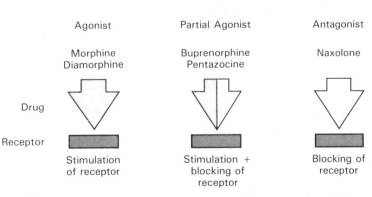

Fig. 8.2 Mode of action of opioid agonists, antagonists and partial agonists.

mother and fetus is an advantage. It is also useful for breakthrough pain in the postoperative period. There is a large first pass effect so that only some 10% of the oral dose reaches the circulation and it is only used for moderate pain by this route. The dose is 75–100 mg i.m. or 200 mg orally.

Nalbuphine is similar. Its analgesic action only lasts about 4 hours and it can only be given by injection. It also shows a 'ceiling effect'. The dose is 10–30 mg i.v. or i.m.

Nefopam

This drug is a non-opioid analgesic. Unlike the narcotic group it does not depress the nervous system and does not appear to produce dependence. It is quite a powerful analgesic, the usual dose being 30–60 mg three times daily orally. Further increase of dose does not increase efficacy (60 mg orally ≡ 20 mg by injection).

Adverse effects include sweating, tachycardia and nausea, particularly with larger doses, and difficulty with micturition. It should not be combined with MAOIs.

MORPHINE ANTAGONISTS

Several substances available antagonize the actions of morphine and other opioids. Generally they resemble morphine in their chemical structure and thus compete with it for receptor sites. Having occupied receptor sites, however, they produce little or no stimulation so that the actions of morphine are reversed (see Fig. 8.2). They are used to treat overdosage by opioids. The most widely used is:

Naloxone is pure antagonist and has no stimulating actions. It reverses the effects of both natural and synthetic opioids but with buprenorphine up to 10 times the usual dose may be required. It has no analgesic action. In the treatment of poisoning the initial dose is 800 micrograms intravenously or subcutaneously and it is very rapidly effective. It can also be used in doses of 100–200 micrograms to terminate the action of narcotic drugs in the postoperative period.

Its action is relatively short (about 1 hour) and if used to reverse the effects of longer-acting opioids repeated doses may be needed.

ANALGESICS FOR ACUTE PAIN

Acute pain in hospital is frequently generated by surgery but may occur as a result of trauma or as part of a medical illness such as coronary thrombosis or some form of colic.

Attitudes to pain relief on the part of both nurses and doctors are still inclined to be complacent, especially towards pain after surgery. Examples are the unimaginative approach of the 4-hourly injection given rigidly to time because no variation is allowed for on the drug sheet; a scheduled dose not given because the patient was not complaining; and a dose forgotten or postponed until extreme pain has produced a tense, sweating and exhausted patient who needs a far higher dose for adequate relief of pain.

The pain relief programme will depend on the severity, nature and cause of the pain. It may include a wide range of analgesics and, in addition, local anaesthetics and drugs that are specific for certain types of pain (e.g. colchicine for gout). It is impossible to specify regimes for all types of pain but certain general rules should be followed:

1. The programme must be flexible and aim at keeping the patient pain free.
2. Many programmes have a continuous background of analgesia with facilities for a top-up (perhaps with a more powerful analgesic) if the pain breaks through.
3. Patients vary considerably in their sensitivity to pain and response to analgesics so the programme should be individualized.
4. Explanation and reassurance are powerful analgesics.
5. In many hospitals there are specialized teams of doctors and nurses dedicated to the relief of acute pain.

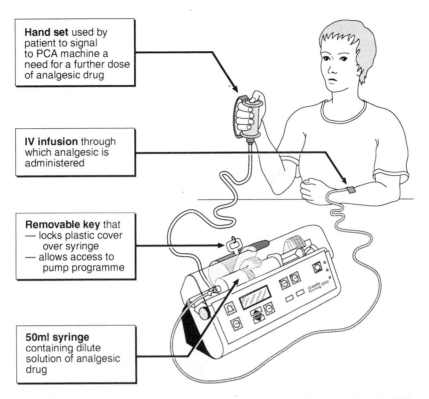

Hand set used by patient to signal to PCA machine a need for a further dose of analgesic drug

IV infusion through which analgesic is administered

Removable key that
— locks plastic cover over syringe
— allows access to pump programme

50ml syringe containing dilute solution of analgesic drug

Fig. 8.3 An example of a machine/syringe pump used for PCA—patient-controlled analgesia. This machine, a specialized syringe pump, enables small bolus injections of analgesic to be given on demand. The minimum time between injections—the 'lock-out period'—is controlled. If required, a background, low dose, continuous infusion is also possible.

These machines contain many safety features. The syringe is locked under a plastic cover and cannot, therefore, be interfered with by any unauthorized person. The pump programme used to control and alter the bolus size, the lock-out period, the continuous infusion rate and other functions, is only accessible using the same key that locks the plastic cover. This key should, therefore, be kept with ward keys or in some other secure place.

Patient-controlled analgesia (PCA)
(Fig. 8.3)

Pain in postoperative and some terminally ill patients can be effectively controlled by the self-administration of analgesia via a syringe pump set up to deliver a pre-set dose of the drug when a delivery button is pressed by the patient. A number of PCA devices are commercially available, all designed so that dose, rate and frequency of administration can be controlled and pre-set. A number of drugs have been used successfully, including morphine and pethidine. Trials have demonstrated high levels of acceptance of PCA among patients in hospital and the community, where small, portable PCA machines have been used. Part of the success of PCA is related to the feeling of control it gives patients and the confidence that they will not have to wait for the nurse to give an injection to relieve pain. Nursing time is saved as, once the device is set up, it obviates the need to prepare and administer routine injections. However, patients must be taught how to use the device before they need it. For surgical patients this should be before their operation as a heavily sedated postoperative patient will not be receptive to lengthy explanations. Patients going home with PCA machines should have the opportunity to become familiar with their use before they are discharged.

ANALGESICS IN TERMINAL DISEASE

Pain is often a prominent feature of terminal disease, particularly cancer. Although the use of drugs is only part of the management of the dying, the correct use of analgesics can play a very important role in the care of these patients.

It must be realized that in this type of patient pain can arise in many ways and the cause should be determined as it may have a specific remedy. It may be related directly to the spread of the cancer; it may be the result of therapeutic measures such as surgery or wound procedures; it may be due to secondary deposits particularly in bone or it may even have some unrelated cause or be due to a combination of these factors.

Whatever the cause of the pain, unresolved fear or anxiety may make it worse. A vicious cycle of pain and distress is thus engendered, relieved only by resolution of the anxiety as well as the alleviation of physical pain. The concept of 'total pain' introduced by Cicely Saunders to incorporate physical, social and emotional factors is crucial if the patient's problems are to be fully addressed (Fig. 8.4).

In this situation the nurse has a fundamental role in the assessment of the patient's pain (Fig. 8.5). Nursing interventions may include regular administration of analgesia and also active listen-

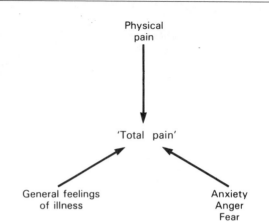

Fig. 8.4 Factors which go to make up the concept of 'total pain' or anguish in the terminally ill patient.

ing to his/her worries and anxieties. Evaluation of the response to such interventions is important in the ongoing care of that individual. Pain cannot be treated in isolation but must be regarded as one facet of the patient's physical and mental state.

For mild pain weak analgesics may be adequate. Paracetamol 500 mg 4 hourly. Co-proxamol (paracetamol + dextroproxyphene) 2 tablets 6 hourly or dihydrocodeine 30 mg 4–6 hourly (a bit constipating) are useful. For pain arising from secondary deposits in bone, anti-inflammatory analgesics (see p. 105) such as aspirin or naproxen are sometimes very effective when combined with opioids.

Moderate to severe pain should be treated by

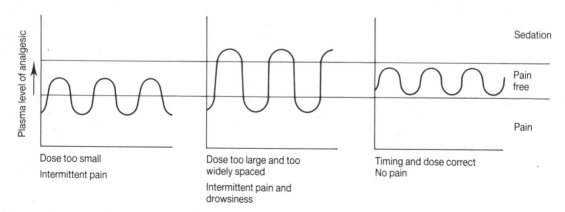

Fig. 8.5 Adjusting the dose to keep the patient free from pain.

giving opioid analgesics regularly, titrated against the patient's pain.

The most effective drugs are morphine or diamorphine. As diamorphine is largely converted to morphine in the body their actions and efficacy are essentially the same. However, diamorphine is more soluble than morphine and is thus better for injection if a small volume is required.

The opioid should be prescribed regularly 4 hourly (2–6–10–14–18–22 hours). The initial dose will depend on the patient's previous analgesic history. Lower doses are required in the elderly, the very ill or those with impaired liver or renal function. For the average patient morphine 10 mg orally as the elixir in chloroform water* or as the immediate release tablets is satisfactory.

At first the patient may need additional doses 'p.r.n.' when the pain breaks through. This should be noted and incorporated in the regular 4-hourly schedule. *The object is to keep the patient pain-free.* It is easier to prevent pain with its attendant fear than to relieve a patient who is already distressed.

Once the correct dose of oral morphine has been established it may be convenient to change to Slow-Release (SR) morphine tablets which are only required twice daily and may be more effective in controlling the pain at night.

If possible the drug should be given orally. This saves repeated injections and also produces a smoother and more prolonged analgesic effect.

Dosage schedules should be reviewed every 24 hours and titrated against the patient's pain and well-being.

Side-effects may develop with the use of narcotic drugs (see Table 8.1). They should be anticipated and treated as necessary.

With this regime tolerance to the analgesic action of the drug does not usually develop. Need to increase the dose of the drug usually indicates advance of the disease.

The risk of dependence is not relevant in the terminally ill patient.

Other routes of administration. Sometimes it is necessary to give narcotics by injection when the dose should be reduced. In very severe pain or when vomiting makes oral administration impossible opioids can be given by *subcutaneous infusion.* Diamorphine is used because of its solubility. The procedure is as follows:

1. A single 4-hour dose is given subcutaneously before the syringe pump is set up.
2. The 24-hour requirement of the analgesic is calculated and dissolved in water.
3. The syringe pump is started at a rate adjusted to give the correct dose over 24 hours. It should not be delivered at more than 1.4 ml/hour or absorption may be incomplete.
4. Haloperidol (5–15 mg/24 h) or metoclopramide (30–150 mg/24 h) can be added to the syringe to prevent vomiting.
5. Careful monitoring of the therapeutic effect and degree of sedation is necessary and adjustment of the dose as required.

Other opioid analgesics

Dextromoramide (p. 98) because of its short and rapid action can be given orally or sublingually before a painful procedure or for 'breakthrough' pain.

Diconal (p. 98) is quite widely used but the cyclizine component causes drowsiness if more than two tablets are required.

Oxycodone suppositories are useful in relieving pain at night, their action lasting for 8 hours, and are particularly useful for patients cared for at home.

Opioid-non-responsive pain

Certain types of pain respond poorly to opioid analgesics. These include pain due to pressure or infiltration affecting a nerve, or bone pain due to secondary deposits where movement may cause an acute exacerbation of pain which breaks through the opioid control. Nerve pain may respond to steroids which reduce surrounding

---

*The shelf-life of morphine in chloroform water is 3 months.

oedema or to anticonvulsants which stabilize the nerve and prevent its stimulation. Bone pain can be helped by radiotherapy (if this is possible), NSAIAs and by preventing movements which cause pain.

Other drugs

Entonox (50% oxygen + 50% nitrous oxide) by inhalation can be used to cover painful procedures.

Chlorpromazine is not only useful as an antiemetic but may increase the effectiveness of analgesics.

Amitriptyline (see p. 125) is a useful antidepressant to combat the psychotic depression which sometimes develops in these patients.

Other methods

The use of analgesics is not the only way to relieve pain in terminal cancer. Radiotherapy is very effective, particularly in treating secondary deposits in bone. In recent years various types of nerve block either at the level of the peripheral nerve or in the spinal cord can relieve pain without any systemic effects. These blocks may be temporary or permanent. Finally, much of the comfort and tranquillity of the patient will depend on the character and understanding of the nurse.

Analgesics in non-painful terminal disease

Many patients with malignant disease or dying from others such as renal failure do not have pain but they may experience considerable malaise and mental anguish. The use of opioids in these circumstances is more controversial. Some people consider that opioids should be used only for pain relief. Others, recognizing their undoubted euphoric action, would give them to reduce the anxieties and discomforts in the terminal stages if necessary, although usually, relatively small doses are required. They are also useful in controlling cough and relieving the sensation of dyspnoea.

Analgesics and chronic non-terminal pain

In some types of chronic pain the cause is obvious (e.g. arthritis), in others it is obscure. Psychological factors play some part in most types of pain but may play a major role in the more obscure varieties. This means that there are many types of treatment depending on the cause and severity of the pain and it is only possible here to make some general statements.

1. Before starting treatment it is very important to listen to the patient and to assess his/her perception of the pain and how it affects his/her daily life.
2. Management with the appropriate drugs will be enhanced by considerable supportive therapy.
3. Alternative methods of pain relief i.e. nerve block, transcutaneous stimulation, which probably acts by closing the relay gate in the spinal cord, etc. may prove very helpful in some patients.
4. Do not forget that *depression* often presents as obscure chronic pain. In this case antidepressants are effective.
5. It is important to avoid drugs with a high risk of dependence. Even so-called 'low-risk' analgesics are not entirely safe, e.g. buprenorphine dependence does occur. In prescribing analgesics therefore, the patient should be assessed carefully and prescriptions should not be repeated endlessly.

The NSAIAs (see p. 105) are free from the risk of dependence but not free from adverse effects.

TERMINAL CARE SERVICES AND THE PAIN CONTROL TEAM

The object of hospice care is to help maintain an acceptable quality of life whilst enabling a patient to die peacefully, with special reference to the person's values, preferences and outlook on life. This may be achieved through a team approach in various settings.

The hospice movement has expanded considerably over the last 25 years. There are over 75 hospices throughout the UK and about 250 domiciliary teams of which over 80 are attached to inpatient units. Referral may be through the general practitioner or district nurse or arranged on hospital discharge.

A more recent development is the hospital support team of which there are now about 20 in the UK. The team is usually multidisciplinary, sometimes working in conjunction with the radiotherapy or oncology departments. The hospital support team provides skills in symptom control and pain relief and can offer emotional support to patients and carers, whilst fulfilling an educational role within the hospital.

Pain control teams have been developed to cope with the problem of those in chronic pain. Although many of these patients have terminal cancer, there are other types of chronic pain such as post-herpetic neuralgia, various long-term pains following injury such as amputation, and pain for which there is no obvious cause but where psychological factors may play a part.

The team usually comprises one or two doctors who are interested in the subject (such as anaesthetists), nursing staff (often a sister who is specially trained) and a psychiatrist. They deal with patients referred to them in hospital; they may run an outpatient service and may also undertake home visiting.

Many types of chronic pain are made worse by depression, fear and anxiety and here the psychiatrist will be able to help by explanation, reassurance and the judicious use of drugs such as antidepressants. As in so many areas of treatment, the control of pain is becoming a team activity.

THE NONSTEROIDAL ANTI-INFLAMMATORY AGENTS (NSAIAs)

This is a large group of drugs. Their chief use is to treat minor pains, i.e. headaches etc., and to control the pain and stiffness in rheumatic conditions and osteoarthritis. They are believed to act by suppressing the formation within the body of *prostaglandins* which occur naturally and are released by cell damage and for various other reasons (see p. 183). One of the actions of prostaglandins is concerned with the production of

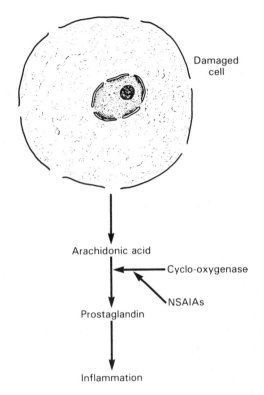

Fig. 8.6 The action of NSAIAs in preventing inflammation.

painful stimuli, and they are also responsible for many of the features of inflammation (i.e. swelling and redness). The NSAIAs, by blocking the action of the enzyme *cyclo-oxygenase*, reduce the production of these substances (Fig. 8.6). The action of these drugs, therefore, is largely in the peripheral tissues rather than in the brain.

The salicylates

The salicylates are an important and widely used group of NSAIAs. They are mild analgesics and also antipyretics. The best known of the group are acetylsalicylic acid or aspirin and sodium salicylate.

Aspirin (acetylsalicylic acid). Aspirin is usually given by mouth and is rapidly absorbed from the intestinal tract. It is rapidly excreted by the kidney partly conjugated with glucuronic acid.

Aspirin is effective against pain of low intensity and particularly that of rheumatoid arthritis and acute rheumatic fever when its anti-inflammatory properties are combined with its analgesic action. It is also useful in other minor pains such as headaches, sore throats, toothache etc.

Aspirin is also antipyretic—that is to say it will lower a raised body temperature. The control of body temperature is regulated by a centre in the hypothalamus which balances heat production resulting from metabolism against heat loss. This is achieved either by increasing heat production by raising metabolism by such means as shivering, or by increasing heat loss by sweating or by dilating blood vessels in the skin. When a patient develops a fever the heat regulating mechanism is set at a higher level than normal. Aspirin acts on this centre and 'resets' it again at the normal level; this results in increased heat loss by sweating, and by dilatation of blood vessels of the skin. These effects are only seen in patients with a raised temperature for aspirin does not lower the normal body temperature to any appreciable degree.

Therapeutics. To relieve pain the dose of aspirin is 300–600 mg given orally, and gastric irritation (see below) may be reduced if it is given with a meal. Aspirin is rapidly metabolized and excreted so that 4-hourly dosage is usually required to keep the patient free of pain. To suppress inflammation rather larger doses are needed, up to 900 mg 4 hourly. Salicylates in high doses are particularly useful in the treatment of acute rheumatic fever. Within 2 or 3 days of starting the drug the temperature should have dropped to normal levels and the swelling and pain in the joints will have disappeared.

In addition to its actions detailed above, aspirin decreases the tendency of platelets to form thrombi (see p. 72).

Soluble aspirin is a mixture of aspirin with calcium carbonate and citric acid. Its actions are similar to those of aspirin. It is more soluble, which aids absorption, and less irritant to the stomach but it may still cause bleeding.

Adverse effects. In large doses aspirin produces effects on the eighth cranial nerve, i.e. dizziness, tinnitus, deafness and vomiting. This is associated with overbreathing due to stimulation of the respiratory centre and to acidosis.

In normal doses aspirin is a gastric irritant and in about 70% of people produces slight bleeding from the stomach. If it is taken continuously over a long period, this may lead to anaemia. More rarely aspirin causes a severe haematemesis, usually from a superficial erosion of the stomach wall. This bleeding may occur with both aspirin and soluble aspirin. Although severe bleeding is rare when considered against the enormous amount of aspirin consumed, it is wise not to use this drug in those with a history of peptic ulcer, haemophilia or liver disease or patients receiving anticoagulants. Occasionally aspirin causes bronchospasm and thus an asthma-like attack, due to reduced production of prostaglandins.

Aspirin should not be given to children under 12 years as it may rarely precipitate *Reye's syndrome* with coma and liver damage which can prove fatal.

Interactions. Aspirin increases the effects of anticoagulants and oral hypoglycaemia agents.

Benorylate is a combination of paracetamol and aspirin which splits into its component drugs after absorption.

Paracetamol is a widely used minor analgesic. Although it has some cyclo-oxygenase inhibiting properties this action is very weak in the peripheral tissues and it has practically no anti-inflammatory action. Its analgesic effect must therefore be mediated by some action on the central nervous system which is not yet understood. Its main advantage is that unlike other drugs in this group, it does not cause indigestion or gastric bleeding.

Therapeutics. The usual dose is 0.5–1.0 g 4 or 6 hourly. It is not very effective in rheumatoid arthritis because of its poor anti-inflammatory action.

It is the preferred mild analgesic for children under 12 years and for this purpose is available as an elixir.

Adverse effects. These are uncommon at normal dosage but in overdose it causes dangerous liver damage (see p. 208).

Mefenamic acid is a mild analgesic but is probably a little more powerful than aspirin. Its action may last longer than that of aspirin, but it may produce diarrhoea. It can also cause acute renal failure in the elderly. The dose is 250–500 mg 8 hourly.

Analgesic mixtures

There are many analgesic mixtures in which aspirin or paracetamol is combined with a small dose of weak opiate, thus the risk of dependence is minimal. These combinations are a little stronger than aspirin or paracetamol alone and are used for more severe pain. Whether in fact they are more effective than the single drugs is debated and certainly the risk of adverse effects and of danger in overdose is increased. Nevertheless, they are very popular and some are available 'over the counter'.

Among those in common use are:

Co-codaprin tablets: codeine phosphate 8 mg + aspirin 400 mg per tablet. This is also available in a dispersible form.
Co-codamol tablets: codeine phosphate 8 mg + paracetamol 500 mg per tablet.
Co-dydramol tablets: dihyrocodeine tartrate 10 mg + paracetamol 500 mg per tablet.
Co-proxamol tablets: dextropropoxyphene 32.5 mg + paracetamol 325 mg per tablet.
Tylex: codeine phosphate 30 mg + paracetamol 500 mg per tablet.

Analgesic nephropathy

Some subjects take large quantities of minor analgesic drugs for recreational rather than therapeutic reasons. The favourite was phenacetin (no longer available) and this led to progressive kidney damage and ultimately, renal failure. Paracetamol, which is related to phenacetin, probably carries the same risk but to a lesser extent. It appears that aspirin and other NSAIAs do not damage the kidneys in this way but see NSAIAs and the kidney (p. 109).

Other nonsteroidal anti-inflammatory agents

Indomethacin. An anti-inflammatory and analgesic agent which is used in various forms of arthritis and in acute gout. It is effective but minor adverse effects are quite common.

Therapeutics. The incidence of side-effects is reduced by starting with a low dose (25 mg daily orally) and increasing the dose slowly. It is not usually helpful to give more than 75 mg daily. If morning stiffness is a problem, a 100 mg suppository at night is useful. In acute gout where a rapid effect is required, the initial dose should be 50 mg 4 hourly for the first 12–24 hours.

Adverse effects:

1. Indigestion and gastric bleeding can occur but are less common than with aspirin. However, it can rarely cause intestinal ulceration and perforation.
2. Headaches and light-headedness can be troublesome particularly if the initial dose is high.
3. Salt and water retention may occur.
4. The action of antihypertensive drugs may be reversed.

Phenylbutazone is a powerful NSAIA. Unfortunately it has a number of serious adverse effects including agranulocytosis, gastric bleeding, salt and water retention and rashes. Its use is therefore restricted to the treatment of ankylosing spondylitis in hospital.

Newer agents

There is now a large number of nonsteroidal anti-inflammatory agents available for use in rheumatoid arthritis and allied conditions. They are also used to reduce the inflammatory element in osteoarthritis though this use is more controversial as there is a suspicion that although they relieve pain they may hasten the degenerative changes in the joint. Some are listed in Table 8.4. They all act by reducing the production of pro-

Table 8.4

Drug	Trade name	Dose	Side-effects and special features
Azapropazine	Rheumox	600 mg–1.2 g daily	Rashes
Diclofenac	Voltarol	25–50 mg t.d.s.	Indigestion, avoid in peptic ulceration. Rashes. Can be given by i.m. injection
Etodolac	Lodine	200–300 mg b.d.	
Fenbufen	Lederfen	600 mg nocte 300 mg mane	Indigestion, avoid in peptic ulceration. Produces a therapeutically active metabolite
Fenoprofen	Fenopron	300–600 mg t.d.s. or q.d.s.	Indigestion, avoid in peptic ulceration. Rashes
Flurbiprofen	Froben	50 mg t.d.s. or q.d.s.	Indigestion, avoid in peptic ulceration. Rashes
Ibuprofen	Brufen Ebufac	400 mg t.d.s. or q.d.s.	Indigestion, avoid in peptic ulceration. Rashes. Low incidence of side-effects but not so active as some of the group. Now available without prescription
Ketoprofen	Orudis	50 mg 2–4 times daily	Indigestion, avoid in peptic ulceration. Rashes
Nabumetone	Reliflex	1–2 g daily	Converted to active metabolite
Naproxen	Naprosyn	250–500 mg b.d.	Indigestion, avoid in peptic ulceration. Rashes. Twice daily dosage
Piroxicam	Feldene	20 mg once daily	Indigestion, avoid in peptic ulceration. Once daily dosage
Sulindac	Clinoral	100–200 mg twice daily with food	Rapidly converted to active metabolite in the body. Indigestion, avoid in peptic ulceration. Rashes. Dizziness

staglandins (see p. 183) and thus reduce inflammation.

There are certain general principles which can be applied to this group:

1. There is no preferred drug—patients vary in their preference and if one drug is ineffective after 2 weeks of treatment a change should be made to another. It is, however, generally accepted that *ibuprofen* in doses usually recommended is rather less likely to produce side-effects but is perhaps less effective. It is available 'over the counter' without a prescription.
2. It is useless to give two drugs of this type concurrently.
3. If a satisfactory response is obtained, use the lowest dose which is effective.
4. All these drugs may cause some gastric irritation and should be given with or after meals.

NSAIAs can also be used to control pain or to reduce the need for opioids after surgery, or for such acute pain as renal colic. Several are available as suppositories (e.g. diclofenac, indomethacin, ketoprofen) or for injection (diclofenac). They are particularly useful after day surgery when undue sedation has to be avoided.

Several NSAIAs are now available to be *massaged into the skin* over a painful joint or soft tissue area. It is claimed that an appreciable amount of the drug reaches the inflamed area and pain is relieved. There is certainly a powerful placebo effect; whether, in fact, the drug achieves a therapeutic action is not yet certain.

Adverse effects are similar for all these drugs. They are:

1. Indigestion.
2. Gastric bleeding and perforation. This is particularly common in the elderly and is believed to be due to the inhibition of the gastric protective action of prostaglandins. They should not be given to patients with peptic ulcers but, if essential, they can be combined with an H_2 blocker or possibly with misoprostol (see p. 81) an oral prostaglandin preparation.
3. Occasionally, salt and water retention.
4. Rarely, bronchospasm.

Interactions. NSAIAs:

- antagonize the actions of diuretics and hypotensive drugs
- increase the effects of anticoagulants

- decrease the excretion and increase the effect of lithium (see p. 128).

NSAIAs and the kidney

NSAIAs do not appear to damage the kidneys in normal subjects. However, in patients with heart failure, cirrhosis of the liver, renal disease or who are taking diuretics they can occasionally precipitate renal failure. This is believed to be due to an alteration of blood flow through the kidneys which follows inhibition of prostaglandin production. It usually recovers on stopping the drug but rarely NSAIAs cause irreversible renal damage. When this group of patients is given regular treatment with NSAIAs their renal function should be checked after a few weeks of treatment.

NSAIAs and the uterus

Prostaglandins can cause contraction of the uterus and are important in the initiation of labour. NSAIAs, by preventing prostaglandin formation, are useful in reducing period pains and have also been used to prevent premature labour.

DISEASE-MODIFYING DRUGS

These drugs are used when NSAIAs fail. In some way they suppress the rheumatoid process.

Chloroquine appears to be of some benefit in rheumatoid arthritis and also in the skin lesions of lupus erythematosus. It is given in doses of 200 mg daily. Unfortunately prolonged treatment may cause corneal opacities and, more serious, retinal damage. The former may be suggested by the patient complaining of haloes round bright lights.

Gold in the form of *sodium aurothiomalate* suppresses the rheumatoid process but its mode of action is unknown. It is usually given weekly by intramuscular injection, starting with 10 mg and increasing gradually to 50 mg per week to a total of 1.0 g. It is then sometimes continued with monthly injections of 50 mg.

Adverse effects are common and can be serious and may require withdrawal of the treatment.

1. Itching followed by rashes which can progress to exfoliation requires treatment to be stopped.
2. Renal damage—urine must be tested for protein at each visit.
3. Bone marrow suppression requires weekly blood counts and the patient should report bleeding, bruising or sore throat.
4. Stomatitis.

An oral form of gold (*auranofin*) is available which is less toxic but less effective than the injection.

Penicillamine (see also p. 311) is used with some success in treating rheumatoid arthritis. Its mode of action is not clear but in some way it suppresses the inflammation. The initial dose is 250 mg daily, which is increased. Its use is not without risk as it can cause nausea, depression of the blood count and, rarely, damage to the kidneys. It is therefore necessary to test the urine for protein and to perform a blood count at regular intervals.

Sulphasalazine (see also p. 197) also suppresses the disease process and is rather less toxic than gold or penicillamine.

All these drugs take a month or more to produce their full therapeutic effect.

Methotrexate and cyclophosphamide are cytotoxic drugs which suppress the immune response. They are used when other drugs have failed and the patient will require careful monitoring with regular blood counts and, with methotrexate, liver function tests.

Special points for patient education

Patients usually take these drugs long term and they must be aware of possible adverse effects and the importance of regular checks and of reporting warning symptoms.

TREATMENT OF RHEUMATOID ARTHRITIS

Rheumatoid arthritis is a common disease but it is difficult to treat. As a rule treatment consists of

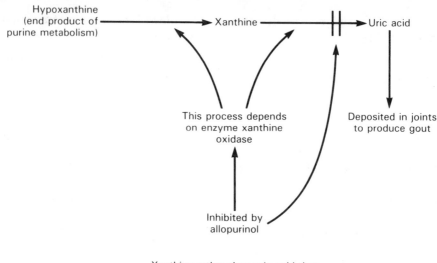

Fig. 8.7 Mode of action of allopurinol.

controlling the symptoms of pain, stiffness and swelling in the joints and preventing deformity. It is usual to start treatment with one of the new NSAIAs, the choice depending on the doctor's previous experience and preference.

It is often necessary to give simple analgesics such as paracetamol in addition to anti-inflammatory agents to minimize pain and these can be used on a regular basis or to cover times when pain is severe.

If these treatments fail recourse should be made to either gold or penicillamine, but both drugs have serious side-effects and care is needed when they are given.

Steroids, though effective, are now rarely used to treat rheumatoid arthritis because of the high incidence of adverse effects which seem particularly common with this disease. They are very much 'last resort' treatment.

Physiotherapy is useful in relieving stiffness and preventing deformity.

GOUT

Gout is a metabolic disorder which tends to run in families. In gout there is an increase in the amount of uric acid in the body, probably due to increased production, and this precipitates around joints (particularly the big toe) producing an acute arthritis. In longstanding cases uric acid may also accumulate in other parts of the body.

Drug treatment is used for two purposes:

1. To relieve the acute attack. Various drugs may be used for this purpose. Indomethacin (see above) is very effective and is the drug of choice. It is used in large doses to produce a rapid effect, i.e. 50 mg 4 hourly until the pain subsides (usually about 12–24 hours) and then at a reduced dose for a week. An older remedy is colchicine.
2. To decrease the amount of uric acid in the body. This can be achieved by increasing its excretion in the urine by uricosuric drugs or by preventing the production of uric acid by giving allopurinol.

Colchicine. An alkaloid obtained from the autumn crocus or meadow saffron.

It is not an analgesic in the strict sense of the word for it relieves only one type of pain, that associated with an acute attack of gout. Its mode of action in gout is complicated and still not entirely understood. It is of interest that colchicine also has the property of arresting the division of cells in plants and animals.

Therapeutics. The pure alkaloid colchicine is used in the treatment of gout. The dose for the acute attack is 500 micrograms two or three times daily to a maximum of 10 mg for the course. Do not repeat for 3 days. Sometimes toxic effects (vomiting and diarrhoea) many cause premature cessation of treatment.

Uricosuric drugs

These drugs increase the excretion of uric acid by the kidney.

Probenecid increases excretion of uric acid by the kidney, probably by an action on the renal tubular cells. It can be given over long periods in doses of 1 g daily. Side-effects are rare but gastro-intestinal upsets and rashes may occur.

Sulphinpyrazone is a very powerful uricosuric agent. Its effects are blocked by simultaneous administration of citrates or salicylates. It can be given over long periods, the dose being 200–400 mg daily.

Drugs preventing the production of uric acid

Allopurinol slows the production of uric acid by inhibiting an enzyme (xanthine oxidase) which is concerned with the synthesis of uric acid within the body. It is given orally, the usual dose being 300 mg daily. It is excreted via the kidneys and care is necessary if it is used in renal failure. Skin rashes are particularly common if retention of the drug occurs. It must not be combined with the anticancer agent *6-mercaptopurine* as it prevents the breakdown of this drug and greatly increases its effect. It has proved particularly useful in the long-term management of gout particularly if the attacks are frequent, and will usually need to be continued for the rest of the patient's life.

Nursing points

1. Uricosuric drugs and allopurinol may cause an acute attack of gout in the first 2 months of treatment, probably because deposits of uric acid are mobilized, and should therefore be combined with a NSAIA during this period.
2. If uricosuric agents are used the patient should be advised to maintain a high fluid intake to prevent the formation of uric acid crystals in the renal tract.

FURTHER READING

Alison M C et al 1992 Gastrointestinal damage associated with the use of NSAI drugs. New England Journal of Medicine 327: 7949
Brooks P M, Day R O 1991 Non-steroidal anti-inflammatory drugs. New England Journal of Medicine 324: 1716
Editorial 1991 Second line drugs in rheumatoid arthritis. British Medical Journal 303: 201
Editorial 1987 Treatment of rheumatoid arthritis. Prescribers Journal 27: 1
Editorial 1991 Post-operative relief of pain and non-opioid analgesics. Lancet 337: 524
Edwards S 1992 Evaluating syringe drivers. Nursing Times 88(3): 46
Farmer M, Harper N J 1992 Unexpected problems with patient-controlled syringe analgesia. British Medical Journal 304: 6826
Hanks G W, Justins D M 1992 Cancer pain management. Lancet 339: 1031
Jordan S, 1992 Drugs update—drugs for severe pain. Nursing Times 88 (2): 24
Laporte J M et al 1991 Upper GI bleeding in relation to previous use of analgesics & NSAIA. Lancet 337: 85
McLintock T et al 1990 Analgesic requirements in patients previously exposed to positive intra-operative suggestion. British Medical Journal 301: 788
Shady P 1992 Patient-controlled analgesia: can education increase outcomes. Journal of Advanced Nursing 17: 408
Wall P D, Melzack R (eds) 1989 Textbook of pain. Churchill Livingstone, Edinburgh

9

Hypnotics

Insomnia

Approximately 20% of the adult population consider they do not get enough sleep. This is a subjective opinion and in very few does their health suffer. However, insomnia can cause feelings of anxiety, inability to concentrate and general debility.

Sleep requirements vary with age. Teenagers need about 10 hours sleep, adults about 8 hours and the elderly about 6 hours but there is also considerable interperson variation.

Hypnotics are drugs which produce sleep that is comparable with normal sleep. They do not relieve pain. Before prescribing hypnotics it is important to ascertain whether the patient is not getting enough sleep, as some people exaggerate their insomnia, and to find out if there is some reason for failing to sleep. Among these reasons may be:

- Anxiety and stress
- Depression
- Physical illness e.g. heart failure, chronic lung disease
- Pain
- Caffeine and alcohol taken before retiring.

If these are remedied sleep should occur naturally. Various simple measures can be tried—a walk or bath before retiring, a rather unexciting book or a glass of milk at bedtime may be sufficient. More sophisticated measures such as audio-cassette programmes can help some people.

Although hypnotic drugs may be required in some circumstances, for example during periods of stress or for certain chronic insomniacs, their use should be discouraged. Tolerance to their action often develops in 2–3 weeks with some degree of dependence. Withdrawal at this stage can lead to increasing wakefulness at night for a few days. This is particularly important in hospital where they are often prescribed much too freely and where a lifetime of habituation to these drugs may start. Patients should not as a general rule be sent home from hospital taking hypnotics.

The nature of sleep

Sleep is not just a state into which one lapses on going to bed and from which one emerges on waking. It is a series of cycles each lasting about 90 minutes. After falling asleep the subject becomes progressively more relaxed with slow pulse and respiration rate; this phase lasts about 80 minutes and ultimately the state of 'deep sleep' is reached. Then follows a phase lasting about 10 minutes with increased muscle tone, rapid eye movements and increased heart rate, known as *rapid eye movement* (REM) sleep. The whole cycle is then repeated about six times per night.

It has been shown that if a subject is deprived of REM sleep he will show psychological changes during waking hours. Many centrally acting drugs and alcohol do in fact suppress REM sleep and thus do not really produce natural sleep.

Chloral hydrate is a colourless crystalline substance soluble in water. It is rapidly absorbed following oral administration and produces its hypnotic action in about 30 minutes. The drug is conjugated with glucuronic acid in the liver and excreted in the urine. The effect of chloral lasts about 4 hours.

Therapeutics. Choral is a useful and safe hypnotic, particularly in the elderly and in children. It is, however, a mild gastrointestinal irritant and may produce vomiting. It also has an unpleasant taste. It is given in a dose of 500 mg to 2 g at bedtime and is commonly dispensed as capsules containing 500 mg which should be taken with

plenty of water or as an elixir with 500 mg in 5 ml.

It is very useful as a hypnotic for children for whom an elixir is available. The usual dose recommended is too low and if real sedation is required the dose for an infant should be 30–50 mg/kg body weight (max 1 g).

Adverse effects and interactions. Chloral is relatively safe but may cause gastric upset. It should be used with caution in liver or renal failure. It reduces the effect of warfarin and oral contraceptives by increasing their rate of metabolism.

Paraldehyde is an oily liquid with a characteristic and unpleasant taste and smell. It is soluble in water. It may be given by mouth, per rectum dissolved in saline or by intramuscular injection. It is quick acting and powerful hypnotic. It is rapidly broken down in the body and a small amount is excreted unchanged via the lungs and its action only lasts a few hours even after a large dose.

Therapeutics. Paraldehyde is occasionally used in status epilepticus or to quieten a noisy patient. It tastes unpleasant and the patient and the ward smell of it for hours after administration. The drug is given intramuscularly and the dose for an

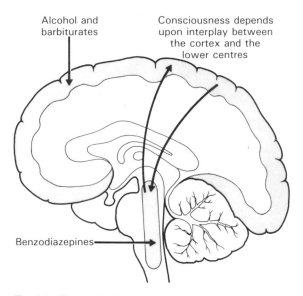

Alcohol and barbiturates

Consciousness depends upon interplay between the cortex and the lower centres

Benzodiazepines

Fig. 9.1 The mode of action of hypnotics and tranquillizers.

adult is 5 ml, repeated after 2 hours if necessary. It can dissolve plastic but is safe with modern plastic syringes provided it is given immediately. However, injections of paraldehyde are painful and may cause abscesses at the site of injection, so it has been largely superseded. It may also be given rectally as a basal narcotic in children before operation. A 1 in 10 solution of the drug in saline is warmed and run into the rectum and will rapidly produce sleep.

Chlormethiazole. This drug, which is related to vitamin B1, can be used both as a sedative or hypnotic. It can be given orally or intravenously. Its action is short-lived.

Therapeutics. Chlormethiazole is used particularly in elderly subjects, for patients who are agitated and confused and for controlling the withdrawal symptoms in alcoholics, although in this circumstance dependence on chlormethiazole may develop. As a hypnotic the usual dose is two capsules (each containing 192 mg base). To control withdrawal symptoms the dose is three capsules four times daily and reduced as necessary. Chlormethiazole can also be given intravenously to terminate status epilepticus or control delirium tremens. It is given as a 0.8% solution, the initial dose being 40–100 ml (320–800 mg) infused over 5–10 minutes and then adjusted as necessary. When given in this way there is a danger of respiratory depression and hypotension and the patient requires careful observation. *The infusion should not usually be continued for more than 18 hours.*

Adverse effects are rare but some patients complain of stuffiness in the nose shortly after taking the drug.

The benzodiazepines (see also p. 123)

Several members of this group of drugs can be given as a hypnotic and there is very little to choose between them. Most of them have quite a long half-life (see p. 4 and Table 9.1) and some are broken down in the liver to demethyldiazepam which also has a prolonged hypnotic action. This means that some hangover into the next day is

Table 9.1 Benzodiazepines used as hypnotics

Drug	Dose	Half-life	Duration of action
Nitrazepam	5–10 mg	20 h	Fairly long
Diazepam	2–10 mg	30 h	Long, also active breakdown product
Temazepam	10–20 mg	5–6 h	Short

quite common if they are used to produce sleep. Their main advantage is their very wide safety margin.

Nitrazepam. This was the first benzodiazepine to be recommended as a hypnotic. Although it has been claimed that this drug is unlikely to confuse the elderly this is not true. In addition, some sedative effect may persist well into the following day.

Diazepam. Although more usually used as a minor tranquillizer, diazepam is quite a good hypnotic if there is some background anxiety and sedation lasting into the next day is needed.

Temazepam. This drug has a rather shorter half-life and length of action than most other benzodiazepines and it does not produce metabolites which are also hypnotics. It is, therefore, less liable to cause drowsiness into the next day.

Adverse effects. The benzodiazepines are remarkably free from adverse effects. The main problem is the development of dependence. This may occur after 2 weeks or less when they are used as hypnotics. Withdrawal then results in considerable difficulty in sleeping for the next few nights and the temptation is to resume taking them. (See also p. 123.)

When stopping treatment with benzodiazepines, particulary if they have been taken for a long time, the dosage should be reduced stepwise, halving it about every 4 days depending on symptoms and finally withdrawing it altogether.

Zopiclone

Zopiclone is chemically distinct from the benzodiazepines but probably acts in a similar way via the GABA mechanism. It is rapidly absorbed and produces sleep lasting a few hours with little, if any hangover. The available evidence suggests that tolerance may develop and dependence occur. In general it is very similar to the short-acting benzodiazepines. The usual dose is 7.5 mg at bedtime.

Adverse reactions. Hallucinations have been reported.

Ethyl alcohol. Alcohol is occasionally used as a sedative at night, particularly in the elderly. It is not a good hypnotic and though it may help patients to get to sleep, they often waken during the night due to rebound insomnia. It is important to remember that patients who take alcohol regularly may become restless and have difficulty in sleeping if it is stopped suddenly.

The use and choice of hypnotics

The first essential is to make certain that a hypnotic drug is necessary to relieve the patient's insomnia. Insomnia may be considered in three categories.

1. Transient insomnia occurs in people who usually have no sleep problem and is due to altered circumstances, i.e. admission to hospital or travel. In these cases a short-acting benzodiazepine such as temazepam is appropriate.

2. Short-term insomnia may be due to anxiety, illness etc. Here a short-acting benzodiazepine can be used but if anxiety is prominent, a drug such as diazepam may be more useful as its effect will last into the next day. It is important that the drug is not given for more than 2 weeks and that intermittent dosing is introduced as early as possible as there is a *definite risk of dependence developing*.

The nurse has an important role to play by listening to the patient's worries and by relieving any physical discomfort if possible.

3. Chronic insomnia. Careful analysis is necessary in these patients. Some will be suffering from psychiatric illness, particularly depression. In other cases an excess of coffee or alcohol may be the cause. If these can be excluded, a change in

lifestyle with regular exercise and reduction of stress (if possible) can be tried.

Diazepam is the most suitable hypnotic, preferably on an intermittent basis, for a month. If this fails, the trial of an antidepressant is appropriate. The long-term management of this type of patient is often difficult.

There is little indication for the use of hypnotics other than the benzodiazepines but if an alternative is required chloral is probably the most satisfactory substitute.

Hypnotics in special circumstances

In renal failure. Some hypnotics are excreted via the kidney so that accumulation occurs in renal failure. Nitrazepam and chloral do not fall in this group and are satisfactory.

In liver failure. Nitrazepam is satisfactory but should be used with care.

In respiratory disease. All hypnotics produce some depression of respiration so they must be used with great care in patients with respiratory failure and during attacks of asthma. Temazepam is as good as any.

In the elderly chloral may be useful and if nocturnal confusion is a problem thioridazine 25–30 mg (see p. 121) is preferred.

(see p. 121)

Nursing points

Dependence can occur with long-term use of all hypnotics. Use the minimum dose for the minimum time.
  Do not forget that depression causes insomnia.

Sedatives prior to minor procedures

Patients often require some sedation before such manoeuvres as gastroscopy, etc. Benzodiazepines are useful for they are both sedative and also produce amnesia for the event. Diazepam is often used intravenously. It is, however, rather irritant to the vein. A specially prepared non-irritant solution of diazepam, Diazemuls, is preferable.

Alternatively, **midazolam** which has an action lasting about 2 hours can be given. The usual dose is 2.5–7.5 mg i.v. (2.5 mg for the elderly) and it is non-irritant.

Following injections of this type the patient should be warned not to drive until the next day and to avoid alcohol or other depressants.

Adverse effects. There have been a number of reports of respiratory depression and cardiac arrest after midazolam, especially in the elderly who do not eliminate the drug so rapidly as younger subjects. This is usually due to excessive dosage and care should be taken.

FURTHER READING

Burton E 1992 Drugs update: something to help you sleep? Nursing Times 88(8): 52

Editorial 1990 The treatment of insomnia. Drug and Therapeutics Bulletin 28: 97

Editorial 1990 Zopiclone. Lancet 335: 507

Hodgson L A 1991 Why do we need sleep? Relating theory to nursing practice. Journal of Advanced Nursing 16: 1503

Lader M 1988 A practical guide to prescribing hypnotic benzodiazepines. British Medical Journal 293: 1048

Prinz P N et al 1990 Sleep disorders and aging. New England Journal of Medicine 323: 520

10

Drugs used in psychiatry

INTRODUCTION

Mental illness is one of the major causes of ill health. During the last 30 years large numbers of drugs have been produced which were hoped to have some therapeutic effect. The chemical abnormalities in the brain which are responsible for mental diseases have not yet been discovered; in fact it is debatable as to whether any such abnormalities exist at all in some mental disorders.

Certain substances appear important in the function of the brain. These are acetylcholine, adrenaline and noradrenaline, dopamine, and 5-hydroxytryptamine (5HT) and GABA (gamma aminobutyric acid). Most of these substances have, in addition, well-defined actions outside the brain (see p. 25). Acetylcholine probably acts as a transmitting agent between nerve cells in the brain. Adrenaline and noradrenaline may act in a similar fashion. If the amounts of adrenaline and noradrenaline are increased in the brain by giving drugs (amine oxidase inhibitors) which retard their breakdown or interfere with their reabsorption (tricyclic antidepressants) an awakening and stimulating effect is produced. If the amount of these substances in the brain is reduced by reserpine, a tranquillizing or depressing effect is produced. 5HT also seems to be concerned with mood. GABA exerts a sedating inhibiting effect.

One further point is worth remembering. Formerly it was considered that the cerebral cortex was the part of the brain largely concerned with consciousness. It is now realized that the reticular formation, a band of tissue running through the brain stem is also important, and it is the interaction between this formation and the cerebral cortex which maintains the state of wakefulness. It seems that some drugs which are used in psychotherapy act on this area of the brain (Fig 9.1). In addition the limbic system is concerned with various emotions entering consciousness.

During the last 30 years many drugs which might be useful in mental disease have been produced but testing them is difficult. At the animal level it is impossible to reproduce exactly in the laboratory psychological disorders which are seen in man and therefore the drugs are put through a battery of tests which it is hoped will pick out those which are potentially useful as therapeutic agents. Trials of these drugs in man are also fraught with difficulty and much of their alleged usefulness will not stand up to scientific examination. The nurse, therefore, must be on guard against extravagant claims for new drugs in this field and should temper enthusiastic claims with careful and impartial observations.

Special points in the administration of drugs to psychiatric patients

1. In hospital many psychiatric patients are not confined to bed and drugs may be given out at a central point rather than having a 'drug round'.
2. Two nurses should always be concerned with drug administration.
3. In psychiatric patients compliance may be a problem and it is necessary to ensure that medication is actually taken.
4. In some patients, especially schizophrenics, drugs may be given by injection as depot preparations to get round the problem of non-compliance.
5. Occasionally a patient's paranoia may extend to drugs they are given.
6. Drug education for when the patient returns home is very important and relatives may have to be involved. It should also be possible for patients or relatives to ring up for information if problems arise.
7. The nurse should observe the effects of drug treatment.

8. On discharge, care should be taken not to prescribe excessive quantities of drugs, particularly if there is a suicide risk.

TRANQUILLIZERS

Tranquillizers are drugs which produce a state of calm without making the patient unduly sleepy. There are now a large number of these drugs.

NEUROLEPTICS

These drugs are particularly useful in controlling the states of agitation found in acute schizophrenia, mania and some other forms of delirium and in paranoia. Their exact mode of action in these conditions is not known but they all block the action of *dopamine* which is a transmitting substance in several areas of the brain and this seems to be important in their antipsychotic and sedative effect. Some of them have other actions such as being anti-emetic. By interfering with the function of dopamine they are liable to produce disorders of posture and movement (see below).

The phenothiazines

These drugs all act on the central nervous system but their actions may differ in detail. They affect mainly the reticular formation and basal ganglia and block both dopamine and acetycholine receptors. As a result they modify behaviour:

1. They have an antipsychotic effect. Restlessness, agitation and hallucinations are reduced and this has made them especially useful in treating schizophrenia.
2. They produce some sedation with a feeling of detachment from external worries and troubles.
3. Many of them have some anti-emetic action.
4. Chlorpromazine is sometimes used to control persistent hiccup.

In addition, peripheral effects include anticholinergic blockade and some blockade of α-adrenergic receptors.

Most of the phenothiazines are well absorbed after oral dosage. They are largely metabolized in the liver to numerous breakdown substances.

A number of phenothiazines are now used in treatment, some are preferred for one type of disorder, some for another. Table 10.1 gives some of the most commonly used drugs in the group.

Table 10.1

Name	Trade name	Salient feature	Dose 24 h
Chlorpromazine	Largactil	Widely used as a sedative in the confused. Occasionally as an anti-emetic or in the anxious	50–800 mg orally. Can be given by injection
Promazine	Sparine	Weaker than chlorpromazine. Otherwise similar	50–200 mg
Prochlorperazine	Stemetil	Used for vomiting and vertigo	5.0–30 mg Can be given by injection
Thioridazine	Melleril	Useful in the agitated elderly. Can cause retinal damage	150–600 mg
Trifluoperazine	Stelazine	Widely used in schizophrenia	5–15 mg
Fluphenazine decanoate	Modecate	Used for depot injection in schizophrenia	12.5–50 mg Single dose

The doses of these drugs are very variable and depend on the disorder being treated and the response of the patient.

Adverse effects are not uncommon and the incidence varies from drug to drug. They include:

1. Jaundice. This is quite common with chlorpromazine and is due to blocking of the bile canaliculi in the liver. It is presumed to be an allergic effect, and recovery occurs when the drug is stopped.
2. Various disorders of movement due directly or indirectly to a dopamine blocking action in the brain. *These may occur with all neuroleptics.*
   a. Parkinson-like syndrome.
   b. Akathisia, which is a feeling of restlessness with inability to stand still.

c. Dystonia, which is uncontrolled movements.

All these may commence soon after starting treatment and require a reduction of the dose if possible. Sometimes the addition of a benzodiazepine may help.

d. *Tardive dyskinesia*, consisting of abnormal movements of the mouth and tongue and sometimes the upper limbs. It develops in about 20% of patients on long-term neuroleptics. Its onset is usually delayed for a while. Control is difficult and it may not stop even if the drug is withdrawn.

3. Depression of white cells in the blood.
4. Skin rashes including light sensitivity and contact dermatitis when the drug is handled.
5. An α blocking effect on the sympathetic nervous system leading to a fall in blood pressure and faintness.
6. In the elderly hypothermia may be precipitated.
7. There may be considerable weight gain and the development of gynaecomastia with these drugs.
8. Dry mouth can be troublesome.
9. Rarely, the *neuroleptic malignant syndrome* with hyperpyrexia, coma and muscular rigidity.

In treating psychotic patients large doses of these drugs are often used and may have to be continued for many months or even longer. This means that a careful watch must be kept for side-effects especially those involving the nervous system.

Therapeutics. The phenothiazines are used in psychiatry to reduce restlessness, anxiety and agitation in psychotic patients and to reduce the severity of hallucinations. They are thus useful in controlling schizophrenics who show these symptoms. They are also used in psychoneurosis with anxiety.

They are, in addition, used as anti-emetics, in severe pruritus and in association with anaesthetic agents.

In the present state of knowledge it is impossible to say which is the best drug of this group. Patients seem to vary in their response to individual drugs and trial and error seems to be the only way to decide which is the best for any particular patient.

The thioxanthenes

These are rather similar to the phenothiazines. They are antipsychotic and anti-emetic and are largely used in the treatment of schizophrenia. They are less sedative than the phenothiazines but akathisia is rather common. Among them are:

Flupenthixol used as an injected depot preparation in doses of 20–40 mg every 2 weeks or as tablets.

The butyrophenones

This group of drugs has actions rather similar to those of the phenothiazines but they are less sedative.

Haloperidol is widely used in doses of 0.5–2 mg three times daily orally and may be increased. It is particularly useful in the management of manic or confused patients when 2–10 mg 6 hourly by intramuscular injection may be used. In doses above 5 mg daily symptoms of Parkinsonism may develop.

Droperidol is similar but acts more rapidly. The dose is 5–10 mg by injection or 5–10 mg orally.

Other neuroleptics

Pimozide. This is another antipsychotic drug similar to the phenothiazines but with a lower incidence of side-effects. The dose is 2–16 mg orally.

Sulpiride has a more specific dopamine-blocking action than the other neuroleptics. However, it can still cause the various disorders of movement. The dose is 200–400 mg twice daily orally.

Clozapine differs in detail from other neuroleptics in its actions on the brain. It causes

little in the way of disorder of movement and posture. It is effective in schizophrenic patients who have proved resistant to other neuroleptics. The initial dose is 25 mg daily which can be increased to a maximum of 300 mg.

Adverse effects. These can be serious. About 3% of patients taking this drug for 1 year develop neutropenia, so monitoring of the blood count is mandatory. Other adverse effects include fits, hypotension, excessive salivation and sedation. It is also very expensive. Because of these problems it should be reserved for specially selected cases.

Depot injections

Several antipsychotic drugs are given as depot injections including fluphenazine and flupenthixol, because patients with severe mental disease often fail to take their pills regularly. Depot preparations given by deep intramuscular injection into the upper and outer part of the buttock or the lateral aspect of the thigh get round this problem. However, this dosage scheme is inflexible and there is difficulty if a patient develops some adverse effect.

Nursing point

Do not forget the adverse effects of this group of drugs, particularly those affecting the nervous system. With long-term use careful surveillance is also required on withdrawal of treatment as the re-emergence of symptoms may be delayed for several weeks.

Nursing point

Special care is needed if neuroleptics are given to:
1. Patients with Parkinson's disease as symptoms may be increased.
2. Epileptics or patients with alcohol withdrawal symptoms as fits may be precipitated.
3. Elderly patients who may get postural hypotension.
4. Pregnant and lactating mothers.

THE DRUG TREATMENT OF SCHIZOPHRENIA

Schizophrenia is a mysterious disease. It may take many forms but the essential feature is a change of personality with disordered thought processes which may be associated with hallucinations, delusions and withdrawal. Once it has developed complete recovery is unusual although considerable improvement is possible. It usually starts in young people.

There are many theories as to its cause; some believe it to be due to a biochemical disorder affecting the brain, others that it is a disorder of personality development related to faulty interaction with the family in early life.

The total management of the schizophrenic patient has many facets but the introduction and use of neuroleptic drugs have greatly improved treatment (Table 10.2). They have enabled many patients who, without treatment, would be confined to a mental hospital, to take their place in the community and lead a reasonable life. The dosage requires individual titration for each patient and drug treatment must be combined with support and management, especially the avoidance of stressful situations.

Table 10.2 Some drugs used in treating schizophrenia

Drug	Sedation	Extra pyramidal effects	Usage
Chlorpromazine	++	++	Acute and long-term
Promazine	+	++	Acute and long-term
Haloperidol	+	+++	Acute, sometimes long-term
Pimozide	+	(+)	Long-term only
Flupenthixol	+	+++	Depot injection

MINOR TRANQUILLIZERS

The benzodiazepines

In addition to their use as hypnotics this group of drugs is widely used as minor tranquillizers in anxious patients. It is believed that they act on the reticular formation in the brain. There are specific receptors for benzodiazepines and they appear to enhance the action of a substance called GABA which is produced by the brain and which depresses brain function.

All the benzodiazepines have much the same effect, being tranquillizing and sedative, but vary in their duration of action. The variation is due to different rates of breakdown in the body and some of them produce breakdown products which are themselves sedative and which thus prolong the action.

Although the benzodiazepines are effective in relieving anxiety they have two disadvantages:

1. They become less effective with prolonged use.
2. If the drug is stopped suddenly, even after a relatively short period of use (e.g. 2–3 weeks), withdrawal symptoms can develop. These are anxiety and sleeplessness for a few days but after prolonged and heavy dosage may include fits, psychotic symptoms, muscle pains and twitching. They usually occur within a week of stopping the drug and earlier if it is short-acting. This suggests that dependence has developed and in severe cases patients may take many weeks to recover. Such patients require slow and stepwise withdrawal of the drug over several weeks.

They should therefore only be used for anxiety if it is severe and disabling, and the treatment should be the lowest effective dose for no more than 2–3 weeks and combined with other therapy.

Previously, they have been used in acute emotional crises but by preventing the patient responding to the painful situation they may delay psychological adjustment.

Diazepam and clonazepam are also given intravenously in treating status epilepticus (see p. 149) and diazepam as a sedative before various investigations.

Diazepam also has some muscle relaxing properties and is used in combination with an analgesic to relieve pain and spasm in lumbago and related disorders.

The benzodiazepines are metabolized in the

liver and often produce further active compounds. For example, diazepam is partially converted to desmethyldiazepam which also has a prolonged sedative action.

Table 10.3 gives some of the benzodiazepines used as tranquillizers (see also table of hypnotics, p. 115).

Table 10.3

Drug	Dose/day	Duration of action (approx)	Special features
Diazepam	4–30 mg	24 h	Can be used i.v. in status epilepticus
Chlordiazepoxide	30–60 mg	24 h	
Oxazepam	45–120 mg	12 h	
Lorazepam	1–4 mg	12 h	May be more liable to cause dependence
Medazepam	15–30 mg	12 h	
Clonazepam	4–8 mg	24 h	Largely used in epilepsy
Clorazepate	15 mg	30 h	

Duration of action is also dependent on the dose and to some degree on the individual. Although the actions of these drugs are very similar the price varies considerably—diazepam is cheap and usually very adequate.

Adverse effects and interactions. The group is very safe generally. Overdose can cause marked sedation, incoordination, memory difficulties and occasionally respiratory depression but this is rarely serious in healthy individuals, even with considerable overdose. Interactions can occur with other CNS depressants (e.g. alcohol) increasing sedation.

The problem of dependence is considered above.

Flumazenil is a benzodiazepine antagonist. It is given intravenously and reverses benzodiazepine-induced sedation in a few minutes. It has been used in overdose and to speed recovery in patients who have been anaesthetized with midazolam (see p. 117). However, its effect only lasts about 1 hour so repeated doses may be required with long-acting benzodiazepines.

Buspirone is the latest attempt to produce an anxiolytic drug without adverse effects. It appears to have no sedative action or risk of dependence, its only adverse effects are occasional nausea and headache. However, its onset of action is delayed and it seems to be ineffective after benzodiazepines have been used. Its place in therapeutics is not yet decided.

THE TREATMENT OF ANXIETY

Anxiety is a universal phenomenon and a certain amount is useful to the individual, acting as a stimulant and increasing efficiency. However, when it becomes disproportionate to the stimulus an anxiety state develops and this degree of anxiety may interfere seriously with the patient's life.

There are three main types of anxiety:

1. *Free floating anxiety* in which the patient feels generally apprehensive and tense.
2. Anxiety producing various *physical symptoms* such as palpitations and dry mouth due to overactivity of the sympathetic nervous system.
3. *Phobic states* in which the patient fears certain situations. The commonest is agoraphobia in which the subject is frightened to go out and acute anxiety is precipitated by supermarkets or travelling on trains and buses, etc.—the syndrome of the homebound housewife.

A great deal of the treatment of anxiety is by psychotherapy with discussion and explanation. Drugs may be useful to help to control the situation in the early stage but generally should only be used for short periods.

Benzodiazepines are rarely indicated as there is the problem of withdrawal symptoms. Perhaps the most effective drug at present is a small dose of an antidepressant such as dothiepin or imipramine. A single dose of a benzodiazepine (e.g. diazepam) can be useful to control a *panic attack* but should not be repeated, and drug treatment should be combined with 'self-help' psychotherpy.

Physical symptoms can be controlled by a β blocker such as propranolol 20 mg three times daily. In phobic states behavioural techniques are very important and drugs play a minor role but monoamine oxidase inhibitors are sometimes used.

THE MANAGEMENT OF ACUTE CONFUSIONAL STATES

Acute confusional states have many causes. They may be part of a psychiatric illness but often develop as a result of a serious 'organic' illness or may be due to drug dependence, e.g. alcohol withdrawal.

1. It is important that such patients are nursed in quiet surroundings. The nurses' approach must be calm and as much explanation given as is feasible.
2. If possible drugs should be given orally. The choice lies between a benzodiazepine such as diazepam, or a neuroleptic such as haloperidol. More seriously disturbed patients can be given lorazepam i.m. or droperidol i.m. *Patients confused as a result of alcohol withdrawal should not be given neuroleptics owing to the risk of fits.*

ANTIDEPRESSANT DRUGS

Depression

Depression is a common and normal emotion and people quite naturally become depressed as a result of unfortunate domestic and social conditions. Sometimes, however, the depression is disproportionate to the precipitating factors or there may be no obvious cause at all. This is an illness called *endogenous* or *psychotic* depression and is common in older people. Some psychiatrists recognize a further type of depressive illness in which environmental factors play a more prominent part and this is sometimes called reactive depression or *depressive neurosis*. Sometimes depression may alternate with attacks of mania. This is known as *bipolar depression* or *manic-depressive psychosis*.

In depression the mood is at its lowest in the morning and improves throughout the day. The patient is disinterested and may be irritable and anxious. The appetite is poor and vague symptoms including headache and odd pains are common. *Suicide is a special risk in depressed patients.*

The cause of depression is not known but there is evidence that a major factor is a reduction in the amount of amines such as 5-hydroxytriptamine or noradrenaline at the junctions between nerve cells in the brain. Many of the drugs used to treat depression increase the amount of these substances in the brain, thus providing some evidence that amines are connected with changes of mood.

The following groups of drugs are used to relieve depression:

- Tricyclic antidepressants
- Tricyclic anxiolytics
- 5HT re-uptake inhibitors
- Other antidepressants
- Monoamine oxidase (MAO) inhibitors
- Lithium

Tricyclic antidepressants

There are several tricyclic antidepressants in use and there is not a great deal of difference between them. They are well absorbed after oral administration and undergo considerable breakdown in the liver; some of these metabolic products are therapeutically active (Table 10.4). It is believed that they produce their therapeutic effect by preventing the re-uptake of amines at nerve endings in the brain which thus increases the concentration of these substances available for receptor uptake (Fig. 10.1).

Some members of the group (i.e. nortriptyline and desipramine) have a greater effect on noradrenaline concentration and others (imipramine

Table 10.4 Other tricyclic antidepressants

Drug	Dose/24 h	Special features
Desipramine	75–150 mg	
Nortriptyline	20–50 mg	
Protriptyline	15–60 mg	Least sedative
Clomipramine	30–100 mg	Particularly useful in obsessional features
Lofepramine	140–210 mg	Least side-effects, sedation minimal

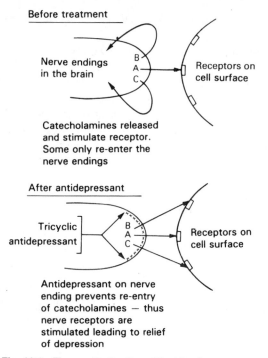

Before treatment

Nerve endings
in the brain

Receptors on
cell surface

Catecholamines released
and stimulate receptor.
Some only re-enter the
nerve endings

After antidepressant

Tricyclic
antidepressant

Receptors on
cell surface

Antidepressant on nerve
ending prevents re-entry
of catecholamines — thus
nerve receptors are
stimulated leading to relief
of depression

Fig. 10.1 The mode of action of the tricyclic antidepressant drugs.

and amitriptyline) on 5-hydroxytryptamine concentration.

Imipramine. The first of these drugs to be used. The dose is 25–150 mg daily and increased as required.

Amitriptyline is very similar to imipramine but is rather more sedating. The usual dose range is 25–150 mg daily.

Both these drugs have a long action and need only be given once a day. If amitriptyline is given in the evening its sedative action will help sleep which is often disturbed in depression.

Therapeutic use. After starting treatment the sleep disorders associated with depression usually respond fairly quickly but it is important to remember that it may take several weeks before the depression itself is relieved.

The drug should therefore be continued for 6 weeks before deciding that treatment has failed. About 80% of depressed patients will ultimately respond.

Blood concentration. Owing to the considerable intersubject variation in the breakdown of these drugs blood levels may vary widely. Extensive investigation has been carried out on the measurement of blood levels to control treatment but it is doubtful whether this is necessary for most patients.

Adverse effects:

1. Anticholinergic effects. Dry mouth can be troublesome and may be mitigated by lemon juice. Elderly male patients may experience difficulty with micturition, and constipation can be a problem particularly in depressed patients already preoccupied with their bowels. Owing to a dilating effect on the pupil of the eye, they should not be given to patients with glaucoma.
2. Fall in blood pressure with occasional faintness especially in the elderly.
3. Weight changes.
4. *The action of sympathomimetic drugs is dangerously increased if given to patients taking tricyclic antidepressants.* This is particularly liable to happen with local anaesthetics containing adrenaline or noradrenaline. They may reverse the effect of some hypotensive drugs and their action is increased by alcohol. *They should not be combined with MAOIs.*
5. In epileptics, the tendency to fits is increased and the dose of anti-epileptic drugs may require alteration if tricyclic anti depressants are used.
6. They depress conduction in the heart, and a number of sudden deaths have been reported in patients with heart disease taking tricyclics. They are therefore best avoided in this group of patients.
7. Tricyclic antidepressants are dangerous in overdose producing cardiovascular disturbance, fits and coma.

Imipramine is also used for *nocturnal enuresis* (bed wetting) in children. The dose is:

7–10 years	25–50 mg	2 hours before
11–16 years	50–75 mg	bedtime.

It is important to explain to the child's parents that:

1. The effect may be delayed for 2–3 weeks.
2. The tablets must be stored in a childproof place.
3. Treatment should not be given for more than 3 months.

Anxiolytic tricyclic antidepressants

Doxepin, dothiepin. These drugs are similar to the tricyclic antidepressants but have a weaker antidepressant action and are particularly useful when anxiety complicates mild depression. They are also more rapidly effective than the standard tricyclics.

Dose:

- Doxepin—50–100 mg at night
- Dothiepin—75–150 mg daily.

Adverse effects. Similar to the tricyclics but generally less marked.

5HT re-uptake inhibitors

5HT is concerned with mood and behaviour and a deficiency in the brain is believed to be a factor in depression. Several drugs have been introduced which specifically inhibit 5HT re-uptake at nerve junctions and thus raise its concentration in the brain. Those available at present are:

Drug	*Daily dose*
Fluvoxamine	100–200 mg
Fluoxetine	20 mg
Sertraline	50 mg
Paroxetine	20 mg

In relieving depression these drugs are about as effective as the tricyclics. Their advantage lies in the lack of many of the adverse effects of the former group.

- They are not cardiotoxic and therefore less dangerous in overdose.
- There are no anticholinergic effects.
- They do not cause weight gain.
- They do, however, sometimes cause nausea and dyspepsia.

Interactions are important. Combination with lithium or MAOI can cause CNS toxicity and fits

and an adequate gap must be left between stopping MAOI and starting these drugs.

It seems likely that ultimately they may replace tricyclic antidepressants on grounds of safety but at present they are much more expensive.

Other antidepressants

There are several other antidepressants which act by modifying the amount of amines in the brain but do not fit the above categories.

Mianserin. This drug, although an antidepressant, differs from the tricyclics in that it does not block the re-uptake of catecholamines. Its mode of action is not known but it may increase noradrenaline release in the brain.

Therapeutic use. The usual daily dose is 30–60 mg. Unlike the tricyclics mianserin does not adversely affect the heart even with overdosage, and it does not interfere with the treatment of hypertension. However, experience suggests that it is not very effective.

Adverse effects. The most common is sedation which can be troublesome. Less common are blood abnormalities particularly liable to occur in the elderly and requiring a monthly blood count for the first 3 months of treatment, and polyarthritis.

Trazodone is rather similar to mianserin.

Therapeutic use. It is an antidepressant and also an anxiolytic, the usual dose being 50–600 mg daily. It is not cardiotoxic and may therefore be useful for those with cardiac disease. It is mildly sedative and at present, much more expensive than the standard tricyclics.

Table 10.5 Comparison of tricyclic and 5HT re-uptake inhibitor antidepressants

	Tricyclics	5HT re-uptake inhibitors
Cardiotoxicity	++	–
Anticholinergic effects	+++	–
Sedation	+++ or +	–
Weight gain	++	–
Nausea	–	++
Price	Low	High

Monoamine oxidase (MAO) inhibitors

These drugs interfere with the breakdown of adrenaline, noradrenaline and 5-hydroxytryptamine in the brain and thus lead to an accumulation of these substances. It is tempting to link this action with the antidepressive action of these drugs but this has not been finally proved.

They produce a mood change with increase in cheerfulness, energy and well-being in about half of patients with depression. The main use for the MAO inhibitors is in atypical depression and phobic anxiety states. The long list of possible adverse effects limits their usefulness and they should only be prescribed by those who are familiar with the problems which may arise. The most important member of the group is:

Phenelzine which is given in doses of 15–60 mg by mouth.

Adverse effects and interactions. Monoamine oxidase inhibitors can cause insomnia and nervousness, difficulties with micturition and, rarely, jaundice.

Interactions are important and can be dangerous. They may exaggerate the effects of such centrally acting drugs as the barbiturates, alcohol, cocaine, morphine and particularly pethidine.

They also lead to over-action by vasopressors such as adrenaline and amphetamine and a number of vasoconstrictor drugs which are included in widely used 'cold-cures' may cause headaches, hypertension, restlessness and even coma and death. Similar effects may also occur if these amine oxidase inhibitors are taken with various articles of food including cheese, meat, yeast extracts, some wines and beers, game, broad bean pods and pickled herrings. Hospitals often have their own cards listing restrictions. This is because these foods contain vasopressor substances which are normally broken down by amine oxidase. If this breakdown is inhibited, the vasopressors accumulate and produce toxic effects. Therefore, the utmost care must be taken in administering these drugs and all those concerned with patients should be informed. If a surgical operation is to be undertaken, when it may be necessary to give such drugs as morphine or pethidine, the amine oxidase inhibitors should be stopped 2 weeks previously. *It is dangerous to combine MAO inhibitors and tricyclic antidepressants.*

Nursing point

A persistent headache is often a warning of rising blood pressure in a patient on MAO inhibitors.

Lithium

Lithium is treated by the body in a similar way to sodium. It is believed to enter the nerve cells of the brain and decrease their excitability. Lithium is used in treating patients with bipolar depression (manic-depressive psychosis). It can either be given to control an attack of mania or used regularly to prevent the extreme swings of mood seen in these patients. Before starting treatment with lithium, renal function must be checked as retention of the drug may occur if it is impaired. The dose usually lies between 0.5–1.2 g daily, and is adjusted to produce a blood level of 0.4–0.9 mmol/litre in a blood sample taken 12 hours after dosing. If the slow release preparation (Priadel) is used, the tablet must be swallowed whole. Because lithium is excreted rather slowly it takes some days of treatment before a steady blood level is reached and it is usual to start measuring blood levels 1 week after starting treatment. Once a satisfactory dose is established monitoring is only required monthly.

Adverse effects can be divided into two groups —those due to overdosage and those which do not appear to be dose related.

Overdose	*Not dose related*
Weakness	Thyroid deficiency
Drowsiness	Increased urine secretion
Confusion	Weight gain
Coma	

Interactions. If a thiazide or loop diuretic is combined with lithium the excretion of lithium by the kidney is reduced and toxicity may develop.Under these circumstances the dose of lithium must be reduced and the blood level carefully monitored.

THE MANAGEMENT OF DEPRESSION

Most patients with mild to moderate depression are managed at home. Indications for hospital admission are severe depression, risk of suicide and those who cannot care for themselves. All patients need support and encouragement.

The main physical methods of treatment are drugs and electroconvulsive therapy (ECT). Tricyclic antidepressants are widely used to treat endogenous depression. If sleep is a problem *amitriptyline* is preferred as it is fairly sedative, otherwise *imipramine* is satisfactory. The other members of this group are used in special circumstances. Because of their long half-life, once daily dosage, usually before retiring, is sufficient. Sleep problems respond promptly but it may take several weeks for the depression to lift. The initial dose of both drugs would be 50–75 mg as a single dose at night for an outpatient but larger doses may be used for inpatients. In the elderly 25 mg is a safer starting dose and twice daily dosing may be necessary if postural hypotension is a problem. In severe depression, especially if there is a serious risk of suicide or antidepressants have failed, ECT is often used. This is given twice weekly to a total of six or eight treatments.

Elderly patients or those with heart disease are at special risk from tricyclic antidepressants; therefore it may be expedient to use another type of antidepressant such as a 5HT re-uptake inhibitor. Some authorities think that the use of 5HT re-uptake inhibitors should largely replace tricyclics on grounds of safety and possibly efficacy.

In depressive neurosis when environmental factors are playing a part monoamine oxidase inhibitors are sometimes used and can be combined with a benzodiazepine. Tricyclic antidepressants must not be combined with MAO inhibitors as this may cause excitement and pyrexia. Normally there should be a 2 week gap when changing from one type of antidepressant to another.

Treatment for depression is usually continued for at least 4 months after recovery. Shorter periods of therapy increase the risk of relapse. The drug should then be phased out over about 6 months otherwise withdrawal symptoms may ensue. These consist of anxiety, diarrhoea, insomnia and restlessness.

In *bipolar depression* (manic-depressive illness) the manic phase can be controlled by a neuroleptic (usually haloperidol, see p. 122) and the depressive phase by a tricyclic antidepressant. The long-term use of lithium to prevent the mood changes has revolutionized the treatment of this condition. Sometimes it is more effective if carbamazepine is combined with lithium (see p. 148).

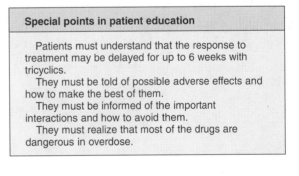

Special points in patient education

Patients must understand that the response to treatment may be delayed for up to 6 weeks with tricyclics.

They must be told of possible adverse effects and how to make the best of them.

They must be informed of the important interactions and how to avoid them.

They must realize that most of the drugs are dangerous in overdose.

Nursing point

Non-compliance is an important cause of treatment failure.

FURTHER READING

Ballinger B R 1990 Hypnotics and anxiolytics. British Medical Journal 300: 456

Batemen D N, Chaplin S 1988 Centrally acting drugs. British Medical Journal 296: 417

Behavioural emergencies 1991 Drug and Therapeutics Bulletin 29: 62

Editorial 1985 Management of patients requiring long-term treatment with neuroleptic drugs. Prescribers Journal 25: 131

Editorial 1988 Benzodiazepines and dependence. Bulletin of the Royal College of Psychiatrists 12: 107

Editorial 1988 Tardive dyskinesia. British Medical Journal 296: 150

Orme M L'E 1984 Antidepressants and heart disease. British Medical Journal 289: 1

Potter W Z et al 1991 The Pharmacologic treatment of depression. New England Journal of Medicine 325: 633

Silverstone T, Turner P 1988 Drug treatment in psychiatry, 4th edn. Routledge, London

Song F et al 1993 Selective serotonin reuptake inhibitors: meta-analysis of efficacy and acceptability. British Medical Journal 306: 683

Szabadi E 1989 Antipsychotic drugs in profile. Prescribers Journal 29: 244

Tyrer P 1988 The Nottingham study of neurotic disorder. Lancet ii: 235

11

Drugs used in anaesthesia, cardiac arrest and resuscitation. Local anaesthetics. Drugs affecting the function of voluntary muscle

GENERAL ANAESTHESIA

HISTORY

General anaesthesia for surgery was first used in 1842 by William E. Clark, of Rochester, New York, for a dental extraction. He used **ether**, a drug that is still in use in parts of the world where more recent and expensive drugs are unavailable. Horace Wells, a dentist in Hartford, Connecticut, introduced **nitrous oxide** in 1844, also for dental extractions (he first persuaded a travelling lecturer in chemistry to give him nitrous oxide whilst a fellow dentist took out one of his teeth before he then used it successfully on his own patients). Nitrous oxide is still widely used as part of almost every general anaesthetic. **Chloroform** was introduced, in 1847, by James Y. Simpson, of Edinburgh, for use in general surgery and obstetrics. It was administered to Queen Victoria, in 1853, at the birth of Prince Leopold. Chloroform remained popular for over 100 years but is no longer used as a general anaesthetic.

PREMEDICATION

Premedication is given for two reasons:

1. To allay anxiety
2. To reduce oral secretions.

Both effects of premedication make the induction of anaesthesia easier and possibly safer. However, premedication is not essential, and the best treatment for anxiety is to listen to the patient, to allow sufficient time for him or her to fully express his or her concerns and worries, and to give clear and simple explanations and reassurance whenever possible. The nurse looking after the patient probably plays a more important role in this respect than anyone else.

Most patients are anxious before anaesthesia and surgery. Some feel a general sense of nervousness or apprehension but have no particular concern or worry. Others may have one or more specific fears which may be of injections, of dying, of waking up in the middle of the operation, of waking up in pain, of talking during the anaesthetic (and perhaps giving away personal secrets), of the embarrassment of nakedness, or of the loss of control over themselves and their environment brought on by the sedative effects of drugs.

Drugs used to reduce anxiety or its effects include the *benzodiazepines,, chlorpromazine derivatives, opioids* and, occasionally, *butyrophenones*. Oral and tracheal secretions are reduced using anticholinergic drugs. See Table 11.1 for a list of the commonly used drugs.

Premedication is given 1–2 hours before anaesthesia and increasingly the oral route is being preferred to the intramuscular route.

Nursing point

Try always to give patients the opportunity and time to ask any questions they wish and to fully express their anxieties before anaesthesia and surgery.

Table 11.1 Drugs used for premedication

Drug	Trade name	Dose	Usual route	Comments
Benzodiazepines				
Diazepam	Valium Diazemuls	10–20 mg	oral, i.m. or i.v.	Potent anxiolytic but has no analgesic action. Good amnesic effect in larger doses. i.v preparation is 'Diazemuls'.
Lorazepam	Ativan	1–3 mg	oral	Similar to diazepam but longer action
Temazepam		10–20 mg	oral	Similar to diazepam but shorter action. A popular drug for premedication
Chlopromazine derivatives				
Promethazine	Phenergan	25–50 mg	i.m.	Used for children only. Can cause marked
Trimeprazine	Vallergan	3 mg per kg	oral	pallor
Opioids				
Morphine		10–15 mg	i.m.	Good euphoric effect. Potent analgesic which may provide useful initial postoperative pain relief. Commonly causes nausea and sometimes vomiting after surgery. May cause respiratory depression in large doses or in combination with other drugs or in sick patients
Papaveretum	Omnopon	10–20 mg	i.m.	Similar to morphine (it is a mixture of alkaloids obtained from the poppy of which 50% is morphine)
Pethidine		50–100 mg	i.m.	Less sedative and shorter action than morphine
Butyrophenones				
Droperidol		5–10 mg	i.m.	Major tranquillizer and potent anti-emetic
Anticholinergic drugs				
Atropine		0.3–0.6 mg	oral or i.m.	Dries mouth by reducing secretion of saliva. Causes marked tachycardia if given i.v. No sedative action
Hyoscine	Scopolamine	0.2–0.4 mg	i.m.	Similar to atropine but also has a potent sedative action

INTRAVENOUS INDUCTION AGENTS

Intravenous drugs, or induction agents, are usually used to start general anaesthesia although a 'gas' induction using any of the inhalational anaesthetic agents is sometimes used, particularly for children. Intravenous induction agents only act for a few minutes and anaesthesia is then continued using inhalational anaesthetics and other intravenous drugs.

Thiopentone was first used in 1934 and is still in widespread use. It is a barbiturate. *Unconsciousness* occurs about 20 seconds after injection and continues for several (5–10) minutes. The termination of its action occurs as the drug is redistributed away from the brain into other tissues, particularly muscle and fat.

It is *metabolized very slowly* (several hours) and thus cannot be used as a continuous intravenous infusion as it would accumulate and lead to prolonged sleepiness or unconsciousness when discontinued (compare propofol).

Loss of muscle tone and therefore of normal airway control occurs immediately after injection as does a short period of *hypoventilation* (respiratory depression) and sometimes *apnoea*. It is therefore important to have facilities for lung ventilation and the delivery of oxygen immediately at hand.

It causes a small *drop in blood pressure* mainly due to a reduction in peripheral resistance; a marked fall in blood pressure may occur if the injection is too rapid, the dose is too large or the patient is sick.

Accidental *intra-arterial injection* results in immediate and severe pain in the arm distal to the site of injection and, if concentrations greater than 2.5% are used, this may be followed by arterial spasm, loss of peripheral pulses and permanent ischaemic damage to parts of the arm. The risk of this occurrence is reduced by injecting the drug into a vein on the dorsum of the hand where arteries are rarely found, although extra-vascular injection can also result in tissue damage.

Methohexitone was first described in 1957. It is also a barbiturate and is similar to thiopen-tone, although it has a slightly shorter duration of action and is metabolized more quickly, but not fast enough to be used as a continuous infusion.

It is commonly *painful on injection* but the pain is along the line of the vein and does not reflect any damage to tissues. *Involuntary muscle movements, twitching* and *hiccups* are a common effect of the drug. Intra-arterial or extra-vascular injection does not lead to tissue damage. It is rarely used except for ECT (electroconvulsive therapy—a treatment for depression).

Etomidate was first used in 1973. It is not a barbiturate. It is metabolized more quickly than either of the barbiturates and recovery is probably faster than from methohexitone. It also causes pain on injection and involuntary muscle movements.

It has *minimal or no effect on blood pressure* and for this reason is sometimes chosen for use in patients with cardiac problems. It is otherwise not commonly used.

Propofol, an increasingly popular agent, was first used in 1977, although it was not released for general use until 1986. It is dissolved in the oil phase of an emulsion of soybean oil and purified egg phosphatide and is white and looks like milk (like Diazemuls).

It is *very rapidly metabolized* (in a few minutes) and can therefore be used as a continuous low dose intravenous infusion to provide prolonged periods of anaesthesia or to sedate patients for hours or days in intensive care wards.

Recovery from its effects is more rapid and complete than from any of the other induction agents; it is therefore commonly used for short procedures and in outpatients.

Like methohexitone and etomidate, it causes pain on injection which can be considerably reduced by mixing it with lignocaine. It possibly causes more hypoventilation, apnoea and hypotension than the other agents (apart from ketamine) particularly if injected rapidly.

Ketamine is unique amongst the induction agents. Some of the differences between ketamine and other induction agents are:

1. It can be given *intramuscularly* as well as intravenously.

2. It has *potent analgesic activity* and produces a state known as dissociative analgesia in which the patient looks dreamily half awake and may move around a little but is, in fact, unaware of his or her surroundings and is free of any pain.

3. *Muscle tone is maintained* and therefore the patient retains the ability to maintain his or her own airways despite being unconscious. It is thus of particular use when adequate access to the head and neck is not possible as occurs in children receiving radiotherapy, some civilian transport disasters and casualties in the field of battle.

4. It causes a *rise in blood pressure* and is therefore popular for use in children with severe congenital heart disease.

5. During recovery *nightmares and hallucinations*, referred to as emergence phenomena, are common, except, apparently, in children. These effects are so unpleasant in adults that the drug is rarely used for adults except in the unusual circumstances mentioned in paragraph 3 above.

Nursing point

After ketamine has been used let the patient wake up peacefully, preferably in a quiet room with subdued lighting, and don't prod and shout at the patient in order to wake him or her up more quickly. This will reduce the incidence and severity of emergence phenomena—nightmares and unpleasant hallucinations.

MAINTENANCE OF ANAESTHESIA

There are three important groups of drugs used to maintain anaesthesia after the effects of the induction agents have worn off:

1. Inhalational anaesthetics
2. Short acting opioids
3. Muscle relaxants.

INHALATIONAL ANAESTHETICS

Nitrous oxide is the original 'gas' or 'laughing gas', so called because it causes some patients to laugh during the induction of anaesthesia if used on its own. It is a faintly smelling gas that is compressed and stored as a liquid in cylinders (coloured blue in the UK). Even in concentrations up to 80% it is only a weak anaesthetic and it needs to be combined with other inhalational agents or intravenous drugs. Unlike the other inhalational anaesthetics, it has a powerful analgesic effect in concentrations less than those required to produce unconsciousness.

Entonox takes advantage of its analgesic properties. It is a 50:50 mixture of nitrous oxide and oxygen, stored as a compressed gas in cylinders (coloured blue and white in the UK). It is used for pain relief in labour, and by ambulance crew and others for pain relief outside hospital.

Halothane, enflurane and isoflurane are potent halogenated hydrocarbons and have very similar structures and effects. Some of the differences between them are listed in Table 11.2. They are volatile liquids that require a carrier gas, usually oxygen and nitrous oxide, to deliver them, and vaporizers capable of delivering accurate concentrations in the range of 0.5–5%. Unlike nitrous oxide, they have no analgesic properties in sub-anaesthetic concentrations. Halothane is the oldest but is now little used as it causes cardiac arrhythmias and, very rarely, severe hepatitis; isoflurane is the most commonly used as it does not cause any cardiac arrhythmias or organ damage, has the least effect on cardiac output and is associated with the most rapid recovery from anaesthesia.

Ether is, of course, an historically important drug, but is no longer used except in a few parts of the developing world where resources and skills are limited. It is cheap, potent, fairly safe and can be used with simple and portable equipment using room air instead of cylinder oxygen. Induction of, and recovery from, anaesthesia are, however, very slow, and it has a pungent and unpleasant smell and is explosive.

SHORT ACTING OPIOIDS

Long acting opioids, such as morphine, are described elsewhere. In patients whose lungs

Table 11.2   Some inhalational anaesthetics

	Halothane	Enflurane	Isoflurane
Trade name	Fluothane	Ethrane	Forane
First use in man	1956	1966	1971
Equipotent concentrations	0.8%	1.6%	1.2%
Boiling point	50°C	56.5°C	48.5°C
Cardiac arrhythmias	+++	+	0
Hypotension	+	+	++
Cost	+	++	+++
Amount of absorbed drug metabolized	20%	2%	0.2%
Potential for organ damage	Very rarely causes severe hepatitis	Causes mild, reversible renal tubular damage in large doses	None

are ventilated by machine during anaesthesia, potent and short acting opioids are commonly used and safe. They have three very useful actions contributing to general anaesthesia:

1. Profound analgesia
2. Sedation and, in large doses, hypnosis
3. Intense respiratory depression (in this situation, a useful effect!).

They have almost no effect on blood pressure and, in large doses, they reduce the need for inhalational anaesthetic agents to a minimum. Of the three commonly available, **fentanyl** is the most popular. The only significant difference between them is the dose required and their duration of action (see Table 11.3).

Table 11.3   Short acting opioids

	Approximate equipotent doses	Approximate duration
Alfentanil	500 micrograms	10 min
Fentanyl	100 micrograms	30 min
Phenoperidine	1 mg	60 min
Morphine	10 mg	4 hours

If necessary, as with the longer acting opioids, their action may be easily reversed at the end of an anaesthetic using **naloxone**. This may be necessary to correct any respiratory depression but, of course, it will also reverse any analgesia and may leave the patient in pain.

MUSCLE RELAXANTS (NEUROMUSCULAR BLOCKING AGENTS)

The introduction of muscle relaxants into anaesthetic practice in the 1940s has been claimed as the greatest single advance in anaesthesia made this century.

Tubocurarine was the first such drug to be used and is an alkaloid extracted from the bark, leaves and vines of the tropical plant, *Chondrodendron tomentosum*, found around the upper reaches of the Amazon. Crude preparations of this plant have long been used by the South American Indians to poison the tips of their arrows. Since the 1940s many new relaxants have been produced and those in current use, and some of the differences between them, are listed in Table 11.4.

Table 11.4 Muscle relaxants

Drug	Type of blocker	Duration of action	Reversal of action	Other points
Alcuronium Gallamine Pancuronium Tubocurarine	Competitive	45–60 minutes	With neostigmine (and atropine or glycopyrrolate)	Renal excretion is significant
Atracurium Vecuronium	Competitive	20–30 minutes	With neostigmine (and atropine or glycopyrrolate)	First choice in renal failure as renal excretion is minimal
Suxamethonium	Depolarizing	2–5 minutes	Cannot be reversed with drugs	1. May cause muscle pains 2. Prolonged action in 1 in 2800 patients

Clinical use

Most anaesthetics involve the use of muscle relaxants for which there are three main indications:

1. To facilitate intubation of the trachea with an endotracheal tube at the start of an anaesthetic.
2. To relax muscles sufficiently to make surgery possible. This applies particularly to abdominal surgery for which relaxed abdominal muscula-

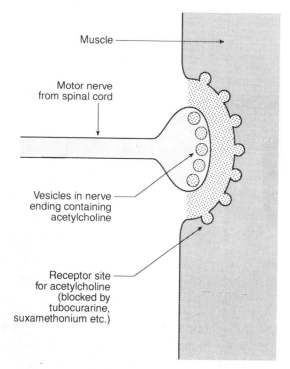

ture is necessary for easy access to, and closure of, the abdomen.
3. To enable easy ventilation of the lungs by machine or hand. There are many situations in anaesthesia when it is better to ventilate lungs mechanically than let patients breathe spontaneously. These include lengthy surgery, chest surgery and severe cardiorespiratory disease.

Mechanism of action

These drugs act at the neuromuscular junction (or motor end plate) by blocking the transmission of nerve impulses from nerve to muscle (see Fig. 11.1). When a nerve supplying a voluntary muscle is stimulated, *acetylcholine* is liberated from vesicles in the nerve ending and acts on special receptor sites on the muscle to produce a change known as depolarization. This is followed by contraction of the muscle fibre. The *acetylcholine* is then rapidly broken down by the enzyme cholinesterase and repolarization occurs. The muscle is now ready to be stimulated again. Should depolarization persist (see Depolarizing muscle relaxants) then the muscle would remain unresponsive to further stimulation.

Competitive muscle relaxants

Two types of block are produced by muscle relaxants. Most are competitive blockers, that is they occupy receptor sites for acetylcholine and so render ineffective the acetylcholine that is released following nerve stimulation.

Muscle

Motor nerve from spinal cord

Vesicles in nerve ending containing acetylcholine

Receptor site for acetylcholine (blocked by tubocurarine, suxamethonium etc.)

Fig. 11.1 The neuromuscular junction.

Atracurium and vecuronium, both released for general use in 1983, have a medium duration of 20–30 minutes, and are now the most commonly used competitive blockers. **Neostigmine** reverses their effects more quickly than the longer acting drugs. Only minimal vecuronium and no atracurium is excreted by the kidney.

Alcuronium, gallamine, pancuronium and tubocurarine have a long duration of action of 45–60 minutes. Their effects may be reversed by the anticholinesterase drug, **neostigmine**. They are predominantly excreted by the kidney.

Depolarizing muscle relaxants

These drugs also occupy receptor sites for acetylcholine. However, they initially stimulate the muscle to contract (visible as the 'twitching' that occurs almost immediately after they are injected) and then produce a state of persistent depolarization during which no further stimulation is possible.

Suxamethonium is the only representative of this group in current use. It has a short duration of action of 2–5 minutes and is mainly used for endotracheal intubation at the beginning of anaesthesia and for very short procedures requiring relaxation.

1 in 2800 of the population will have a prolonged period of paralysis of up to 2 or 3 hours (suxamethonium apnoea) due to a genetically determined and familial abnormality of the enzyme cholinesterase that is normally responsible for the rapid breakdown of this drug.

A common side-effect is muscle pain and tenderness, particularly in the chest and abdomen, often severe, and occurring about 24 hours after it has been given.

Nursing point

'Suxamethonium pains'. Look out for patients, mostly young adults, who complain, about 24 hours after surgery, of pain and tenderness in their muscles, usually of the abdomen and chest. These symptoms may follow the use of suxamethonium and can sometimes be very severe.

ANTICHOLINESTERASES

These drugs have two main uses:

1. Reversal of muscle relaxants
2. Myasthenia gravis.

Reversal of muscle relaxants

The effects of the competitive, non-depolarizing, muscle relaxants may be allowed to wear off spontaneously. However, the effects can be reversed more quickly by using one of the anticholinesterase drugs. (Compare the depolarizing muscle relaxant, suxamethonium, whose effects cannot be reversed with drugs.) Anticholinesterases act at the neuromuscular junction where they temporarily inhibit the enzyme *cholinesterase*, which normally breaks down acetylcholine, and so allow *acetylcholine* to rise in concentration and therefore increase its duration of action. This helps the return of normal neuromuscular transmission and muscle strength.

Neostigmine is the drug of this group most commonly used to reverse muscle relaxants.

Edrophonium is also effective in reversing muscle relaxants, although, possibly, less so than neostigmine when used to reverse the effects of the long acting muscle relaxants.

Myasthenia gravis

This disease is due to progressive destruction of the neuromuscular junction of voluntary muscles by antibodies and is characterized by muscle weakness and fatigue. *Acetylcholine* is no longer as effective as normal as a transmitter at the neuromuscular junction and, so, the symptoms of weakness and fatigue may be completely or partially relieved with anticholinesterases which, by inhibiting the enzyme, *cholinesterase*, increase the amount of *acetylcholine* available.

Pyridostigmine is the longest acting anticholinesterase and probably has the least side-effects. It can only be given orally.

Neostigmine, given orally, acts for up to 4 hours. It can be given intravenously for the emergency management of myasthenia gravis but side-effects are common by this route and it must be given with atropine.

Edrophonium is the shortest acting, can only given intravenously and is mostly used to establish the diagnosis of myasthenia gravis.

Corticosteroids, because of their immunosuppressive action, improve a majority of patients. It is important to start with a low dose which is slowly increased until optimal results are obtained. Occasionally patients get temporarily worse after starting steroids.

Side-effects of anticholinesterases

Unfortunately these drugs also have cholinergic effects at sites other than the neuromuscular junction, namely, at peripheral parasympathetic nerve endings. The most important effects of this are:

1. A bradycardia—this can be very marked and therefore dangerous
2. An increase in salivation and tracheobronchial secretions
3. An increase in peristaltic activity in the gut causing colic and diarrhoea.

Fortunately these effects can be prevented by giving one of the anticholinergic drugs (atropine or glycopyrrolate—see below) at the same time as the anticholinesterase.

ANTICHOLINERGIC DRUGS

These drugs temporarily block the effects of acetylcholine, particularly at postganglionic parasympathetic nerve endings, and have three uses during anaesthesia:

1. To reduce tracheobronchial and salivary secretions. They may be included as part of premedication for this purpose.
2. To increase the pulse rate.
3. To prevent the unwanted effects of the anticholinesterases.

Atropine, glycopyrrolate and hyoscine are the drugs for these purposes. Glycopyrrolate has a longer duration of action than atropine and causes less temporary tachycardia when given with neostigmine. Hyoscine also causes marked sedation and can therefore *only* be used as part of premedication.

MALIGNANT HYPERPYREXIA

Susceptibility to this extremely rare condition is familial and genetically determined. It occurs following exposure to *suxamethonium*, *halothane*, *enflurane* or *isoflurane* but, curiously, almost no other drug. It starts with excessive metabolic activity in muscle cells which leads to muscular rigidity, a high temperature and widespread severe metabolic disturbances. It used to have a high mortality.

Dantrolene, if given promptly and combined with aggressive treatment of the metabolic problems, markedly reduces mortality from this condition. It acts at an intracellular level and reduces the excessive metabolic activity in the muscle cells. Every operating department should stock sufficient of this drug to treat one patient although, of course, it will very rarely be required. It is very expensive.

Miscellaneous relaxants

Patients with various disorders of the musculoskeletal system and of the central nervous system suffer from muscle spasm. This spasm may produce pain and deformity, and, if the spasm could be relieved without altering normal muscle function, the patient could be helped considerably.

There are now several drugs which claim to relax such spasm, probably by damping down reflexes in the spinal cord.

Diazepam acts on the spinal cord and has some antispasmodic effects. Rather large doses, i.e. 10 mg t.d.s. are usually required and sedation can be a problem.

Baclofen is rather similar to diazepam but is

less sedating. The dose is 5–20 mg t.d.s. but this may cause nausea, particularly with the larger doses.

Dantrolene has a direct inhibiting effect on skeletal muscle and reduces spasm in this way. However, muscle power is reduced in parallel with the decrease in spasticity and this limits dosage. The initial dose of 25 mg daily is slowly increased.

LOCAL ANAESTHETICS

Local anaesthesia for surgery was first used in 1884 when **cocaine** was used for ophthalmic surgery by Carl Koller, in Vienna. The use of cocaine for nerve blocks was first described by William S. Halstead in 1885; unfortunately Halstead soon became addicted to cocaine after he had experimented on himself with too many nerve blocks.

Local anaesthetics produce a reversible inhibition of conduction along nerves and, in a sufficient concentration, produce a complete sensory and motor blockade.

However, the fine, unmyelinated, nerve fibres that conduct pain sensation are more easily blocked by local anaesthetics than the thicker, heavily myelinated, motor fibres to muscle, and so, if an appropriate low dose or concentration of local anaesthetic is used, it is possible to provide good analgesia without loss of too much motor function. This is best illustrated by observing the effects of an epidural during labour in which there is good pain relief and yet the patient is still able to move her legs.

There are several ways of giving local anaesthetics:

1. Direct application to mucous membranes
2. Direct application to the skin
3. Intradermal injection
4. Local infiltration of subcutaneous tissues, or deeper to involve muscles, other soft tissues or periosteum
5. Local nerve blocks
6. Extradural injection (an 'extradural', 'epidural' or 'caudal')
7. Subarachnoid injection (a 'spinal')
8. Intravenous injection (a 'Bier's block').

A **Bier's block**, otherwise called intravenous analgesia, is established as follows. The arm is elevated for a few minutes to encourage drainage of as much blood as possible. Further exsanguination may be achieved by applying an Esmarch bandage. A previously applied blood pressure cuff is inflated to above arterial blood pressure. 40 ml of 0.5% prilocaine are then injected into a previously inserted cannula in a vein in the dorsum of the hand. The prilocaine now spreads through all the vessels in the arm below the blood pressure cuff and after a few minutes this will produce complete analgesia of the arm below the cuff. A similar procedure can be undertaken in the leg but requires 100 ml of 0.5% prilocaine.

Nursing point

Do not forget that the patient will be conscious during procedures done under local anaesthesia. Conversation between staff should be at a minimum but the patient should be reassured throughout.

Vasoconstrictors and local anaesthetics

Some local anaesthetics are vasodilators which, by increasing local blood flow, hasten the removal of the drug from the site of action. If **adrenaline** is mixed with the drug, then the vasoconstriction it produces will delay the removal of the drug and so prolong the duration of its action.

Felypressin (Octapressin), is a safer alternative to adrenaline. It is an analogue of vasopressin and is a powerful vasocstrictor but has none of the potentially serious effects that adrenaline has on the heart.

Adrenaline must never be used with local anaesthetics given intravenously, as in a Bier's block, because of its obvious dangerous effects on the heart. Neither should vasoconstrictors be used for blocks around the base of the penis or for 'ring' blocks of the fingers or toes; they may severely interrupt the blood supply and cause permanent ischaemic damage to the penis or digit.

Toxicity of local anaesthetics

All local anaesthetics have dangerous side-effects at doses only a little above those used for the more extensive blocks. Care must therefore be taken to calculate the total dose used when establishing any block. See Table 11.5 for maximum doses.

Nursing point

A 1% solution equals 1 g in 100 ml
or 10 mg in 1 ml

Only by knowing this can the amount of drug given be calculated.

Signs of toxicity start with tinnitus, tremor and restlessness and progress to convulsions and cardiac and respiratory depression.

Lignocaine is the most commonly used local anaesthetic. It has a rapid onset of action and a duration of action of approximately 1–2 hours. It is a mild vasodilator and so has a much longer duration of action if mixed with adrenaline.

It is available in various concentrations and preparations including an aerosol spray for use on mucous membranes, most commonly in the mouth, pharynx or trachea.

Lignocaine also depresses myocardial excitability and so is used to suppress ventricular arrhythmias such as may follow myocardial infarction or cardiac arrest. For this purpose it is given as a bolus injection or as a continuous, low dose, intravenous infusion. (It will, of course, like all local anaesthetics, cause myocardial depression in overdose.)

Prilocaine is similar to lignocaine although it has a slightly longer duration of action, is less potent and less toxic. Because it is less toxic than lignocaine, it is the preferred drug for intravenous analgesia, a 'Biers block'. It is commonly used, with felypressin, for dental blocks. In doses greater than twice the recommended maximum, it causes cyanosis due to the formation of methaemoglobinaemia.

Table 11.5 Summary of important local anaesthetics

Drug	Trade name	Maximum dose plain	with adrenaline	Main uses
Lignocaine	Xylocaine Xylocard Xylotox	200 mg	500 mg	ALL local anaesthetic techniques Cardiac arrhythmias
Bupivicaine	Marcaine	150 mg	150 mg	All infiltration techniques Epidurals, caudals and spinals (NEVER for intravenous analgesia—Bier's blocks)
Prilocaine	Citanest	400 mg	600 mg	Intravenous analygesia (Bier's blocks) Dental blocks (often mixed with felypressin) Constituent (with lignocaine) of EMLA cream
Amethocaine				Surface analgesia in the eye
Benoxinate (oxybuprocaine)				Surface analgesia in the eye
Cocaine		100 mg	—	Surface analgesia for intranasal surgery Surface analgesia in the eye

Bupivicaine has a slower onset of action than lignocaine but about twice the duration of action. It is particularly popular and suitable for continuous epidural analgesia in labour and for postoperative pain relief. It is probably markedly more toxic on the heart than other local anaesthetics and must therefore never be used for intravenous analgesia, a 'Bier's block'.

Amethocaine has a slow onset and a long duration of action. It is a vasodilator. It is, however, very toxic and can therefore never be given by injection. It provides excellent surface analgesia and almost its only use is for conjunctival analgesia in the eye.

Oxybuprocaine is only used as a local anaesthetic in the eye. It causes less initial stinging sensation, and has a shorter duration of action, than amethocaine.

Cocaine, the first of the local anaesthetics, is a very different drug.

It is an alkaloid obtained from the leaves of a tree, *Erythroxylon coca*, found in Bolivia, Brazil, Peru and other South American countries. For centuries it has been chewed by the peoples of these countries to produce euphoria and to increase their capacity for physical work.

It is absorbed well by mucous membranes and is used to provide surface analgesia in eye surgery and nose and throat surgery where its intense local vasoconstrictor action is also a useful feature. It is available as a paste, and as solutions of various concentrations, for these purposes.

It is too toxic for use by injection.

It has widespread sympathomimetic actions causing mydriasis (dilatation of the pupil), marked vasoconstriction, hypertension, tachycardia and ventricular arrhythmias; in overdose, sudden death due to ventricular fibrillation occurs. Headache, nausea, vomiting and abdominal pain are common. It causes excitement, restlessness, euphoria and confusion, and with increasing dosage, central nervous system depression, coma and convulsions.

It is a drug of addiction, which occurs after only a few doses. Not surprisingly, it is a Controlled Drug.

Eutectic mixture of local anaesthetics. Better known as **EMLA cream**, this is a unique preparation. If powders of lignocaine and prilocaine are mixed together, a eutectic mixture is formed, that is, the consistency changes from a powder to a paste. Substances are then added to this paste to make a cream, containing 2.5% lignocaine and 2.5% prilocaine, suitable for application to the skin.

Absorption through the skin is slow but application for at least 45 minutes produces adequate analgesia, and EMLA cream is now used extensively to permit pain free venepuncture, particularly in children.

There are many other local anaesthetics, old and new, amongst which are **procaine**, **mepivicaine** and **benzocaine**, all of which are still available, although they are rarely used. They are sometimes used as constituents of proprietary drug mixtures.

DRUGS USED FOR CARDIO-PULMONARY RESUSCITATION

Useful guidelines to basic life support and advanced life support are given by the Resuscitation Council (UK) in *Resuscitation* (1992) 24: 104.

Basic life support

Once it is established that a patient is unconscious and unresponsive, then basic life support may be needed and consists of three parts:

1. *Airway.* The patients airway should be cleared and kept open.
2. *Breathing*. If the patient is not breathing then the lungs should be ventilated using mouth to mouth, or other, techniques as appropriate.
3. *Circulation*. If there is no pulse then cardiac massage should be started.

ADVANCED CARDIAC LIFE SUPPORT

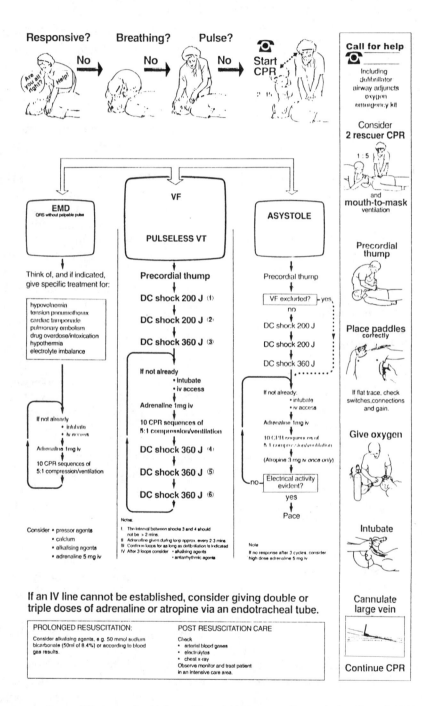

Fig. 11.2 Summary of advanced life support guidelines. (Copyright European Resuscitation Council 1992; reproduced with permission.)

Advanced life support

If the appropriate drugs, equipment and skills are available, as they are in any hospital, then advanced life support is now started. Initially three things are done:

1. *Oxygen*, instead of the resuscitator's expired gas, is used to ventilate the lungs and, often, *tracheal intubation* is undertaken to facilitate efficient lung ventilation.
2. An *intravenous infusion* is established, preferably into a central vein, i.e. a large vein in the neck or groin, from where drugs will reach the heart quickly in an arrested circulation.
3. An *EGG machine is connected* so that the exact rhythm disturbance and the effects of treatment can be seen.

Treatment is now aimed at reversing the life-threatening arrhythmia using drugs and defibrillation as indicated in the algorithm in Figure 11.2.

Adrenaline is used to convert asystole to ventricular fibrillation, which may then be converted to sinus rhythm by defibrillation. Adrenaline does not, of course, convert VF to sinus rhythm. Adrenaline is also important because it raises peripheral resistance and, therefore, blood pressure and so improves coronary and cerebral circulation. It also increases myocardial contractility. It should be given every 5 minutes during resuscitation in a dose of 1 mg (1 ml of 1 in 1000 or 10 ml of l in 10 000).

Large doses of adrenaline cause dilatation of the pupils and this effect may be misinterpreted as evidence of persistent and severe brain damage during and shortly after resuscitation.

Nursing point

1 mg of adrenaline = 1 ml of 'l in 1000'
or 10 ml of '1 in 10 000'

This information is important during cardio-pulmonary resuscitation. (It is unfortunate that the concentration of adrenaline is still given in such a curious manner —1 in 1000 means 1 g in 1000 ml. The concentration of NO other drug is indicated in this way.)

Atropine is given to increase cardiac rate. Bradycardia is common during recovery from cardiac arrest. Atropine, like adrenaline, causes dilatation of the pupils.

Lignocaine reduces the excitability of myocardial cell membrane and so reduces the incidence of abnormal rhythms that appear during resuscitation. It also reduces the incidence of reversion of sinus rhythm back to VF that sometimes occurs after successful defibrillation. Dosage must, however, be limited as it is also a potent myocardial depressant.

Bretylium is occasionally used and is recommended for the treatment of VF resistant to lignocaine and defibrillation. Its effect is slow and resuscitation may need to be continued for 30 minutes before it is effective. It is an anti-arrhythmic drug.

Calcium chloride, once popular, is no longer recommended for routine use during resuscitation except when there is a specific indication, e.g. hypocalcaemia, hyperkalaemia or calcium antagonist toxicity. Nevertheless, it is still sometimes used, and is effective, during electromechanical dissociation in an otherwise normal heart.

Sodium bicarbonate is used to correct the metabolic acidosis that occurs following prolonged inadequate tissue perfusion. Over enthusiastic use can cause serious hypernatraemia and, paradoxically, intracellular acidosis. It should therefore be withheld for the first 30 minutes of resuscitation and then be given in small amounts (e.g. 50 mmol) or in response to the measurement of blood acid–base status.

Route of administration of drugs during CPR

The ideal route for the administration of drugs is via a *central vein*, i.e. a vein in the neck or the groin, from where drugs can easily reach the coronary circulation where they are required. If a *peripheral vein* is used then the drug should be flushed generously through the vein with saline or 5% glucose since the peripheral circulation will be very sluggish.

Lignocaine and atropine are also absorbed fairly reliably through the *lungs*, if given in twice the normal dose down the endotracheal tube. This route may thus be worthwhile using if intravenous access has not been established. However, it is doubtful if sufficient adrenaline can be absorbed via this route.

Intra-osseous administration is effective and is gaining popularity in children. Finally, the use of the long *intracardiac needle* to administer drugs is dangerous and should rarely, if ever, be used: there is a danger of intramyocardial injection, intrapericardial haemorrhage and pneumo-thorax.

FURTHER READING

Adams A P, Cashman J N 1991 Anaesthesia, analgesia and intensive care. Edward Arnold, London

Nieman J T 1992 Cardiopulmonary Resuscitation. New England Journal of Medicine 327: 1075

12

Respiratory stimulants, antiepileptics, and drugs used in Parkinson's disease

RESPIRATORY STIMULANTS

Respiratory failure may occur in patients who have chronic bronchitis with emphysema. In this condition the amount of air reaching the alveoli may be insufficient and the uptake of oxygen and excretion of carbon dioxide may be impaired. Respiratory failure is diagnosed when there is not enough oxygen and/or too much carbon dioxide in the blood.

Hypoxaemia can be relieved by giving oxygen which returns the blood oxygen concentration towards normal. In certain patients, however, this leads to a decrease in respiration and alveolar ventilation so that carbon dioxide is inadequately excreted and accumulates in the body causing the patient to become disorientated and finally, comatose. To some extent this situation can be avoided by giving low concentrations of oxygen (24–28%) and thus maintaining adequate alveolar ventilation.

Respiratory stimulants have a limited role in these circumstances. Given intravenously they can increase respiration and alveolar ventilation for a short time and allow more oxygen to be absorbed without carbon dioxide retention.

Doxapram is the most effective drug and is given by intravenous infusion at a rate of 1.4–4 mg/minute, the dose being adjusted depending on response. This treatment requires careful monitoring and every effort should be made to get rid of retained secretions in the respiratory tract by physiotherapy. In overdose, doxapram can cause convulsions.

Methylxanthines

These drugs are weak respiratory stimulants but are not used for this purpose. They inhibit the enzyme phosphodiesterase and are powerful relaxants of smooth muscle.

Aminophylline and theophylline. Aminophylline is theophylline plus ethylene diamine. Both drugs have identical actions, the most important being to relax the smooth muscle of the bronchial tree; therefore they are used to relieve bronchospasm in asthma and sometimes in bronchitis or acute pulmonary oedema. Although they are effective, these drugs require careful use as there is only a small difference between a therapeutic and a toxic dose. In addition, their elimination rate depends on a number of factors including weight, sex, age, concurrent disease and other medication (Fig. 12.1).

Therapeutics. Aminophylline is given intravenously as a single dose of 250 mg to terminate an acute attack of asthma. The injection should be given over 10 minutes. It can also be given as a loading dose of 5 mg/kg intravenously, followed by an infusion of 500 micrograms/kg/hour preferably by an infusion pump or a micropipette. If the infusion is prolonged, plasma levels (therapeutic range 10–20 mg/l) should be measured after 24 hours to control further dosage rate. The high plasma levels achieved by the combination of oral and intravenous administration can be dangerous. *Therefore before giving intravenous aminophylline it is important to enquire whether the patient is already taking methylxanthines by mouth.* Aminophylline and theophylline can both be given orally but are liable to provoke nausea and vomiting. However, several slow release preparations are available which only need to be given twice daily and because peaks in the plasma levels are avoided, they are less likely to cause side-effects. They may be useful at night to *prevent* nocturnal attacks or morning dipping in asthmatics. Because of interindividual variation, fixed dose regimes are not very satisfactory and it is better to control oral dosage by measuring blood levels for optimal results. In practice, however, this is rarely possible. *These preparations must be swallowed whole to avoid interfering with the slow delivery system.* Available preparations include:

Phyllocontin: Aminophylline 100 mg or 225 mg/tablet
Theo-Dur: Theophylline 200 mg tablet
Slo-Phyllin: Theophylline 60 mg, 125 mg or 250 mg/capsule.

Slo-phyllin contains granules in the capsule and these can be sprinkled on food for easier administration to children and this does not interfere with the slow release delivery system.

Interactions. Effects are increased by cimetidine, erythromycin and oral contraceptives.

Adverse effects are dose related and consist of anxiety, tachycardia with arrhythmias and convulsions.

Caffeine is very similar to aminophylline being a mild central stimulant. It is not used therapeutically (see p. 278).

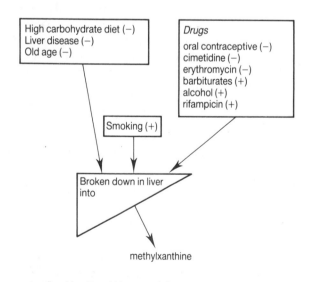

+ = (low blood levels) increased clearance,
− = (high blood levels) decreased clearance

Fig. 12.1 Factors altering the blood level and activity of methylxanthines.

ANTIEPILEPTICS

Antiepileptic drugs are used in the treatment of epilepsy. There are several varieties of epilepsy and they vary in their response to drugs. In focal epilepsy the attack arises from a focal electrical discharge in the brain. This may produce a brief *aura* which is a feeling or movement. If the discharge becomes generalized the patient falls unconscious and passes through the typical tonic and clonic phases, regaining consciousness after a varying interval. This is known as a *tonic–clonic (grand mal) seizure*. Sometimes the spread of the discharge is limited (*partial seizure*) producing psychological disturbances (*psychomotor seizure*) or various involuntary movements. Alternatively, the electrical discharge is widespread from the start, and causes *absence (petit mal) seizure* which is a brief interference with consciousness. These attack are common in childhood. The object in treating epilepsy is to completely abolish the attacks by means of drugs. Although there are now a number of drugs which are useful in controlling epilepsy, it is usually best to start treatment with one drug and only use multiple drug regimes in resistant cases. Treatment should be continued until the patient has had no attacks for at least 3 and preferably 5 years, when the dose can be slowly cut down and finally all treatment stopped.

Epileptic patients should be warned against driving vehicles, swimming, and working under conditions where a fit could produce disaster. The most useful drugs employed in the treatment of epilepsy are:

DRUGS USED IN TONIC–CLONIC AND PARTIAL SEIZURES

Phenytoin. Phenytoin sodium is well absorbed by mouth and does not produce drowsiness or sleep. It probably acts by preventing the abnormal discharge from spreading in the brain.

Therapeutics. Its effectiveness as an anticonvulsant and the incidence of side-effects depend on the blood level of the drug which should be 10–20 mg/litre. Finding the correct dose may be difficult for several reasons:

1. Patients vary considerably in the rate at which they break down phenytoin so there is a wide variation of dose requirements between patients.
2. The relationship between dose and blood level is not linear: this means that a small increase in the dose may cause a considerable rise in the blood level (Fig. 12.2).
3. Because phenytoin is slowly broken down, once daily dosage is adequate. It takes about a week for the blood level to become steady, this means that the dose should not be altered at less than fortnightly intervals.

The initial dose is usually 150 mg once daily and increased by 50 mg fortnightly until the correct dose is found as judged by the control of fits, the absence of toxicity and the blood level.

Adverse effects. These are rather common with phenytoin and include:

1. If dosage is too high the patient is sedated, ataxic and may show nystagmus.
2. Greasy skin and hirsutism may cause problems in women.
3. Macrocytic anaemia due to folic acid deficiency.
4. Gum hypertrophy—dental care is important.
5. Lymph node enlargement.
6. A variety of rashes.

Interactions. These are common and indicate the need for regular measurement of plasma levels of phenytoin.

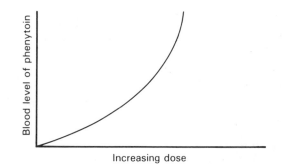

Fig. 12.2 Relationship between dosage and blood level of phenytoin.

Phenytoin levels are altered by chlorpromazine, carbamazepine, diazepam, ethanol, isoniazid and sodium valproate.

Phenytoin alters the levels of hydrocortisone, oral contraceptives, theophylline, tricyclic antidepressants and thyroxine among others.

Carbamazepine. This drug has been used for many years in the treatment of trigeminal neuralgia (see p. 152). It is also useful in controlling tonic–clonic epilepsy and is rather similar in its action to phenytoin. Carbamazepine is given orally and is rather slowly absorbed from the intestine. It is interesting that its rate of breakdown in the body increases with prolonged use. The usual initial dose is 100 mg twice daily and this is increased until the fits are controlled.

Children may break down the drug rapidly so they may require three or four doses daily.

Adverse effects include dizziness and drowsiness, depression of the white cells of the blood and occasionally jaundice and rashes and excessive salivary secretion.

Phenobarbitone is one of the barbiturate group of drugs. It is slowly absorbed, the major portion is broken down in the body and the rest slowly excreted by the kidneys. Its action is therefore prolonged over about 12 hours.

Therapeutics. Phenobarbitone is particularly effective in the treatment of tonic–clonic seizures but may also be used in other types of epilepsy. The usual dosage is 60 mg twice daily, but requirements vary.

Adverse effects are not uncommon. Drowsiness and ataxia may be troublesome and occasionally a rash resembling measles is seen. Phenobarbitone is a powerful inducer of enzymes in the liver, particularly those which break down other drugs. For example, phenobarbitone increases the rate of breakdown of anticoagulants and steroid hormones whose effects are therefore reduced.

Primidone is in many ways similar to phenobarbitone and is effective against both grand and petit mal attacks. It is important to start treatment with low dosage and gradually increase the dose,

otherwise *adverse effects* such as drowsiness, vertigo and vomiting may occur.

The usual dosage scheme for an adult is to commence treatment with 125 mg daily for a few days and then gradually increase to between 750 mg and 1 g daily.

Sodium valproate. This drug increases the amount of GABA in the brain. GABA is a naturally occurring inhibitory substance and sodium valproate is effective in both tonic–clonic and absence seizures. The initial dose is 400 mg daily and may be increased.

Children usually require 20–30 mg/kg/day.

Adverse effects. Sodium valproate quite commonly causes a modest fall in the platelet count. Occasionally this is severe and the patient should be warned to report any bruising or bleeding. It is advisable to do a platelet count before major surgery. Very rarely it causes serious liver damage particularly in those with pre-existing liver disease or in mentally retarded children. Drowsiness, thinning of the hair and weight gain are not uncommon.

Vigabatrin inhibits the breakdown in the brain of GABA which accumulates and suppresses fits. It is particularly effective in partial seizures and is also used in tonic–clonic seizures. It is taken orally and, although fairly rapidly excreted, its action lasts for 24 hours so once daily dosage is possible.

Therapeutic use. Vigabatrin is used when the older antiepileptic drugs have proved unsuccessful. The initial dose is 2 g daily.

Adverse effects. Sedation may occur and occasionally, gastric upsets and headaches. Behavioural problems such as irritation, aggression, hallucination and memory faults occur in about 15% of patients.

Lamotrigine inhibits the release in the brain of the exciting substance glutamate and thus prevents fits. It is effective in partial and tonic–clonic fits and should be used when other drugs have failed.

Therapeutic use. The initial dose for an adult is

50 mg twice daily. Higher doses may be required if it is combined with phenytoin or carbamazepine and lower doses with sodium valproate.

Adverse effects. Ataxia, headaches, nausea and rashes.

Clonazepam is related to the benzodiazepine drugs and may act by enhancing the inhibiting effect of GABA (see above). It is effective in all forms of epilepsy and the initial dose is 1 mg daily which may be increased. It is also useful in treating status epilepticus (see below).

Outcome of treatment

About 80% of patients with grand mal epilepsy are controlled by a single drug. When the patient has been free of fits for 5 years, the treatment can be slowly withdrawn. Many subjects will have no further fits but about 40% (rather less in children) will relapse.

It is important that anticonvulsants are not discontinued too suddenly as this may precipitate fits.

DRUGS USED IN ABSENCE SEIZURES

Ethosuximide is the drug of choice. It may aggravate tonic–clonic seizures and may, if necessary, be combined with a drug which controls this type of attack. *Adverse effects* include sleepiness, gastric upsets and headaches.

Dose: Ethosuximide 0.5–2.0 g daily.
Children—30–50 mg/kg once daily.
Sodium valproate (see above) is also effective.

DRUG COMBINATIONS

In most patients with epilepsy, complete control can be obtained with a single drug. This is desirable as it minimizes adverse affects and there is no problem with interactions between the drugs. Sometimes, however, a combination of drugs is required to achieve better control.

STATUS EPILEPTICUS

In status epilepticus the patient has a series of fits,

rapidly following each other. These patients require careful nursing so that they do not injure themselves. They should be nursed in the lateral semi-prone position, false teeth removed and the airway established; oxygen should be given by mask. *The patient should not be left unattended until the fits have ceased.* The most effective drugs are *diazepam* (as *Diazemuls*) in a dose of 10 mg intravenously or *clonazepam* 1 mg slowly intravenously. In young children rectal diazepam using rectal tubes (*Stesolid*) in a dose of 5 mg for those aged 1–3 years and 10 mg for older children, is rapidly effective and useful particularly if intravenous injection is difficult. Diazepam should be effective within 10 minutes and if the fits persist the dose may be repeated. Although diapezam will usually stop the fits, relapse quite commonly occurs within the next hour. To prevent this *phenytoin* 15 mg/kg is injected intravenously, no faster than 50 mg/minute. Phenytoin has some action on the heart so should not be given via a central line and should be monitored by ECG and blood pressure measurements. If the fits persist *chlormethiazole* should be given intravenously and the dose adjusted to produce a satisfactory therapeutic effect. Finally, if all else fails, *thiopentone* (see p. 133) can be given by intravenous injection. When this drug is used *it is essential to have an anaesthetist* to help as intubation may be necessary and the procedure is not without risk.

Nursing point

The use of chlormethiazole and thiopentone requires considerable expertise and should, if possible, be carried out in an intensive care unit with expert guidance.

FEBRILE CONVULSIONS

About 3% of infants and young children have a fit when feverish. Of these some 3% will ultimately develop true epilepsy.

The *immediate treatment* is to lie the child semi-prone and most convulsions stop within a few minutes. If the fit persists, rectal diazepam as for status epilepticus (above) is the safest and easiest treatment. Hospital admission may be necessary to exclude serious infection.

Prevention. The parents should be taught to reduce fever. If attacks recur with fever the alternatives are:

1. To give rectal diazepam when the child develops a fever.
2. To give continuous medication. Phenobarbitone in doses of 5 mg/kg/day is effective in most children but side-effects may limit its use.

Finally, parents will require reassurance as the majority of convulsions of this type are short-lived and cause no long-term problems.

ANTIEPILEPTICS AND PREGNANCY

There is evidence that antiepileptics given during pregnancy are associated with an increased incidence of fetal malformation. This certainly seems to be the case with phenytoin and sodium valproate. Carbamazepine appears to be the safest agent. If possible a single antiepileptic should be used and the dosage controlled by repeated measurement of blood levels.

Antiepileptics are some of the few drugs which should be prescribed by trade name so that the patient always has exactly the same preparation. This is because the same drug from different manufacturers is not always equivalent.

DRUGS USED IN PARKINSON'S DISEASE

Parkinson's disease is characterized by rigidity of muscle, by tremor and by slowness of movement. It is due to changes in nerve cells in the basal nuclei of the brain.

The essential feature of these changes appears to be a considerable decrease in the concentration of *dopamine* in the basal ganglia and thus the balance between *acetylcholine* and *dopamine* in this region of the brain is upset (Fig. 12.3). It can be seen, therefore, that relief of symptoms can be

achieved by reducing cholinergic activity or by increasing the amount of dopamine.

> **Nursing point**
>
> The nurse should remember that the symptoms of Parkinson's disease can be caused by treatment with neuroleptic drugs. In the majority of patients these symptoms will disappear when the drug is stopped.

DRUGS WHICH DECREASE CHOLINERGIC ACTIVITY

Originally drugs of the belladonna group were used for this purpose but they have now been replaced by synthetic substitutes.

Benzhexol is used in the treatment of Parkinson's disease. It has some effect on both rigidity and tremor.

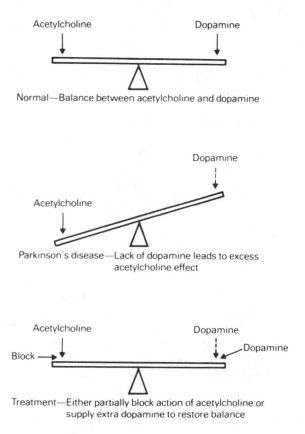

Fig. 12.3 The use of drugs in Parkinson's disease.

It is given orally in doses of 2 mg daily and this is gradually increased until a satisfactory response is obtained or the limit of tolerance is reached.

Orphenadrine has the advantage of having a general stimulating effect as well as relieving the symptoms of Parkinsonism. This is useful as these patients are often depressed. The dose lies between 50–300 mg daily.

Benztropine is in many ways similar to atropine. It is particularly useful in the excessive salivation often found in Parkinsonism and in muscular rigidity.

It is liable to cause drowsiness and is best given as a single dose of 1–4 mg at bedtime.

Adverse effects of these drugs include nausea, constipation, giddiness, dry mouth, urinary retention and glaucoma; in overdose, confusion and hallucinations may also occur.

DRUGS WHICH INCREASE DOPAMINE (Fig. 12.4)

Levodopa. It is not possible to restore the deficiency in the brain by giving dopamine, as this substance will not enter the brain. Therefore levodopa is used. This is a precursor of dopamine which passes freely into the brain where it is converted to dopamine. It is particularly useful in reducing rigidity but has less effect on tremor.

Levodopa and a decarboxylase inhibitor. Levodopa is broken down by an enzyme called *dopa decarboxylase* which is found particularly in the gut wall and liver. If this enzyme is inhibited by a drug which can be administered in combination with levodopa, the effects of levodopa are enhanced and prolonged and a much smaller dose of levodopa is required. This reduces the incidence of some side-effects. Two preparations which are widely used are:

- Levodopa + carbidopa (Sinemet co-careldopa)
- Levodopa + benserazide (Madopar co-beneldopa).

Therapeutics. Adverse effects are very troublesome when levodopa is used alone so treatment is usually started with a small dose—either half a tablet of Sinemet Plus (levodopa 50 mg) or Madopar 125 (levodopa 50 mg) three times daily after food. This is gradually increased until a satisfactory control of symptoms is obtained, usually 3–6 Sinemet Plus tablets (levodopa 300–600 mg) daily.

Adverse effects. Nausea and vomiting are very common but can be minimized by giving the drug in divided doses with meals and using an anti-emetic such as cyclizine, if necessary.

Some postural fall in blood pressure is common but rarely causes symptoms. Blood pressure should be measured before and during treatment.

A few patients become restless, and at higher dose levels involuntary movements, usually affecting the face, may occur.

Constipation will require a good fluid and fibre intake.

Interactions. Levodopa/decarboxylase inhibitor combinations should not be combined with monoamine oxidase inhibitors. Concomitant use of halothane, cyclopropane or trichlorethylene carries an increased risk of cardiac arrhythmias and the drug should be stopped 8 hours before an operation.

Selegiline inhibits the breakdown of levodopa in the brain. It is often used in combination with levodopa with or without a decarboxylase inhibitor and this allows a smaller dose of levodopa to be used. The usual dose is 10 mg each morning.

Amantadine increases the concentration of dopamine in the basal ganglia and thus relieves the symptoms of Parkinson's disease. It is not so effective as levodopa but can be used when that drug is contraindicated. The initial dose is 100 mg daily which may be increased after 1 week to 200 mg daily.

Dopamine receptor agonists

Bromocriptine has a dopamine-like action and is used if patients become resistant to other drugs. The initial dose is 1.0 mg daily and increased as necessary.

Lysuride and Pergolide have similar actions.

Adverse effects. A few patients develop postural hypotension but the most common problem is nausea which can be controlled by domperidone (see p. 89).

THE TREATMENT OF PARKINSON'S DISEASE

As can be seen from the above there are a number of drugs which are useful in relieving the symptoms of this disease. There is no unanimous opinion as to the order in which these drugs should be given. In mild cases a start may be made with an anticholinergic drug such as benzhexol. If this is ineffective or tolerance develops it can be changed to amantadine or levodopa. Some experts believe that selegiline slows the progression of Parkinson's disease and that it should be included in any regime from the start of treatment. In those with more severe disability it is usual to start with levodopa and a decarboxylase inhibitor.

About three-quarters of patients with Parkinson's disease respond to drugs. Rigidity is usually most amenable to treatment and tremor less so.

Unfortunately, in more than half the patients being treated by levodopa the effectiveness of the drug decreases after about 5 years. These patients may develop the 'on-off' phenomenon. In this state the therapeutic effect of the drug wears off very quickly and thus more and more frequent dosage is required. At this stage the addition of selegiline to the regime may be useful. Finally, if levodopa becomes ineffective or intolerable because of side-effects, bromocriptine or one of the new dopamine receptor agonists may be used.

TRIGEMINAL NEURALGIA

This is an unpleasant disorder of unknown aetiology which produces attacks of severe pain in the face (i.e. in the distribution of the trigeminal nerve).

Treatment has been considerably improved by the use of **carbamazepine**. The initial dose is 100 mg two times daily and is subsequently modified according to the response of the patient. About 70% of patients are relieved. If drug treatment fails, it may be necessary to destroy the trigeminal nerve ganglion by injection or surgical section. This has the disadvantage of leaving the side of the face numb.

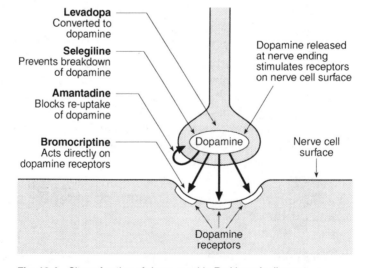

Fig. 12.4 Sites of action of drugs used in Parkinson's disease.

FURTHER READING

Brodie M J 1990 Established anticonvulsants and the treatment of refractory epilepsy. Lancet 336: 350

Chadwick D 1988 Management of adult epilepsy. Prescribers Journal 28: 130

Editorial 1984 Parkinson's disease. Lancet i: 829

Editorial 1989 Withdrawing anti-epileptic drugs. Drug and Therapeutics Bulletin 27: 29

Editorial 1991 Dopamine agonists for Parkinson's disease. Drug and Therapeutics Bulletin 29: 7

Mawer G 1987 Drugs for epilepsy. Update 35: 274

O'Brien M D 1990 Management of major status epilepticus in the adult. British Medical Journal 301: 918

Remy C, Beaumont D 1989 Efficacy and safety of vigabatrin in the long-term treatment of epilepsy. British Journal of Clinical Pharmacology 27: 1255

Rylance G 1986 Practical problems in using anticonvulsants in children. Prescribers Journal 26: 9

13

The endocrine system

The endocrine or ductless glands are small islands of tissue in various parts of the body (Fig. 13.1). Each gland secretes a substance, and in some cases, several substances called *hormones*. These are released into the blood stream and circulate through the body. Their speed of action is variable; the effects of some hormones are seen immediately after release, whereas others may take hours or even days to show their effect. After release, these hormones act upon a receptor mechanism in the organ or organs which they influence, thus producing their specific actions. The actions of the various hormones differ widely, one group being concerned with metabolic processes, another with secondary sexual characteristics and so on. Sometimes a hormone will act on another endocrine gland and stimulate it to produce a further hormone. This two stage, or even three stage series of events is particularly likely to involve the anterior lobe of the pituitary gland (see below).

Most of these hormones have been isolated and their structure determined. This has made it possible to prepare synthetically either the hormones or analogues which are sometimes more active than the hormones themselves.

The endocrine glands can be divided roughly into three groups:

1. The pituitary, which secretes hormones that exercise a controlling influence over the rest of the endocrine system
2. Those affecting metabolism
3. Those affecting the reproductive system.

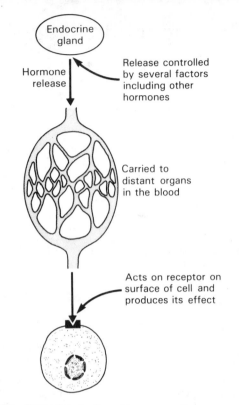

Hormone release

Endocrine gland

Release controlled by several factors including other hormones

Carried to distant organs in the blood

Acts on receptor on surface of cell and produces its effect

Fig. 13.1 Endocrine glands and hormone action.

SECTION I: THE PITUITARY

The pituitary is a small endocrine gland attached to the brain by a stalk and lying, almost surrounded by bone, in the base of the skull. It consists of anterior and posterior lobes (Fig. 13.2). In spite of its small size, it is of great importance. It secretes a number of hormones which not only affect various processes in the body, but also the activity of nearly all the other endocrine glands. It is of interest that the activity of the pituitary itself may be influenced by other hormones, so that a balance is maintained between the pituitary and other endocrine glands.

The release of pituitary hormones is a complex function and it appears that for many of them there is a specific *releasing hormone* which is probably produced in the brain. Thus thyrotrophic hormone is released into the circulation after the pituitary has been stimulated by thyrotrophic releasing hormones. Releasing hormones are only just becoming available on a commercial scale for general use.

POSTERIOR LOBE

Two hormones can be extracted from the posterior lobe of the pituitary.

Oxytocin. This hormone causes contraction of the uterus and is considered on page 183.

Vasopressin, Argipressin (synthetic vasopressin). Vasopressin has two actions. In large doses it causes vasoconstriction with a concomitant rise in blood pressure, but its more important effect from the therapeutic aspect is concerned with water balance as it is the *antidiuretic hormone.*

If the intake of water is limited, the blood becomes slightly more concentrated. This affects special receptors in the base of the brain, which in turn stimulate the posterior pituitary to secret more vasopressin. The vasopressin increases the reabsorption of water by the renal tubules and thus decreases the amount of urine and conserves the body water. If the intake of water is increased the production of vasopressin drops and the output of urine by the kidneys is increased; thus balancing the intake and output of water by the body.

Therapeutics. Occasionally damage to the posterior pituitary or closely related structures produces a disease called *diabetes insipidus*, in which little or no vasopressin is produced. There is thus a continuous high output of urine which in turn requires the drinking of vast quantities of water if dehydration is to be avoided.

The condition can be controlled by the administration of vasopressin which is given as an injection of 5–20 units two or three times daily. It was previously used as a snuff but has now been replaced by desmopressin (see below).

Desmopressin is a synthetic drug allied to vasopressin. It can be given nasally (5–10 micrograms) or intramuscularly (1–4 micrograms). It has a very long action so that one or two doses

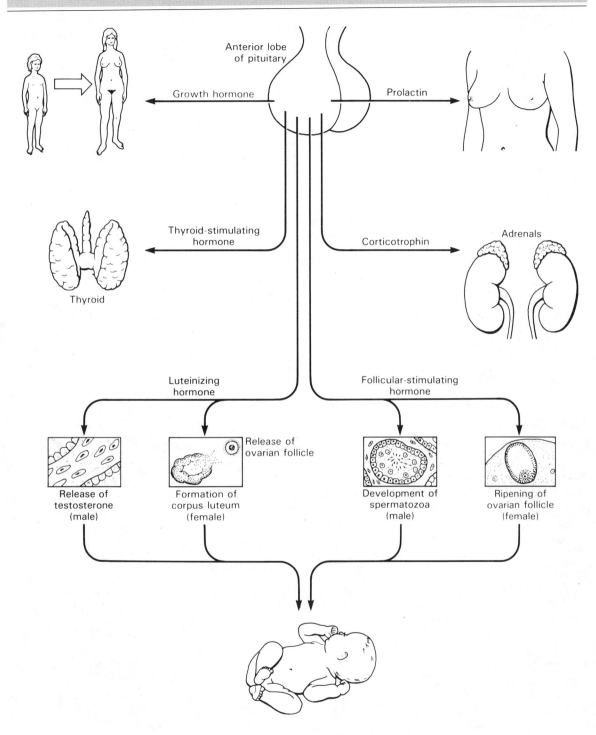

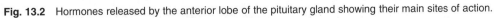

Fig. 13.2 Hormones released by the anterior lobe of the pituitary gland showing their main sites of action.

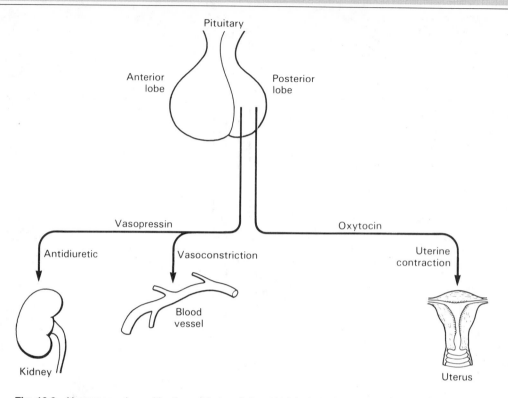

Fig. 13.3 Hormones released by the posterior pituitary and their sites.

daily suffice to control diabetes insipidus and it is now the preferred preparation. Unlike vasopressin it does not cause vasoconstriction. Treatment should aim at reducing the patient's output to about 2 litres a day.

The vasoconstrictive properties of vasopressin are used in the treatment of bleeding from oesophageal varices. The vasoconstriction lowers pressure in the portal vein and allows the bleeding vein to clot. 20 units are given very slowly intravenously (over 10 minutes); the patient may complain of abdominal colic.

Lypressin is similar to the above and is given by nasal spray.

The preparations available are:

Vasopressin—Argipressin (synthetic vasopressin)
Dose: Diabetes   — 5–20 units several times
   insipidus   daily by i.m. injection,
                     (20 units/ml).
   Bleeding varices — 5–20 units by infusion.

Desmopressin: Injection—4 micrograms/ml
               Dose 1–4 micrograms daily
               Intranasal solution—
               100 micrograms/ml. Dose
               10–20 micrograms once or
               twice daily.

ANTERIOR LOBE

Several hormones are produced by the anterior lobe of the pituitary. They may be divided into:

1. Those which stimulate the release of other hormones.
2. Those which inhibit hormone release.
3. Those which act directly on their target organs. These include luteinizing hormone and follicular stimulating hormone (see p. 177).

Those releasing other hormones

Corticotrophin (adrenocorticotrophic hormone, ACTH). Corticotrophin is a protein and is destroyed in the stomach if given orally; it must therefore be given by injection. Its action is to stimulate the production of cortisol (hydrocortisone) and certain other steroid hormones by the adrenal cortex. It is largely used to produce a cortisone-like effect, and those effects and their therapeutic application will be considered in the section on cortisone.

The rate of release of corticotrophin is partially controlled by the circulating level of cortisol and other similar hormones from the adrenal gland. High levels of cortisol suppress corticotrophin production and vice versa. There is thus a self-regulating mechanism between the pituitary and the adrenal gland. If large amounts of cortisol or similar hormones are given to a patient the production of corticotrophin is decreased and the adrenal glands atrophy.

It is therefore important not to stop steroid treatment suddenly but to tail it off, so that corticotrophin production may start up again and thus stimulate a return of normal adrenal hormone production.

Methods of administration. Corticotrophin is rapidly inactivated in the body. It may be given by intramuscular injection four times daily; the total daily dose varies considerably, but usually lies between 10–100 units. A more prolonged effect may be obtained by giving the drug dissolved in gelatin or as a corticotrophin–zinc complex.

The preparations available are: Corticotrophin gelatin injection (BP). Strength 20 or 40 units/ml. Corticotrophin carmellose injection (BP). Strength 60 units/ml.

Tetracosactrin. This synthetic analogue of corticotrophin is much less likely to cause allergic reactions than corticotrophin which it has now replaced. It is available as a rapidly acting preparation for intramuscular or intravenous use, or as a depot preparation which is given intramuscularly on alternate days or twice weekly for long-term maintenance treatment.

The rapidly acting preparation is used to test adrenal function. A dose of 250 micrograms is injected intramuscularly. Blood levels of cortisol are measured before and 30 minutes after injec-tion. If the adrenals are working properly the injection is followed by a release of cortisol and a rise in the blood level.

The slow release preparation *(Synacthen Gel)* is used as an alternative to corticotrophin in the long-term treatment of rheumatoid arthritis and asthma. However, the response to both these drugs is variable and they are now used mainly for diagnostic testing.

Gonadotrophins. The pituitary secretes two hormones which affect the gonads. They are concerned with reproduction and are considered on page 177.

Thyroid stimulating hormone thyrotrophic hormone (TSH). The stimulation of the thyroid gland by this hormone indirectly increases the metabolism of the body.

If the thyroid function is depressed by drugs or other means the pituitary secretes large amounts of TSH.

It is used in various tests of thyroid function, the dose being 2.5–10 units intramuscularly daily.

Those which act directly on target organs

Somatotrophin (growth hormone). This hormone stimulates growth both in soft tissue and in bone. Its release from the pituitary is complicated as there are at least two substances from the brain which control its secretion. Unfortunately, most animal somatotrophin is ineffective in man so human growth hormone must be used. This has now been synthesized by using biological technology and the product is called **somatotropin**. In patients with dwarfism due to hormone deficiency, treatment must be started before epiphyseal fusion has occurred and continued until growth is complete. Somatotropin is given subcutaneously in doses of 0.5–0.7 units/kg/week. It is expensive.

Overproduction of somatotrophin by the pituitary gland will produce *gigantism* in children and *acromegaly* in adults.

Somatostatin is a naturally occuring hormone which inhibits the release of somatotrophin from the pituitary, a synthetic analogue **octreotide** is being used increasingly in various conditions.

Therapeutics. By suppressing the release of somatotrophin in acromegaly octreotide can control the symptoms when surgery is impossible or incomplete. The main problem in its use is the need for dosage several times daily by injection and it is expensive. Octreotide suppresses the release of several hormones in the stomach and intestine and reduces the blood flow to the gut. As a result of these actions it can be given to control certain types of diarrhoea including that due to AIDS and it is also used to reduce the bleeding from oesophageal varices. It seems likely that further therapeutic uses will be found in the future.

Adverse effects. Gastritis and gallstone formation.

Lactogenic hormone. Prolactin, the lactogenic hormone, produces its maximum effect on the breast which has already been prepared throughout pregnancy by oestrogens and progesterone. Its production by the pituitary can be suppressed by bromocriptine (see below) which is used when it is necessary to suppress lactation.

Prolactin also has a powerful inhibitory effect on ovarian function and high blood levels during the period of lactation are probably responsible for the delayed return of menstruation after pregnancy. Overproduction is also a cause of infertility in women.

Bromocriptine. This interesting drug is related to ergot. It acts on the pituitary in the same way as the naturally occurring substance dopamine and inhibits the release of various hormones, particularly prolactin and growth hormone. It also stimulates dopamine receptors in the basal ganglia and thus relieves the symptoms of Parkinson's disease (see p. 151).

Therapeutics. Bromocriptine has been used to suppress lactation following childbirth. The dose is 2.5 mg b.d. for 2 weeks.

Increased production of prolactin by the pituitary can cause impotence in men and amenorrhoea in women. By suppressing the production of prolactin, bromocriptine is successful in re-versing these symptoms though treatment may have to be continued for some time. The initial dose is 1.25 mg at night with food to decrease nausea and *slowly* increased.

By inhibiting growth hormone release, it is of some value in the management of acromegaly. It has also been used in the treatment of Parkinson's disease.

It is important to start with a small dose which can be increased gradually, otherwise the side-effects, nausea, vomiting, low blood pressure and drowsiness, are troublesome.

FURTHER READING

Editorial 1992 Octreotide-steams ahead. British Medical Journal 339: 837
Editorial 1992 Cyclical breast pain—what works and what doesn't. Drug and Therapeutics Bulletin 30: 1
Smail P 1991 The GP, specialist and HGH. Prescriber Issue 38: 28

SECTION II: HORMONES AFFECTING METABOLISM

THE THYROID

The thyroid consists of two lobes connected by an isthmus and is situated in the neck, in front of the trachea. Circulating iodine is picked up by the cells of the thyroid gland and incorporated to form two hormones, thyroxine (T_4) and triiodothyronine (T_3). These are stored in the thyroid as thyroglobulin. With appropriate stimulation both thyroxine and triiodothyronine are released into the blood stream. On reaching certain tissues thyroxine is converted to triiodothyronine which is the more active hormone.

The effect of these thyroid hormones is to increase tissue metabolism and thus to raise the basal metabolic rate. They are also important in promoting growth. The release of thyroid hormone is controlled by the thyroid stimulating hormone (TSH) from the pituitary which, in turn, is controlled by thyroid releasing hormone (TRH). In normal people the release of thyroid hormone is nicely adjusted to maintain the metabolic rate at a satisfactory level. Under certain

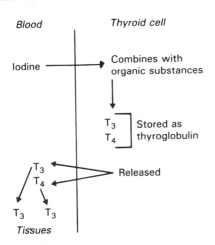

Fig. 13.4 Production, storage and release of thyroid hormones.

conditions, a considerable excess of thyroid hormone is produced and metabolism is greatly increased which, together with overactivity of the sympathetic nervous system, give rise to the clinical condition known as *thyrotoxicosis* or *Graves' disease*. Exophthalmos which is a characteristic sign of thyrotoxicosis is not due to thyroid hormone or to TSH but is partially due to sympathetic overactivity and also to a rather mysterious hormone called 'long-acting thyroid stimulator' (LATS). Suppression of the thyroid by drugs or by surgery (see below) will not therefore relieve exophthalmos.

Conversely, the thyroid may produce little or no hormone, with a resulting fall in metabolic rate and the appearance of the state known as *cretinism* in infants or *myxoedema* in adults. Both these conditions may be treated by replacement with thyroxine.

THYROID DEFICIENCY

There are two preparations which are effective in treating thyroid deficiency. They are *thyroxine* (BP), which is the pure hormone synthetically prepared and is used for long-term treatment, and *liothyronine*.

Thyroxine. Thyroxine tablets given orally are absorbed from the intestinal tract, but their full effects are not seen for about 10 days. If they are given to a patient with cretinism or myxoedema they will cause them to return to normal. Large dosage will cause excessive rise in metabolic rate and the symptoms of thyrotoxicosis with loss of weight, tachycardia, nervousness and tremors.

Therapeutics. It is important to start treating cretins as soon as possible because if they are left in a hypothyroid state too long, the change may be irreversible. The usual dosage of thyroxine for infants with cretinism is 25 micrograms daily, which is subsequently modified according to the response of the patient.

In myxoedema it is very important to start with a small dose or the undue stimulating effect on the heart may cause untoward effects, including anginal pain. Treatment should be started with 50 micrograms of thyroxine and this is cautiously increased until the desired effect is produced, the usual maintenance dose being 100–400 micrograms daily.

Early in treatment the patient should be kept warm, hypnotics should be avoided and constipation, which is common, should be relieved.

In both cretinism and myxoedema it is usually necessary to continue treatment for the rest of the patient's life.

Although the dose can be monitored by the clinical response of the patient, it is preferable to measure the plasma T_4 and TSH occasionally to ensure that the correct amount of hormone is being given.

Thyroxine is sometimes used to stimulate the metabolism of fat patients and thereby cause a loss of weight. It should not be used for this purpose as dangerous amounts of the drug are required to cause much weight loss.

Liothyronine is the official name of tri-iodothyronine. Its actions are similar to those of thyroxine but are much more rapid in onset, the maximum effect being seen after 3 days.

Therapeutics. Liothyronine is not so useful as thyroxine in treating myxoedema as the control of the disease is apt to be uneven but it is useful if a rapid effect is required.

In treating myxoedema coma the dose is 10–20 micrograms i.v. repeated at 4-hourly intervals as required. The initial oral dose is 10–20 micrograms daily, increasing to 20–100 micrograms daily.

EXCESS THYROID HORMONE (THYROTOXICOSIS)

Overproduction of hormone by the thyroid gland may be treated by surgical excision of most of the thyroid gland or by drugs. There are several drugs which decrease thyroid hormone production. Some of the most important are discussed.

Iodine. Iodine will temporarily depress thyroid function and relieve the symptoms of thyrotoxicosis.

It is usually given orally as *aqueous iodine solution (Lugol's iodine)*.The maximum effect is seen after about 2 weeks and is not maintained. It is therefore not used for the long-term treatment of thyrotoxicosis, but is valuable in preparing thyrotoxic patients for operation. The dose of aqueous iodine solution is 0.3–1.0 ml daily and it may be given in milk to improve the taste. Rarely it can cause sensitivity reactions.

Radioactive iodine (^{131}I) is used both diagnostically and therapeutically. It is given by mouth and rapidly absorbed from the stomach and intestines. Small doses are given and their uptake by the thyroid measured, thus providing an index of the 'iodine turnover' in the gland. Larger doses are used for their radiation effect on the thyroid, and will produce a permanent decrease in hormone production in cases of thyrotoxicosis. It will also destroy malignant cells in certain patients with carcinoma of the thyroid. ^{132}I is another isotope of iodine which is radioactive for a shorter time than ^{131}I and may therefore be preferred for certain diagnostic tests.

Special care will be required in the handling of and disposal of urine, etc. from these patients.

Carbimazole. Carbimazole suppresses the overproduction of thyroid hormones and is most commonly used in the treatment of thyrotoxicosis.

Therapeutics. The initial dose is 30–60 mg daily by mouth and it usually takes 1–2 months to return the thyroid function to normal although the thyroid gland itself often enlarges. The dose is then reduced to 5–15 mg daily and continued for about 18 months after which treatment may be stopped. About 60% of patients will remain well but 40% will relapse and either require further drug treatment or surgery.

Adverse effects include rashes, joint pains, enlarged lymph nodes and fever. Transient depression of the white cell count develops in around 10% of patients and rarely dangerous agranulocytosis; therefore severe sore throats should be reported.

Carbimazole should be given with care to pregnant women as excessive dosage may suppress the fetal thyroid causing goitre and hypothyroidism. It is also excreted in maternal milk and may have similar effects on the newborn.

Propylthiouracil may be used in a similar way.

β **blockers** (see p. 35). These drugs reduce those symptoms of thyrotoxicosis due to sympathetic overactivity including tachycardia, tremor, sweating and anxiety. They are useful for the rapid control of these symptoms particularly in the preparation for operation and may be continued with digitalis if atrial fibrillation develops. It must be remembered, however, that they do not cure thyrotoxicosis, so that if they are stopped the symptoms will return.

The treatment of thyrotoxicosis

For otherwise healthy young or middle-aged patients with thyrotoxicosis either surgery or drug treatment with carbimazole produces satisfactory results, and the complications and failure rates are about equal for both methods of treatment. Surgery has the advantage of getting a quick result, but some patients prefer to avoid an operation. For nodular goitres surgery is indicated. Prior to operation it is usual to make the patient euthyroid with carbimazole and to follow this with a short course of aqueous iodine solution which in addition to keeping the patient euthyroid, makes the thyroid less vascular and easier for the surgeon to handle. β blockers can also be used to prepare patients for operations.

Patient education in the recognition of the symptoms of thyroid disorders and the adverse effects of drugs used in treatment is important.

If β blockers are used alone the drug must be continued for 10 days after operation to prevent a thyroid crisis.

In the elderly or those with some other complicating disease ^{131}I is very satisfactory, but a definite proportion of patients subsequently develop myxoedema, and this proportion increases over the ensuing years.

THE ADRENAL GLANDS

The two adrenal glands are situated at the upper pole of the kidneys. They consist of an outer layer or cortex and a central portion or medulla. These two parts of the adrenal glands produce hormones of very different composition and function and they will therefore be considered separately.

THE CORTEX

There are a number of hormones produced by the adrenal cortex. They also belong to the class of chemical substances known as steroids and three main groups may be defined.

1. Mineralocorticoid hormones

These are concerned with salt (sodium) and water control; the most important is aldosterone.

Aldosterone increases reabsorption of sodium by the kidney, thus raising the amount of sodium in the body which in turn causes water retention. The main trigger to the release of aldosterone is the renin mechanism (see p. 57) and its main function is to ensure that the volume of fluid in the body is kept constant.

Excess of aldosterone gives rise to hypertension and sometimes oedema. It is not available for clinical use as a drug, but very rarely aldo-sterone-producing tumours arise in the adrenal gland causing *Conn's syndrome* which is characterized by hypertension and low plasma potassium with muscle weakness.

2. Sex corticoid hormones

Normally these are only secreted in small amounts and are of little importance. Excessive secretion leads to virilism.

Disorders may occur as a result of deficiency of these hormones following disease of the adrenal gland or from overproduction of one or more of their hormones by hyperplasia or tumour of the adrenals.

Although these conditions may affect only one group of hormones, it is common for a mixed picture to be produced.

3. Glucocorticoid hormones

The glucocorticoids are concerned with metabolism of carbohydrate, fat and protein and will also modify the response of the body to injury.

The chief glucocorticoid released from the adrenal is *cortisol*. Its release is controlled by corticotrophin which is in turn produced by the pituitary. The mechanism is such that when the amount of cortisol in the blood increases it 'switches off' the release of corticotrophin by the pituitary (negative feedback) and this prevents large changes in the blood cortisol concentration (see Fig. 13.5). In addition to cortisol there are a number of synthetic hormones with similar actions and the whole group is sometimes called the *corticosteroid* or *steroid hormones*.

Cortisone and cortisol (hydrocortisone). The actions of these two hormones are essentially the same and they will be considered together. Cortisol is the naturally occurring hormone and cortisone is a synthetic substitute. They are carried in the blood to their various sites of action; they penetrate the plasma membrane and act on intracellular structures. Their main actions are:

Carbohydrate metabolism. They stimulate the production of glucose from protein and decrease

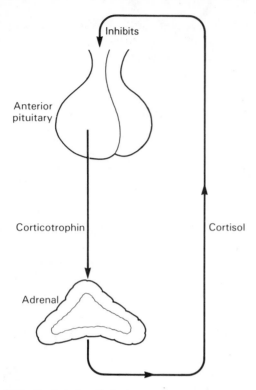

Fig. 13.5 Control of cortisol release.

Effect on the stomach. They may increase gastric acidity, and at times appear to exacerbate ulcers which are already present. It is doubtful if enteric coated tablets have any advantage and their absorption can be erratic. If perforation of the ulcer occurs, their effect on inflammation may mask the symptoms of the perforation with disastrous results.

Effects on immunity. The immune reaction is suppressed and patients become more vulnerable to infections. This is partly due to damping down the antigen–antibody response and possibly also to the reduced production of antibodies. For the same reasons allergic reactions of various types are inhibited.

Psychological effects. They usually produce a feeling of well-being; however, occasionally serious mental disease may follow their administration; it usually occurs in those with a background of mental ill health.

Effect and response to stress. Stress causes an increased secretion of cortisol. Failure of this response leads to a shock-like state.

Miscellaneous effects. In large doses they will produce a picture similar to that of Cushing's disease, with a round 'moon-like' face, hair on the face and body, a tendency to acne and purple striae on the trunk. Occasionally muscle weakness and wasting occur and the skin becomes thin and very susceptible to bruising.

Prolonged treatment will also lead to atrophy of the adrenal gland, and after such treatment the dosage should be reduced slowly to allow the patient's adrenal gland to start functioning again.

Prednisolone; prednisone; dexamethasone; betamethasone; triamcinolone; beclomethasone. These synthetic substances have powerful anti-inflammatory actions, but less sodium-retaining properties than cortisone. They are therefore used when an anti-inflammatory action is required. Side-effects are similar to those produced by cortisone. In addition, marked muscle wasting has been reported with triamcinolone. Beclomethasone can be given by inhalation in doses of 100 micrograms in treating asthma.

sensitivity to insulin. Prolonged treatment may rarely give rise to diabetes mellitus.

Effect on electrolytes. They cause retention of sodium and water and loss of potassium via the kidneys though they are not so powerful as aldosterone. The retention of sodium and water may lead to oedema and hypertension in some patients. Potassium loss may be replaced by potassium supplements (see p. 192) in patients who are receiving large doses over long periods.

Effect on inflammation. They suppress all inflammatory processes and also the generalized reactions of inflammation such as pyrexia and malaise. This action may be very dangerous, for inflammation is the body's method of dealing with infections. If no inflammatory reaction occurs the bacteria can spread widely without the seriousness of the position being apparent to the doctor or the patient. Such patients require urgent treatment with antibiotics and an *increase* in steroid dosage.

Fludrocortisone has very powerful sodium-retaining properties with minimal anti-inflammatory action.

Therapeutics. The therapeutic uses of corticosteroids may be considered under two headings:

a) Suppression of some disease process when relatively large doses are required.
b) Replacement of steroid hormones which, for some reason, are deficient. In this situation small (physiological) doses are needed.

Suppression of disease processes.

Anti-inflammatory actions. This effect is used in treating certain patients with systemic lupus, polyarteritis nodosa, temporal arteritis and, rarely, rheumatoid arthritis. In these conditions, much higher concentrations of the drugs are required than those which occur naturally, in order to suppress the inflammation and thus relieve the patients of their symptoms. It must again be stressed that these drugs are only useful in certain types of inflammation; in inflammation due to bacterial infection they may actually favour spread of infections and are thus dangerous.

The best drugs to use when anti-inflammatory effects are required are those with little sodium-retaining actions such as prednisolone.

Anti-allergic actions. By suppressing allergic reaction these drugs are useful in such conditions as asthma, hay fever and eczema.

In asthma they are reserved for those patients who do not respond to more usual measures, particularly status asthmaticus when 100 mg of cortisol (hydrocortisone) intravenously and repeated three hourly may be life saving. In long-term treatment of asthma steroids (beclomethasone) can be given by inhalation to produce a maximal local action with minimal systemic effect. In hay fever and eczema cortisol (hydrocortisone) may be applied locally and it is also used as eye drops.

They are also used to suppress immunity and thus prevent rejection after organ transplant.

Antitumour actions. Steroids have some antilymphocyte action and are used in combination with cytotoxic drugs to treat lymphomas and some leukaemias. Large doses (i.e. prednisolone 30–60 mg daily) are given over 1 or 2 weeks. Dexamethasone in doses of 16 mg daily is given in the palliative treatment of either primary or secondary cerebral tumours. It probably acts by reducing oedema.

Miscellaneous uses. Steroids produce an improvement in idiopathic thrombocytopenic purpura, in certain acute haemolytic anaemias and in certain types of the nephrotic syndrome. In these conditions large doses are usually required.

Dose. The dose required in treating the above condition is the smallest amount which produces a satisfactory therapeutic effect. This varies considerably.

Table 13.1 Potencies of various steroids

Drug	Anti-inflammatory effect	Salt retaining effect	Equivalent dose
Cortisol (Hydrocortisone)	+	+	100 mg
Cortisone	+	+	125 mg
Prednisolone	++	+	25 mg
Prednisone	++	+	25 mg
Methyl-prednisolone	++	(+)	20 mg
Betamethasone	++	0	4 mg
Dexamethasone	++	0	4 mg
Triamcinolone	++	0	20 mg
Fludrocortisone	(+)	++	—

If *rapid action* is required hydrocortisone hemisuccinate can be given intravenously.

Ideally, steroids should be given with food at breakfast. At this time natural steroid production is maximal so least suppression of adrenal function results. In children, long-term treatment with steroids retards growth. This may be minimized by giving the hormone on alternate days. Evening dosage should be avoided as this may keep the patient awake at night.

Replacement therapy. In these circumstances steroid hormones are used to replace the normal secretions of the adrenal glands because the adrenals have either been destroyed by disease (Addison's disease) or removed at operation.

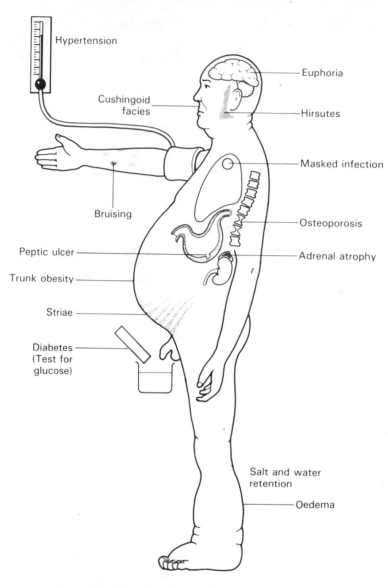

Fig. 13.6 Side-effects of the steroids.

When this occurs, the kidneys are no longer able to retain sodium, which is excreted in the urine and the body thus becomes depleted of sodium. This in turn leads to collapse with vomiting and low blood pressure. A curious feature of Addison's disease is the widespread pigmentation, particularly characteristic in the mouth.

The aim of treatment in this condition is to replace the missing hormones. In an acute Addisonian crisis with a collapsed and severely ill patient, cortisol (hydrocortisone) is given intravenously in doses of 100 mg and repeated as required. Saline and glucose are infused and any concurrent infection is treated vigorously.

For maintenance treatment it is important to use a steroid with sodium-retaining properties. Cortisol (hydrocortisone) 20 mg in the morning and 10 mg at night is satisfactory and may be combined with fludrocortisone 50–200 micrograms daily to further reduce salt loss. A rough check of adequate replacement can be achieved by measuring the blood pressure supine and erect. If inadequate, there will be a large postural fall in blood pressure. Other indications are the weight and well-being of the patient.

Any stress such as an acute infection will increase the requirements of steroids by these patients and the dose should be *increased* over the period of the acute episode.

Topical steroids

Steroids may be applied to the skin in the treatment of various dermatological conditions. The best vehicle for the drug is soft white paraffin and between 5–10% of the applied dose is absorbed through the skin. The most active steroids for this purpose include betamethasone, triamcinolone, beclomethasone and fluocinolone. Prolonged application can produce atrophy of the skin and a tendency to bacterial or fungal infection.

Nursing point

The nurse should wear gloves when applying topical steroids otherwise she will absorb the drug herself.

Adverse effects of steroid therapy. These hormones produce some potentially dangerous side-effects; they are summarized below (Fig. 13.6):

1. *General appearance*. With large doses the patient may develop a moon face and acne and oedema may be troublesome. The skin becomes atrophic and purpura may occur.
2. *Blood pressure*. This may become raised and should be measured at regular intervals.
3. *Blood electrolytes*. These may become deranged, particularly in those with renal disease and should be measured with particular attention to sodium retention and potassium loss. Occasionally, supplementary potassium, or sodium restriction is required.
4. *Urine*. Rarely these drugs precipitate *diabetes* and the urine should be tested for glucose.

5. *Symptoms of peptic ulcer* may occur and require the withdrawal of the drug.
6. Any infective disease may spread rapidly and yet produce minimal signs in these patients. Such an infection requires prompt treatment with antibiotics, together with an *increase* in the dose of steroid (see (11) below).
7. With large doses *decalcification of bone* occurs and vertebrae may collapse.
8. *Avascular necrosis of bone*, producing severe pain and affecting usually the hips is a very troublesome complication.
9. *Psychological disturbances* can occur.
10. The *eyes* may be affected with the development of cataracts or glaucoma.
11. *Prolonged treatment* with steroids causes suppression of normal adrenal cortical functions so that the adrenals cannot respond to stress by producing more hormone.
12. *Growth is retarded* in children.

Nursing points .

1. Patients on long-term steroids will require double their usual dose if they develop a moderate illness and treble their usual dose for a severe one. They must be taught to recognize stress situations.
2. Before an operation the surgeon and anaesthetist must be informed if the patient is on steroids. Patients must also inform their doctor and dentist if they are having steroids.
3. If treatment with steroids lasts more than 10 days withdrawal must be gradual as adrenal suppression will have occurred. Patients must be taught not to stop taking steroids suddenly.
4. All patients on long-term steroids should carry a card detailing their treatment.
5. Careful monitoring of adverse effects (see Fig. 13.6) is important.

Drugs reducing steroid action

Spironolactone blocks the action of *aldosterone* on the kidney and may be used as a diuretic (see p. 163).

Metyrapone. The production of hydrocortisone and aldosterone by the adrenal gland is blocked by this drug. This in turn stimulates an increase in production of corticotrophin (see p. 158). Metyrapone is thus used to test the ability of the pituitary to produce corticotrophin and to reduce the production of adrenal hormones in Cushing's syndrome. The dose is 500 mg–4 g daily in divided doses and the chief side-effect is nausea.

THE ADRENAL MEDULLA

The adrenal medulla produces both adrenaline and noradrenaline which are released into the circulation. The prageoperties of these substances are discussed on page 28.

Tumours of the medulla occur rarely and may produce both these substances in excessive amounts.

THE PARATHYROID GLANDS AND CALCIUM

The parathyroid glands are situated in the neck in close relationship with the thyroid gland. They are concerned with the levels of calcium and phosphorus in the blood and their excretion by the kidney. A fall in the level of blood calcium concentration stimulates the parathyroids to produce more hormone which mobilizes calcium from bone and decreases its loss through the kidney, thus returning the blood calcium level to normal.

Deficiency in parathyroid hormones results in an increase in blood phosphorus and a decrease in blood calcium levels. Lowering of the blood calcium causes a condition known as *tetany*, which is characterized by increased irritability of muscles with spasm of the hands and feet (carpo-pedal spasm) and of the larynx. A decrease in blood calcium may result from parathyroid deficiency, from lack of calcium in the diet particularly if the patient is also deficient in vitamin D and from alkalosis. The latter condition, although not necessarily associated with low blood calcium, causes a decrease of ionized calcium in the blood and it is the ionized fraction which is important in preventing tetany.

In cases of tetany due to parathyroid defi-ciency, several drugs are available to treat the condition.

Calcium. Acute attacks of tetany due to low blood calcium may be quickly relieved by giving calcium salts. They are usually administered as the gluconate or chloride. Calcium gluconate 10 ml of a 10% solution given slowly intravenously (2 ml/minute) produces rapid but short-lived relief. Calcium salts can also be given orally, not only to relieve tetany, but to prevent chronic calcium deficiency developing particularly in those who absorb calcium poorly. This occurs in rickets (vitamin D deficiency), following gastrectomy, in steatorrhoea and in the elderly. Calcium is also required in those with excessive loss due to lactation. Prolonged calcium deficiency may lead to decalcification of bones which may become bent or may fracture. Calcium supplements in deficiency states should contain at least 20 mmol of calcium. This could be obtained from:

- 2 tablets of Sandocal 400, an effervescent preparation
- 5 tablets of calcium gluconate twice daily.

For pregnancy supplements lower doses are used.

Nursing point

Calcium salts should never be mixed with sodium bicarbonate in a syringe or infusion as the calcium will precipitate. Note that they may both be used intravenously in cardiac arrest.

Parathyroid hormone is obtained from the parathyroid of animals. It is destroyed in the intestinal tract and should be given by injection. Its maximum effect appears about 6 hours after injection.

It causes a rise in the blood calcium and a decrease in blood phosphorus levels. It is not satisfactory for long-term treatment, as increasing doses are required to produce the desired effect and it may cause allergic reactions.

Vitamin D (see also p. 237). The plasma calcium level can also be raised by vitamin D which increases the absorption of calcium from the intestine. Vitamin D may be required if the diet is deficient in the vitamin, in various conditions in which resistance to the action of vitamin D occurs and in parathyroid hormone deficiency.

Vitamin D (calciferol) itself can be used or substances which have a similar action such as **dihydrotachysterol** or **alfacalcidol**. These drugs are considered on page 238.

Calcitonin. Calcitonin is a hormone which is produced in the thyroid gland but is concerned with calcium balance. It lowers the concentration of calcium in the blood and increases its deposition in bone. It is used in disorders where there is a rapid breakdown of bone, such as Paget's disease or to control malignant deposits in bone where they release excessive amounts of calcium into the blood causing hypercalcaemia. It is prepared from either pig or salmon and is given by injection.

Salcatonin (salmon calcitonin) is given by subcutaneous or intramuscular injection. The dose and frequency of administration depend on the condition being treated.

Adverse effects include nausea, vomiting and flushing after the injection.

The bisphosphonates. These substances are absorbed onto the calcium-containing crystals in bone and slow both their rate of formation and dissolution. It must be realized that bone is not an inert structure but is always being broken down and reformed. In Paget's disease and in malignant disease involving bone, this process accelerates resulting in pain and in the release of calcium into the blood with consequent hypercalcaemia.

Bisphosphonates, by slowing bone 'turnover', relieve pain and control hypercalcaemia.

Disodium etidronate is given orally in doses of 5 mg/kg daily. Food should not be taken for 2 hours before and after treatment.

Disodium pamidronate is used for hypercalcaemia due to malignancy and is given over 2 hours by intravenous infusion.

Adverse effects include nausea and diarrhoea.

Plicamycin is an antibiotic with cytotoxic effects. In malignant disease involving bone there may be mobilization of calcium with release into the blood; this can cause a dangerous hypercalcaemia. Plicamycin inhibits this release. The dosage must be carefully controlled as it causes damage to the bone marrow with low white cell and platelet counts in blood.

Treatment of hypercalcaemia due to malignancy

Malignant disease involving bone can cause a dangerous rise in the plasma calcium concentration which can be a medical emergency. It is treated as follows:

1. 0.9% sodium chloride solution is infused to correct the loss of water and salt through the kidney.
2. When this deficiency has been corrected frusemide can be given to increase calcium excretion.
3. Disodium pamidronate is infused to prevent further bone breakdown.

Other drugs which can be given are steroids, calcitonin and plicamycin.

Prevention of calcium absorption

Sometimes it is necessary to lower a raised blood calcium concentration which is dangerous by reducing calcium absorption from the gut. This is achieved by giving phosphate in the form of **Phosphate-Sandoz** which binds to calcium in the intestine and prevents its absorption.

Sodium cellulose phosphate acts in a similar way and is used in a disorder called hypercalciuria in which the patient absorbs from the gut and excretes in the urine excessive amounts of calcium which may cause recurrent kidney stones.

THE PANCREAS

The pancreas is a relatively large gland lying across the upper part of the posterior abdominal

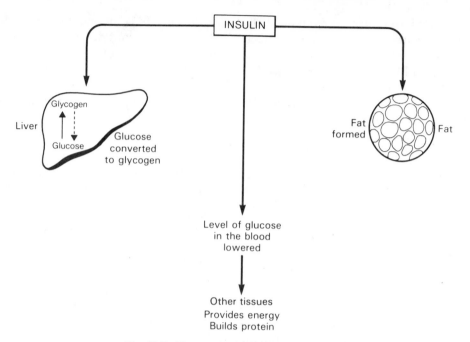

Fig. 13.7 The metabolic effects of insulin.

wall. It produces a number of digestive enzymes which drain into the duodenum and help digestion.

Scattered throughout the gland are small collections of tissue known as the islets of Langerhans. These islets contain two types of cell called alpha and beta cells and from the beta cells is produced the important hormone called insulin.

INSULIN AND DIABETES MELLITUS

Insulin is a hormone which lowers the concentration of glucose in the blood by:

1. Stimulating the uptake of glucose by the tissues.
2. Converting glucose to glycogen in the liver where it is stored.
3. Increasing the production of fat and protein.

In *diabetes mellitus* there are two types of insulin deficiency. The first type is known as *insulin-dependent diabetes* or Type I in which there is a true deficiency of insulin due to atrophy of the islets of Langerhans and which occurs predominantly in young people. This deficiency leads to a rapid rise in the blood glucose concentration with subsequent loss of large amounts of glucose with water and salt in the urine. In addition, fats in the body are broken down releasing ketoacids which cause acidosis. Weight loss may be marked. If not treated, the patient will lapse into a coma *(hyperglycaemic ketoacidosis)*.

The second type of diabetes, known as *non-insulin-dependent* or Type II, occurs in middle-aged or elderly people who are frequently overweight. In this type there appears to be resistance to the action of insulin rather than a true deficiency. The blood glucose concentration is raised with glycosuria but ketoacidosis is not common and the symptoms are often those of the late complications of diabetes see below.

These complications occur with both types of diabetes. Disease of the small arteries leads to damage to the retina of the eye, declining renal function and serious interference with the circulation to the legs, sometimes requiring amputation, and various peripheral nerves may be damaged. Diabetic patients are particularly prone to infection and these infections may, in turn, exacerbate the diabetes, sometimes leading to ketoacidosis and coma. Good control of the diabetes reduces the severity of the complications but does not entirely prevent them.

Sources of insulin

Insulin is available in many preparations which vary in both their duration of action and their purity. Until recently insulin was extracted from the pancreas of cows (bovine) or pigs (porcine). Bovine insulin differs in its structure from human insulin and is thus inherently immunogenic. Porcine insulin is very similar to human insulin and is not much more liable to produce immunological reactions.

It has now become possible to produce *human insulins* either by modifying porcine insulin or by an ingenious method involving bacteria. The code for synthesizing human insulin can be inserted into bacteria (*Esch. coli*) which then multiply and produce human insulin.

Purification

All insulins are now highly purified to remove traces of other substances and make them less immunogenic. Non-human insulins can stimulate the production of anti-insulin antibodies (AIA) which occasionally give rise to local and systemic allergic reactions and to insulin resistance.

Short acting insulins

These are available as human or purified animal insulins. The blood glucose begins to fall within an hour of injection and their action lasts about 8 hours. They are used in the treatment of diabetic coma (ketoacidosis), to cover operations and illnesses in diabetic subjects and sometimes in the long-term control of diabetes, perhaps combined with a longer acting insulin.

Intermediate acting insulins

Insulin zinc suspension (IZS). It was found that if insulin was buffered with acetate its action was prolonged, and a further two types of insulin could be prepared: amorphous, in which the particles were small, and a crystalline form with larger particles. The action of amorphous insulin is rapid and short-lived but that of crystalline insulin is more prolonged. By using a mixture of these insulins a smooth and prolonged effect can be achieved.

There are several mixtures of this type and they are shown in Table 13.2. They are available both as purified porcine insulin or as human insulin (Human Monotard).

Table 13.2 Some commonly used insulins

Preparation of insulin	Purified	Source	Onset of action in hours	Duration of effect in hours	
Human Actrapid	Yes	Human	$\frac{1}{2}$	8	Short acting soluble insulins
Humulin S	Yes	Human	$\frac{1}{2}$	7	
Humulin 1	Yes	Human	1	20	
Human Protaphane	Yes	Human	$1\frac{1}{2}$	24	
Human Monotard	Yes	Human	2	24	Intermediate-acting insulins
Initard	Yes	Porcine	$\frac{1}{2}$	24	
Human Initard	Yes	Human	$\frac{1}{2}$	24	
Mixtard	Yes	Porcine	$\frac{1}{2}$	24	
Human Mixtard	Yes	Human	$\frac{1}{2}$	24	
Humulin Zinc	Yes	Human	2	36	Long-acting insulins
Hypurin Protamine Zinc	Yes	Bovine	4	35	

Isophane insulin is a combination of insulin and protamine; its action lasts for 8–12 hours.

Long acting insulins

Protamine zinc insulin (PZI). This is produced by adding protamine and zinc to insulin. Its action is prolonged, starting after 6 hours and lasting for 24–30 hours. It is a bovine insulin and may give rise to skin rashes and painful lumps at the site of injection. If soluble and PZI insulin are mixed in the syringe before injection, some of the soluble insulin becomes PZI insulin. To minimize this, the soluble insulin should be drawn up first and the mixture of insulins injected immediately. Alternatively, the crystalline form of human insulin zinc suspension also has a prolonged action and is not immunogenic.

TREATMENT OF DIABETES MELLITUS

Management of insulin-dependent diabetics

These patients require insulin replacement and the object of treatment is to give them a diet suited to their lifestyle and work, then give enough insulin to replace the deficiency and maintain them in good health as judged by their subjective feelings, their weight (which should be

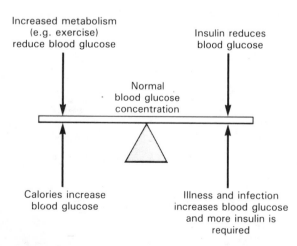

Fig. 13.8 Balancing the diabetic.

kept at the correct level for their age and height) and keep their blood glucose levels near normal.

There are many dietary schemes and with changing fashions it is too lengthy a subject to discuss here in detail. Briefly, about 50% of the calories in the diet should be from carbohydrate in forms which are slowly absorbed such as wholemeal bread, potatoes and various vegetables, but not rapidly digestible sugars such as sweets and cakes. About 35% of the calories may come from fat and the rest from protein.

Choice of insulin

If a patient is satisfactorily controlled on a certain type of insulin, that preparation should usually be continued. Human insulin is the least immunogenic and it should be used in the following circumstances.

1. For patients starting treatment.
2. If the patient develops generalized allergies to an unpurified insulin.
3. If injection causes severe local reactions.
4. If very large doses are required, a situation which suggests that antibodies have been produced by the impure insulin and are interfering with its action.
5. If the patient is pregnant because impurities in the older types of insulin can cross the placenta and affect the islet tissue of the fetus.

If a change is made from animal to human insulin it should be remembered that human insulin acts a little more rapidly and its effect lasts a shorter time so that some readjustment of dosage may be necessary. Also, only 80–90% of the previous dose may be needed.

Giving insulin

Because insulin is broken down in the stomach it has to be given by injection usually 15–30 minutes before breakfast and before the evening meal, often using a mixture of short and medium acting insulins. Some patients will require three injections daily particularly if they are difficult to control or increased flexibility is required. Whilst for others, provided the dose is small, a single

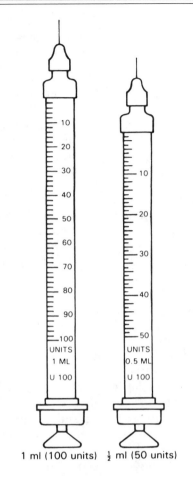

1 ml (100 units)   ½ ml (50 units)

Fig. 13.9 The U100 syringe marked in units of insulin.

injection of long acting insulin is adequate. The type of insulin, dosage and frequency of administration are modified in the light of the patient's response until optimum control is obtained.

Strength of insulin preparations. The introduction of U100 insulin has greatly simplified insulin dosage. All insulins are now of standard strength—100 units in 1 ml. The U100 syringes are marked in units of insulin and so it only is necessary to draw up the required number of units (Fig. 13.9).

Insulin should be stored in the refrigerator (not the freezing compartment) but the bottle in current use can safely be kept at room temperature.

Injection of insulin. Most patients receiving insulin are instructed how to inject themselves and this instruction is usually given by the nurse.

The best sites for injection are the front of the thighs, the abdomen and the outer side of the upper arm and the insulin is given subcutaneously. A different site should be used each time but it must be remembered that the rate of absorption of insulin into the circulation varies with different part of the body. Therefore, it is better to use the same area but not exactly the same site at the same time of day, for example, the morning dose into the thigh and the evening dose into the arm. Other points of note about injecting insulin are:

1. A microfine i.v. needle and syringe or a 25 G x ⅝″ should be used and should be introduced into the skin at an angle of 90°.
2. No spirit should be used for skin cleaning as it hardens the skin and the injection site should not be massaged after injection.
3. Special syringes are available for those with poor eyesight or other infirmities.

Insulin pens are devices which contain a cartridge of insulin which is automatically injected. A wide range of insulins are available in cartridges and they may be more convenient for the patient.

Syringe pumps give a continuous subcutaneous infusion of insulin. The pump is worn by the patient and the rate of infusion modified to the patient's needs thus producing a very fine control of the diabetes.

Monitoring treatment

Patients should be taught to monitor their response to treatment by measuring glucose levels in the blood or urine.

In normal subjects the blood glucose concentration varies from 3–7 mmol/l. The object of treatment is to keep the blood glucose as near as possible to these levels. In patients on insulin this is best achieved by measuring the blood glucose using the drop of blood from a finger prick which is applied to a special indicator strip. The resulting colour change can be read against a colour chart or by a meter. This enables patients to measure their own blood glucose levels and is usually carried out once daily at different times of day. The blood glucose concentration should be kept between 4–9 mmol/l.

In patients not on insulin or for whom strict control is not considered practical, the urine is tested for glucose before breakfast, before the midday meal, before retiring, using some dipstick method or Clinitest tablets. This gives a less precise picture of how the blood glucose level is being controlled as glucose does not appear in the urine until the blood level is 10 mmol/l which is higher than normal. Also it gives no indication if the blood glucose is too low. Nevertheless, it is easy to perform and adequate for many patients, particularly the non-insulin-dependent diabetics.

If the diabetes is seriously out of control, the urine will show the presence of ketones as well as glucose. This means a dangerous situation is developing and immediate treatment is required (see below).

Hypoglycaemia. Overdosage with insulin causes an undue decrease in the blood sugar. This leads to faintness, dizziness, tremor, sweating and abnormal behaviour which may be mistaken for drunkenness. If no treatment is given convulsions, coma and death may occur. It can quickly be relieved by giving sugar or glucose, 4 teaspoonfuls of sugar in half a glass of fruit juice being effective. Glucagon (see p. 176) by injection is also effective and is useful if the patient is too drowsy to swallow.

About a quarter of long-term diabetics may not be aware that they are becoming hypoglycaemic. Alcohol and β blockers may aggravate this and it has been suggested that it is more likely to occur when human insulin is used, but proof is lacking.

Insulin in special circumstances

Details of the methods used under these circumstances vary but the general principles are the same.

Pregnancy. Human insulin is preferable (see p. 172). It is necessary to control the diabetes as well as possible, usually giving insulin two or three times daily. Poor control increases the incidence of fetal abnormality and perinatal problems.

Serious intercurrent illness. The patient's insulin requirement will rise and this situation is a potent cause of diabetic coma. 6 units/hour of soluble insulin should be given by intravenous infusion or by multiple small intramuscular injections together with fluid and glucose as determined by blood glucose estimations.

Major surgery. It is easiest if the patient is first on the morning operating list. The morning dose of insulin is not given but at least an hour before surgery an infusion of 5% glucose with 10 mmol of potassium in each 500 ml is started at 100 ml/hour. Human Actrapid is commenced at the same time at a rate of 4 units/hour. The rate of insulin infusion is subsequently adjusted depending on the blood glucose levels.

Diabetic coma (hyperglycaemic ketoacidosis). Patients with diabetes who are not treated, or develop some infection during treatment, may pass into diabetic coma. These patients have not only a very high blood and urinary glucose level, but are producing large quantities of ketone bodies which can be detected in the urine and which being acids, lead to an acidosis. The excessive diuresis produced by the glucose in the urine leads to severe depletion of sodium, potassium and water.

Soluble human insulin (Humulin S or Human Actrapid) is given *intravenously* by an infusion pump. An initial bolus of 5 units is followed by 3–6 units per hour and adjusted as necessary. If no pump is available, 20 units can be given *intramuscularly* followed by 6 units per hour. At the same time water and electrolyte imbalance is corrected by giving an infusion of normal saline containing 20 mmol of potassium chloride per litre. Restoration of electrolyte and water balance is usually sufficient and the kidneys will correct the acidosis by secreting an acid urine. Occasionally, however, the acidosis is so severe that it is necessary to infuse sodium bicarbonate until the degree of acidosis is improved. Frequent examination of the urine for sugar and ketones and of the blood sugar hourly and of the electrolytes is important in controlling treatment. Subsequent doses of insulin are determined by the blood glucose concentration.

The possibility of infection as a cause of diabetic coma should not be forgotten, and if this is found it is treated by the appropriate antibiotic.

Deep vein thrombosis is a common complication and prophylactic subcutaneous heparin is often given.

Management of non-insulin-dependent diabetics

These patients are usually managed in the first instance by diet. This should contain between 1000–2000 kcal daily depending on activity. The obese should reduce their weight to correct levels. If these measures fail, an oral hypoglycaemic agent should be added to the regime. These drugs are no substitutes for dieting and if used without dietary restriction the patient will gain weight rapidly.

ORAL HYPOGLYCAEMIC AGENTS
The sulphonylureas

This group of drugs is related to the sulphonamides. They lower blood glucose levels by:

1. Increasing insulin production by the pancreas
2. Increasing the peripheral uptake of glucose by the tissues.

They are all given orally and differ largely in their duration of action. They are used in non-insulin-dependent diabetics who are usually middle-aged or elderly and obese, and supplement treatment by diet. They have no place in the treatment of the young insulin-requiring diabetic or of diabetic coma. There are several drugs in the group which are in common use.

Tolbutamide has been used for many years and is very safe and satisfactory if used correctly. Its duration of action is about 6 hours and for this reason it is particularly recommended in the elderly as the risk of hypoglycaemia is reduced

and it is given orally two or three times daily. The dose is 0.5–1.5 g/day and if no satisfactory response is achieved with this dose, larger amounts are unlikely to be successful.

Chlorpropamide is similar to tolbutamide but its action lasts a full 24 hours and 125–250 mg once daily is the usual dose. Because of adverse effects it should only be used for patients who have been successfully treated with it for some time.

With both these drugs gastrointestinal upsets, rashes or rarely blood dyscrasias and fluid retention can occur. Both tolbutamide and chlorpropamide can produce hypoglycaemia but it is much more common after chlorpropamide because of its longer action and because accumulation can occur with impaired renal function. It usually follows a prolonged fast while taking the drug or may occur at the night. In some patients chlorpropamide can cause flushing after taking alcohol.

Glibenclamide has been widely used. Its action lasts about 12 hours and it can be given once daily. With a large single dose, hypoglycaemia can occur and in these circumstances it is best to split the dose and give it twice daily. The initial dose is 5 mg (2.5 mg for the elderly) taken with breakfast and increased as required to a maximum dose of 15 mg daily. However, because of its lengthy action with the attendant risk of hypoglycaemia, its use should now be restricted to patients who have already been successfully treated with it.

Glipizide has a shorter action (6 hours) and serious hypoglycaemia is less likely. The initial dose is 2.5–5.0 mg before breakfast and the dose adjusted. Doses above 15 mg daily should be divided and the maximum is 40 mg daily.

Other sulphonylureas

	Single dose	Duration of action	Max. in 24 hours in divided doses
Gliquidone	15–60 mg	3 hours	180 mg
Gliclazide	40–80 mg	12 hours	320 mg

At present the choice usually lies between tolbutamide which is relatively cheap and glipizide.

Acarbose

This drug, taken orally, inhibits the digestion of sugars and starch and thus reduces the formation and absorption of glucose. The dose is 50 mg before meals. It may cause flatulence and diarrhoea.

The biguanides

This group differs from the sulphonylureas both in chemical structure and mode of action. They stimulate the uptake of glucose by muscles by direct action; they do not, however, prevent the production of ketone bodies. Their main use is combined with one of the sulphonylureas when the patient is not responding satisfactorily to these drugs alone. The biguanides are also occasionally used combined with insulin in insulin-dependent diabetics who are proving difficult to control. They decrease appetite and this may be useful in treating the obese diabetic. They do not cause hypoglycaemia.

Metformin is the only biguanide in common use at present. The usual daily dose is 0.5–3.0 g divided into two or three doses.

Adverse effects. Anorexia and nausea are troublesome and may lead to the abandonment of this form of treatment. More serious is *lactic acidosis* with drowsiness, abdominal pain, vomiting and shock. The mechanism of this side-effect is not understood but it is more liable to occur in alcoholics and those with liver, renal and cardiac failure. It was particularly likely to occur with the biguanide phenformin which has now been withdrawn.

Glucagon

Glucagon is a substance which mobilizes the liver glycogen and thus releases glucose into the blood. It is used to raise the blood sugar in patients who are hypoglycaemic, for instance after an overdose of insulin. The dose is 0.5–1.0 mg i.m. and the effect is seen in about 10 minutes.

The nurse and the diabetic patient at home

The management of the diabetic is a team activity involving the patient, the doctor, the nurse, the dietician and often laboratory staff. Diabetics may be managed by a hospital diabetic clinic but may also be stabilized and controlled in the community. Nurses are trained to supervise treatment in the home with the back-up of the hospital or family doctor. This has the advantage that treatment can be geared to the patient's lifestyle and, most important, the family can be involved particularly in planning meals etc.

Education is very important for the patients who must realize as far as possible the implications of their illness and its treatment.

APPETITE SUPPRESSION AND OBESITY

In the past several drugs related to amphetamine were used to suppress appetite and thus reduce weight. These drugs suffered from the disadvantage that they stimulated the central nervous system and were not entirely safe to use for this purpose.

The treatment of obesity by drugs is of limited value and should be accompanied by a suitable diet. When the drug is stopped weight is usually regained unless it has been possible to induce a change in the patient's eating habits.

Fenfluramine suppresses the appetite and also has a peripheral action on metabolism which may be significant in weight reduction.

Therapeutics. The initial dose of fenfluramine is 60 mg daily. It is important not to stop the drug suddenly as this may cause depression; the dose should be reduced gradually. Other side-effects include nausea, drowsiness and a tendency to dream.

Dexfenfluramine. Fenfluramine is a mixture of a d and **i** isomers (the same molecules but mirror images of each other). The d isomer is dexfenfluramine and is responsible for the anorectic effect which is due to 5HT blockade in areas of the brain. It has less adverse effects than fenfluramine.

Therapeutics. The dose is 15 mg twice daily with meals. It should not be used with MAOIs and has several other interactions.

FURTHER READING

Boyle I, Ralston S 1990 The treatment of hypercalcaemia. Prescribers Journal 30: 180

Brownlow I 1992 Transformed by thyroxine. Nursing Times 88 (8): 40

Chain A W, Macfarlane I 1988 The pharmacology of oral agents used in treating diabetes. Practical Diabetes 5: 59

Editorial 1990 Corticosteroids—Getting replacement right. Prescribers Journal 28: 71

Editorial 1990 Insulin injection technique. British Medical Journal 301: 3

Editorial 1991 Hypoglycaemic and diabetic control. Lancet 338: 853

Editorial 1991 Dexfenfluramine. Lancet 337: 1315

Editorial 1991 Treating obesity. British Medical Journal 302: 803

Fernez R E, Alberti K G 1989 Sulphonylurea treatment of non-insulin dependent diabetes. Quarterly Journal of Medicine 73: 987

Low H 1985 Stable in the community. Nursing Times — Community Outlook 81(7): 27

Schuldham C 1985 Diabetic ketoacidosis: an endocrine emergency. Nursing 2nd series 42: 1246

SECTION III: HORMONES AFFECTING REPRODUCTION

THE FEMALE SEX HORMONES

It is important to understand the hormone background of the normal menstrual cycle and of pregnancy before considering the individual hormones.

At the commencement of the menstrual cycle, the *follicular stimulating hormone* from the pituitary causes ripening of the ovarian follicle which releases oestrogenic hormones. The oestrogens in turn cause proliferation of the mucosa

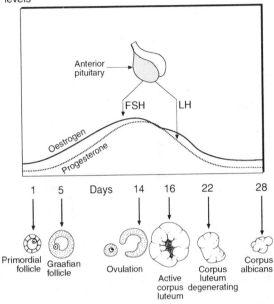

Fig. 13.10   Events of the 'average' menstrual cycle. Reproduced with permission from Prentice Hall.

lining the uterus. Ovulation occurs about half-way through the menstrual cycle and the pituitary now releases *luteinizing hormone* which helps the development of the corpus luteum when the ovum has been discharged from the ovary. The corpus luteum produces the hormone progesterone which causes further thickening of the endometrium. If implantation of the fertilized ovum does not occur, the corpus luteum regresses and the superficial part of the endometrium breaks down and is discharged as the menstrual flow.

If a fertilized ovum is implanted in the uterus the corpus luteum does not immediately regress. Throughout pregnancy large quantities of progesterone and oestrogens are produced, probably by the placenta and can be recovered from the urine. Gonadotrophic hormone is also produced by the human placenta during the early months of pregnancy and its presence in the urine forms the basis of various tests for pregnancy.

Just before parturition the production of progestrone ceases and this may be concerned with the start of labour.

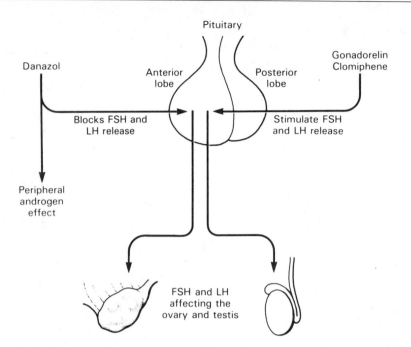

Fig. 13.11 Drugs modifying the release of FSH and LH and thus modifying gonadal activity.

Both oestrogens and progesterone are used therapeutically and will now be considered in detail.

GONADOTROPHINS

Both these pituitary hormones are used therapeutically and will be considered in detail.

Follicular stimulating hormone (FSH) is available as *urofollitrophin*. In the female it causes ripening of the ovarian follicles and the production of oestrogen, and in the male it is necessary for the production of spermatozoa. It is given by injection.

Luteinizing hormone (LH) is available as chorionic gonadotrophin. In the female it produces the corpus luteum and in the male it stimulates the interstitial cells of the testis. It is given by injection.

Menotrophin is a combination of FSH and LH.

Therapeutics. In female infertility these hormones are used to induce normal ovarian function. FSH is given first to produce an ovarian follicle followed by LH to induce ovulation.

Clomiphene stimulates increased secretion of gonadotrophins and is used in the treatment of infertility due to failure of ovulation; 50 mg is given daily for 5 days early in the menstrual cycle. It may be so successful that it results in twins but multiple pregnancies can be avoided by careful dosing.

Adverse effects include flushing, headaches, nausea, weight gain and visual disturbances.

Gonadorelin releases gonadotrophins and induces ovulation. It is given as a pulsed injection every 90 minutes.

Danazol and Gestrinone inhibit gonadotrophin release. They are used in treating endometriosis and various benign breast disorders in doses of 100–400 mg daily orally.

Adverse effects reflect that they are androgen derivatives and cause abnormal hair growth, greasy skin, acne, fluid retention and nausea.

THE OESTROGENS

The oestrogen hormones have a variety of effects, the most important being proliferation of the endometrium, sensitization of the uterine muscle to certain stimulating agents, increase in duct tissue in the breast and inhibition of production of prolactin by the pituitary.

There are a number of oestrogens both naturally occurring and synthetic. Their actions are similar.

Ethinyloestradiol is effective orally and is the oestrogen of choice. The dose is 10–100 micrograms daily depending on the disorder being treated.

Mestranol is inactive as an oestrogen but is converted to ethinyloestradiol in the liver.

Stilboestrol is used in large doses to control some forms of cancer.

Other oestrogens include:

Preparation	Dose
Oestradiol	1–2 mg daily orally
Oestriol	250–500 micrograms daily orally.

Therapeutic uses. Oestrogens are used for replacement therapy or for other actions.

Menopausal symptoms. The menopause is associated with a number of symptoms:

1. Those due to oestrogen deficiency include some atrophy of the uterus and dryness of the vagina which may cause dyspareunia.

Osteoporosis. Loss of protein from bone, with subsequent risk of fracture, is a serious problem in postmenopausal women. Oestrogen treatment is the most effective way of preventing this and there is a strongly argued case that most postmenopausal women should receive hormone replacement therapy (HRT). In addition, HRT appears to give some protection against coronary artery disease and stroke.

Hot flushes. Their cause is unknown but they respond to treatment with oestrogen.
2. Vague emotional symptoms of varying and ill-defined aetiology.

Symptoms in group 1 respond to hormone replacement therapy with an oestrogen but in group 2 the response is variable.

Most patients having HRT will have an intact uterus. The unopposed action of oestrogens stimulates the endometrium and may ultimately cause a carcinoma of the uterus. To prevent this happening, the oestrogen is combined with a progestogen to mimic the normal menstrual cycle with regular shedding of the endometrium. A monthly course consists of an oestrogen given for 3 weeks followed by a progestogen for 5 days which is restarted after 2 days' rest. A convenient alternative is Prempak C in which an oestrogen is given throughout the cycle and a progestogen (norgestrel) for the last 12 days. It is presented in a more or less foolproof pack. Other similar preparations are available.

Tibolone is a synthetic hormone which will control postmenopausal symptoms and limit osteoporosis without stimulating the endometrium, and thus eliminates the risk of causing uterine cancer. There is therefore no need for a progestogen and no monthly bleeding.

Oestrogens can also be given as a patch applied to the skin. The patch available in the UK contains oestradiol which diffuses through the skin and is effective for 3–4 days when the patch is replaced. Cyclical progestogen treatment causing monthly bleeding is still required.

If the patient has had a hysterectomy the progestogen is not needed and replacement can be with an oestrogen alone, e.g. ethinyloestradiol 5–15 micrograms, or conjugated oestrogens (Premarin) 625 micrograms daily orally.

On balance it appears that HRT is ideal for postmenopausal women particularly if they have symptoms; however, there are possible problems:

1. There may be a slightly increased risk of carcinoma of the breast.
2. Adverse effects include nausea, weight gain, headache and the growth of facial hair.
3. Before starting treatment a full examination is necessary to exclude cancer, gynaecological abnormalities and thrombotic disease which may be made worse by HRT, and the patient should be given a full explanation of the implications of the treatment. It is not necessarily an 'elixir of youth'.

Menstrual disturbances. In patients who are deficient in natural ovarian hormones it is possi-

> **Nursing point**
>
> HRT patches should be replaced every 3–4 days. They should be applied to clean, dry, unbroken skin on the trunk below the waist and not near the breasts.

ble to produce uterine bleeding by giving oestrogens for a time and then stopping the hormone. This is, of course, not a normal menstrual cycle, and it is difficult to see any real therapeutic use in the manoeuvre except for its psychological value.

Neoplastic disease. Oestrogens have been used with some success in two types of neoplasm.

In *carcinoma of the prostate* oestrogens probably act by suppressing the production of male hormone which stimulates the neoplasm. Large doses are required. Stilboestrol 15–100 mg daily is given by mouth or pellets of the hormone may be implanted subcutaneously. Some patients complain of nausea and hypertrophy of the breasts with pigmentation of the nipple, but results are often very good, even in widespread disease. An alternative is *cyproterone* which directly blocks the action of androgens on the prostate and thereby induces a remission.

A proportion of patients with advanced *carcinoma of the breast* obtain temporary, but sometimes striking remission of their disease with oestrogens. They are most successful in post-menopausal patients.

Although oestrogens were formerly used to suppress lactation they have now been replaced by bromocriptine (see p. 160).

Oestrogens can also be applied locally. They are used in atrophic vaginitis which occurs in post-menopausal women due to oestrogen deficiency. Dienoestrol cream (0.01%) applied daily for 2–3 weeks is satisfactory.

PROGESTERONE

Progesterone causes further thickening and development of the secretory phase in the endometrium which has been induced by oestrogen and 'damps down' the excitability of the uterine muscle. It probably plays a large part in maintaining the fetus in the uterus until the time is ripe for labour to commence.

Therapeutics. Progesterone derivatives are used, dysmenorrhoea, menorrhagia or endometriosis which is due to ectopic areas of the endometrium. *Medroxyprogesterone* is used in doses of 5 mg daily by mouth on the 16th–21st days of the menstrual cycle for menorrhagia or as intramuscular injections of 50 mg weekly for endometriosis. Dydrogesterone can be used in a similar way.

The newer progesterones (progestogens). There are now a number of steroid hormones which are effective by mouth and which have similar actions to progesterone. They are used either alone or in combination with an oestrogen as an oral contraceptive or for HRT and include **norethisterone, levonorgestrel** and **desogestrel.**

ORAL CONTRACEPTIVES

Most oral contraceptives are a mixture of an oestrogen and a progestogen. They prevent conception in several ways:

1. By inhibiting ovulation—this is the consequence of reducing the output of pituitary gonadotrophins.
2. By changing the character of the mucus of the uterine cervix, and making penetration to the uterus by sperms more difficult.
3. By making the endometrium less suitable for implantation of the ovum.

The oestrogen used is usually *ethinyloesteradiol* and the progestogen is *norethisterone, levonorgestrel, desogestrel* or *gestodene.* There is some evidence that gestodene and desogestrel are less likely to cause changes in the plasma lipids associated with vascular disease. Usually the composition of the pill is unaltered throughout the full monthly course but there are a few preparations in which pills of varying composition are given sequentially—the biphasic and triphasic preparations. Of the many preparations now available the most effective and widely used are those in which both an oestrogen and a progestogen are given throughout the course, with a failure rate of less than 0.5 per 100 women years.

Table 13.3 shows the oestrogenic and progestogenic content of some of the preparations in use at the time of writing.

It is also possible to give preparations which only contain a progestogen but although they impair fertility, they only prevent ovulation in about half the menstrual cycles so are less efficient as contraceptives.

If used correctly, these combinations provide the most effective contraceptives available and failure rarely occurs.

Table 13.3 Oral contraceptives

Progestogen only			
Norethisterone	Microner	350 micrograms	oral
Levonorgestrel	Microval	30 micrograms	
Medroxyprogesterone		150 mg	depot
Norethisterone		200 mg	

Combined preparations		
	Oestrogen	Progestogen
	micrograms	micrograms
Ethinyloestradiol + norethisterone		
Loestrin 20	20	1000
Ovysmen	35	500
Brevinor	35	500
Neocon 1/35	35	1000
Norimin	35	1000
Ethinyloestradiol + levonorgestrel		
Microgynon 30	30	150
Ovranette	30	150
Eugynon 30	30	250
Ovran 30	30	250
Ovran	50	250
Ethinyloestradiol + desogestrel		
Mercilon	20	150
Marvelon	30	150
Ethinyloestradiol + gestodene		
Femodene	30	75
Minulet	30	75
Ethinyloestradiol + norgestimate		
Cilest	35	250

Triphasic preparations		
Ethinyloestradiol + norethisterone		
Trinovum	(7 days) 35	500
	(7 days) 35	750
	(7 days) 35	1000
Ethinyloestradiol + levonorgestrel		
Trinordiol	(6 days) 30	50
	(5 days) 40	75
	(10 days) 30	125
Logynon	(6 days) 30	50
	(5 days) 40	75
	(10 days) 30	125

Using the combined pill

1. It is usual to start with the lowest dose formulation because the risk of thrombosis (see below) is related to the oestrogen content. Preparations containing 20–35 micrograms of ethinyloestradiol are usually prescribed.
2. The 'Pill' is started on the fifth day after the commencement of menstruation and continued for 21 days. Ovulation which occurs about halfway through the cycle is suppressed and withdrawal bleeding starts a few days after the end of the course. It is important that other contraceptive precautions are taken for the first 7 days of the first cycle.
3. The 'Pill' must be taken regularly. If the dose is taken 12 hours late, other contraceptive precautions should be used for the next 7 days.
4. If a low dose combination 'Pill' fails to control the cycle after 3 months, alternatives such as triphasic preparations should be tried.

Nurses working in family planning clinics and health centres have an important role in teaching women about taking oral contraceptives and allaying anxieties, as scares relating to cancer have appeared in the national press and caused alarm. At present, evidence that oral contraceptives may be implicated remains tentative. If concerned, women should be advised to seek medical advice. Stopping the 'Pill' may result in an unplanned pregnancy.

Using progestogens only

This method which inhibits ovulation and changes the character of the cervical mucus is less safe than the combined pill but has virtually no risk of thrombotic disease (see below) and may be preferred in older women or those at special risk from thrombosis.

The pill is started on day 1 and taken at the *same time* each day throughout the cycle with no break.

Progestogens can also be given as depot injections lasting 2–3 months.

The main side-effects of the progestogen-only 'Pill'

Amenorrhoea is common in women taking this form of the 'Pill' and it is essential to teach them the early signs and symptoms of pregnancy to avoid anxiety.

Spotting—slight blood loss—may occur through much of the cycle.

Postcoital contraception

The risk of pregnancy after unprotected sexual intercourse is about 1:30. It is possible to reduce the risk of pregnancy by using the oral contraceptive as a 'morning after' pill. Two tablets of Ovran or Eugynon 50 are taken immediately and repeated after 12 hours. These measures must be instituted within 72 hours of intercourse. Nausea may be a problem. Postcoital contraception can be obtained in family planning clinics.

The main side-effects of the 'Pill'

Nausea is probably related to the oestrogen dosage and can usually be relieved by changing to a preparation with less oestrogen.

Weight gain usually settles after a few cycles.

The menstrual cycle is induced to be more regular and menstrual loss is often decreased.

Thrombosis. There is now clear evidence that taking oral contraceptives carries an increased risk of venous and cerebral thrombosis. Taking the 'Pill' makes it about nine times as likely that the subject will be admitted to hospital with an episode of thrombosis. In addition, there is a slightly increased risk of coronary and cerebral arterial disease. The overall mortality is about 2 per 100 000. Older women who smoke heavily are especially at risk from thromboembolic complications. Heavy smokers in the 40–44 age group have an excess mortality of 54 per 100 000 women, and they should therefore use some other form of contraception. Thrombosis is believed to be due to the oestrogen in the 'Pill'. For this reason the oestrogen content of these preparations is kept as low as possible.

The associated arterial disease is due to the progestogen fraction of the Pill which alters the blood lipids. It is possible, but not proven, that the newer progestogens which do not have this effect on the blood will be safer.

Occasionally patients taking oral contraceptives develop *hypertension*. This is common in older women but usually improves on stopping the 'Pill'.

Many studies have been undertaken to determine whether oral contraceptives could cause cancer.

Breast. There is no clear evidence over all the groups that oral contraceptives increase the risk of breast cancer, but it is possible that their long-term use (> 8 years) carries a slightly higher risk of cancer developing under the age of 36 years.

Cervix. There is some evidence that cancer of the cervix is more common in those taking oral contraceptives. There are many complicating factors and the case is not proven. However, women who have taken oral contraceptives for more than 5 years should have an annual cervical smear.

Ovary/uterus. The use of oral contraceptives reduces the risk of endometrial and ovarian cancer.

Older women may find that conception is delayed after stopping the 'Pill'.

Other side-effects, real or imaginary, of oral conception must be set against the fact that many women feel better while taking these preparations, and also the potential reduction in abortion and unwanted and uncared-for children.

Contraindications to the use of oral contraceptives

- Thromboembolic disease, past or present
- Carcinoma of the breast or uterus

- Severe liver disease or recent viral hepatitis, previous cholestatic jaundice of pregnancy
- Pregnancy
- Hypertension (diastolic pressure >100 mmHg)
- Porphyria
- Herpes gestationis (previous)
- Focal migraine
- Progressive otosclerosis in pregnancy.

In addition to these contraindications the following may be made worse:

- Migraine
- Epilepsy
- Depression

Drugs which interfere with oral contraceptives

Certain drugs when taken with oral contraceptives will increase the rate of breakdown of the oestrogen they contain and thus decrease their efficiency and may occasionally lead to unwanted pregnancy. The most troublesome drug in this respect is *rifampicin* but *phenobarbitone* and *phenytoin*, *isoniazid* and *griseofulvin* have also been implicated. In addition, *broad spectrum antibiotics* may interfere with oestrogen absorption. The occurrence of breakthrough bleeding may give a warning that the contraceptive is ineffective. If this occurs a preparation containing 50 micrograms of oestrogen can be tried or an alternative contraceptive method used.

THE PROSTAGLANDINS

These interesting substances are formed by most cells of the body and are released as a result of a number of stimuli. They usually produce their effects locally rather than at distant sites in the body, and many of them are removed from the circulation when they pass through the lung.

Prostaglandins have been implicated in a number of pathological processes:

1. Inflammation. It seems probable that prostaglandins of the E series are the mediators in some of the changes (swelling, redness and pain) which are seen in inflammation. This is important as drugs which block the production of prostaglandins, such as aspirin, and other NSAIAs reduce the symptoms and signs of inflammation.

2. Thrombosis. Two types of prostaglandins appear to be involved in thrombosis. Thromboxanes stimulate clumping of platelets and constriction of blood vessels and thus encourage thrombosis whereas prostacycline has the reverse effect. It seems possible therefore that increasing the availability of prostacycline and decreasing that of thromboxanes would guard against thrombosis and a great deal of research is being done in an attempt to achieve this effect.

3. Effects on uterine muscle. Prostaglandins cause contraction of the uterine muscle and are concerned with both menstruation and childbirth. Prostaglandin E_2 can be used to induce labour or terminate pregnancy by causing the uterus to contract (see below).

ERGOMETRINE AND OTHER DRUGS AFFECTING UTERINE MUSCLE

Ergometrine is soluble in water. It is rapidly absorbed either from the intestinal tract or from the site of injection. Its chief action is to cause contractions of the uterus. With small doses these contractions are rhythmic but with larger doses they become very powerful and more or less continuous. They are brought about by a direct action of ergometrine on the uterine muscle. The uterus is especially sensitive to ergometrine at the time of childbirth. Ergometrine has little effect on other plain muscle throughout the body.

Therapeutics. Ergometrine is given after childbirth to cause the uterus to contract and thus prevent bleeding. It should not be given before delivery, even if the uterus is sluggish as it may produce such powerful contractions that the uterus is ruptured, or the fetus asphyxiated. The usual dose is 500 micrograms orally or by intramuscular injection or 250 micrograms intravenously. The increased contractions of the uterus are seen within 5 minutes of taking the drug by mouth.

A number of other drugs cause the uterus to contract.

Oxytocin causes contraction of the muscle of the uterus. This effect is not marked until the later stages of pregnancy, and at parturition, when extremely small amounts will cause powerful uterine contractions.

Therapeutics. Oxytocin is used to induce labour. For this purpose it is usual to use synthetic oxytocin (Syntocinon), for the naturally prepared oxytocin contains a small amount of vasopressin. The oxytocin is given by intravenous drip and the rate of infusion is regulated according to the response of the patient. There is a risk of rupture of the uterus with oxytocin and it should only be used to induce labour under expert supervision. Oxytocin is also used after delivery of the placenta to cause uterine contraction, but its effects are not as prolonged as those of ergometrine. For this reason it is sometimes combined with ergometrine as *Syntometrine* (see below). Whole posterior pituitary extract should not be used, because of its vasopressor effects.

Adverse effects. In addition to producing powerful uterine contractions which may be inappropriate in certain circumstances, oxytocin can cause a rise in blood pressure and water retention. It should not usually be combined with prostaglandins to induce labour.

Syntometrine is a mixture of ergometrine 500 micrograms and oxytocin 5 units in 1 ml. It is given intramuscularly in doses of 1 ml, and combines the rapid action of oxytocin on the uterus with the prolonged contraction caused by ergometrine. It is commonly used after the expulsion of the placenta to prevent bleeding.

Prostaglandins (see p. 183) may also activate the uterus.

Dinoprostone (prostaglandin E$_2$), is used to terminate pregnancy and to induce labour. It can be given by several routes.

1. Intravenous infusion. Higher doses are required to cause termination.
2. Extra-amniotic injection to terminate pregnancy.
3. Vaginal tablets, to induce labour.

Gemeprost (Prostaglandin E$_1$ analogue) pessaries are inserted into the vagina to soften the cervix and thus facilitate abortion during the first 3 months of pregnancy.

Adverse effects include nausea, vomiting, diarrhoea, headache and fever.

Interactions. Dinoprostone increases the effects of oxytocin and these drugs should never be given together.

Carboprost is given by intramuscular injection. It is used to treat postpartum haemorrhage when ergometrine and oxytocin have failed to control bleeding. It should only be used in specialist units.

Mifepristone is a progesterone antagonist. In pregnancy, the uterus is prevented from contracting before term by progesterone. If this inhibition is blocked the uterus can be induced to contract and thus abort the fetus.

Therapeutics. Mifepristone is used for the medical termination of pregnancy up to 63 days from the start of the last period. A single dose of 600 mg is given orally followed after 48 hours by a gemeprost vaginal pessary. This procedure must be under medical supervision.

Nursing point

Dinoprostone sterile solutions for intravenous or extra-amniotic administration must be diluted before use.
  Dinoprostone vaginal tablets should be dipped in water or saline before insertion and must not be combined with chlorhexidine cream or KY jelly. Gemeprost pessaries should be warmed to room temperature for 30 minutes before insertion and kept away from direct heat or sunlight.

Drugs inhibiting uterine contractions

Stimulation of β_2 receptors in the uterine muscles will diminish uterine activity. The β_2 agonists *salbutamol* and *ritodrine* are used in the management of premature labour and are usually given by intravenous infusion for this purpose.

A Primary   B Secondary

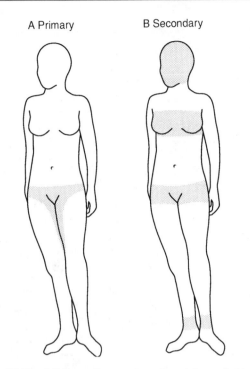

Fig. 13.12   A Primary, **B** secondary sites of discomfort in primary and secondary dysmenorrhoea. Reproduced with permission of Prentice Hall.

Dysmenorrhoea

Dysmenorrhoea is experienced by most women at some time but occasionally periods become so painful and heavy that they disrupt everyday life. Most women manage with a hot water bottle and mild analgesics. However, a nurse may be approached for advice so the type of dysmenorrhoea must be established.

Primary dysmenorrhoea is common in young women whose usual complaint is of low backache and colicky pain in the pelvic area. This is due to the cyclical release of prostaglandins in the uterus, leading to contraction of the uterine muscle and constriction of the arteries supplying the muscle, with consequent ischaemia. Other symptoms include nausea, vomiting, diarrhoea and faintness. NSAIAs (p. 105) e.g. ibuprofen or mefenamic acid, by inhibiting prostaglandins, relieve pain in most cases. They should ideally be taken after menstrual bleeding has commenced to avoid the ingestion of drugs by a possibly pregnant subject. If this fails, oral contraceptives

(oestrogen + progestogen) are frequently effective.

Secondary dysmenorrhoea affects women in their late twenties and thirties, causing a dragging pain often preceded by headaches. As its name implies, this occurs in response to some pathological condition (fibroids, endometriosis) and treatment is by removal of the cause.

Premenstrual tension syndrome (PMS)

The cyclical appearance of a cluster of symptoms in the second half of the menstrual cycle which terminate abruptly with the onset of menstruation is known as the premenstrual tension syndrome (PMS). It is very common but in only about 25% is it severe enough to require medical advice and in about 4% of women is it incapacitating.

The symptoms are legion and are both emotional and physical.

Emotional	*Physical*
Depression	Headache
Tension	Breast swelling and discomfort
Crying	Fluid retention and bloating
Aggression	Backache
Failure to concentrate	

The range of these symptoms suggests that there is more than one cause and, in keeping with this theory, women respond differently to prescribed treatments, but its relationship to the menstrual cycle indicates that it is probably related to the hormonal and metabolic changes which occur.

A selection of possible aetiological factors and treatments is given below.

1. *Changes in water and salt balance.* Levels of aldosterone which is a mineraloid hormone released by the adrenal cortex may be abnormal and fluid retention a marked feature in some cases. *Diuretics* are quite often prescribed with benefit to some patients.

2. *Elevated prolactin levels.* Prolactin is released from the anterior pituitary and stimulates lacta-

tion. When a women is not lactating its secretion is suppressed by a hormone inhibitor. Some women with PMS have raised prolactin levels. *Bromocriptine* which inhibits prolactin release has been found useful for some symptoms especially breast discomfort, but adverse effects may be troublesome.

3. *Diminished progesterone levels* have been suggested as an aetiological agent but injection of progesterone or of a synthetic substitute has not been shown to be beneficial.

4. *Changes in prostaglandin E_1 levels.* This appears important in hormone balance and it has been suggested that PMS is a manifestation of deficiency. *Gamolenic acid* (evening primrose oil) is converted into prostaglandin E_1 and, given as Efamol, it has been shown to be effective sometimes. Conversely, prostaglandin synthesis inhibition by *mefenamic acid* can improve headaches and aches and pains.

5. *Suppression of ovulation* either with the 'Pill' or with gonadotrophin releasing hormone analogues such as goserelin are again successful in a few sufferers.

6. *Various dietary modifications* have been tried. Fluctuation in blood glucose levels can be avoided by giving a 3-hourly high starch diet which may relieve symptoms but weight gain can be a problem. *Pyridoxine* has been used but with high doses there is a danger of neuropathy.

In summary, there is no overall regime to control PMS. It is probably best to treat the leading symptom and drug therapy may be a matter of trial and error.

Self-help measures

The nurse can do much to help the individual to gain insight into her problem. Keeping a diary of the menstrual cycle with daily accounts of the main symptoms and when they occur is useful. It can be used to predict the appearance of PMS in subsequent months, confirm a physical basis for the symptoms and exclude suggestions of neuroticism. It can also allow the patient to plan her life so that PMS does not clash with events such as holidays.

MALE SEX HORMONES

A hormone called *testosterone* is produced by the interstitial cells of the testis. It is responsible for the secondary male sex characteristics, including distribution of hair, deepening of the voice and enlargement of the penis and seminal vesicle.

It can be isolated from the testis, but is usually prepared synthetically.

Its release from the testis is controlled by the luteinizing hormone (LH) of the pituitary.

Therapeutics. Testosterone is used in the treatment of testicular hormone deficiency. This may be of an unknown origin or due to injury, or disease of the testis or may be secondary to lack of gonadotrophic hormone following pituitary gland disease.

Mesterolone which is similar to testosterone, is given orally in doses of 25 mg three to four times daily. Unlike testosterone it does not cause jaundice or depress spermatogenesis.

Esters of testosterone (Sustanon) can be given intramuscularly in doses of 1.0 ml 3 weekly and are released slowly from the injection site, or as an implant which is only needed 6 monthly.

Testosterone is effective in about 30% of premenopausal patients with advanced carcinoma of the breast in relieving symptoms and causing temporary regression of secondary deposits. When given to women, testosterone causes the growth of facial hair, deepening of the voice and acne.

Sex hormone antagonists

Cyproterone acetate and spironolactone block the action of male hormones at the cell receptor. They are used in various endocrine disorders where there is overproduction of male hormone causing hirsutism in the female (when it may be combined with an oestrogen) and hypersexuality in the male.

ANABOLIC HORMONES

The structure of these male sex hormones has been modified so that they have little masculinizing effect but have considerable anabolic action and are capable of building up protein in bone and other tissues. They are used occasionally to hasten convalescence and in senile osteoporosis which is due to lack of protein in bone. Their effectiveness in these conditions is not proven.

They also produce an increase in muscle bulk and have been used by athletes to improve their performance. This is undesirable since it is not only dishonest but also carries the possibility of adverse effects.

Among those used are:

Nandrolone phenylpropionate 0.75–1.0 mg/ kg weekly by intramuscular injection.

FURTHER READING

Drive J O 1989 The menopause. Medicine International 64: 2660

Editorial 1987 Contraception. Prescribers Journal 27: 1

Editorial 1989 Cancer risks from oral contraception. Lancet 1: 21

Editorial 1989 Hormone replacement therapy and cancer. Lancet 1: 368

Editorial 1990 Medical termination of pregnancy. British Medical Journal 301: 352

Editorial 1992 New gonadotropins for old? Lancet 340: 1442

Editorial 1992 Managing the premenstrual syndrome. Drug and Therapeutics Bulletin 30: 69

Editorial 1993 Treating hypoglycaemia in general practice. British Medical Journal 306: 600

Knowledon H A 1990 The Pill and cancer. Journal of Advanced Nursing 15: 1016

Prince R L et al 1991 The prevention of post-menopausal osteoporosis. New England Journal of Medicine 325: 1189

Riggs B L , Melton L J 1992 The prevention and treatment of osteoporosis. New England Journal of Medicine 327: 620

14

Drugs affecting renal function

DIURETICS

Diuretics are drugs which cause increased secretion of urine by the kidneys. They are useful in patients who are suffering from retention of water and sodium chloride (salt) which usually accumulates in the tissue spaces and is called oedema. Diuretics are not used in patients who cannot empty their bladders; this is called urinary retention.

Oedema occurs most commonly in heart failure, the nephrotic syndrome and cirrhosis of the liver.

The factors which cause fluid retention are various and depend on the underlying disease. They include:

1. Lowered cardiac output resulting in underfilling of the arterial system. This causes the kidney to excrete less salt and water and occurs in cardiac failure.

2. Raised pressure in the veins and capillaries. This leads to increased exudation of fluid from the blood to the tissue spaces, and occurs in *heart failure* and *liver cirrhosis*.

3. Low plasma proteins. This is found in the *nephrotic syndrome* where it is due to protein loss in the urine and *cirrhosis of the liver* where there is a failure to make protein.

4. Increased secretion of a hormone, *aldosterone*, by the adrenal glands which causes the kidney to retain more water and salt. This may complicate *nephrotic syndrome, cirrhosis* and occasionally *heart failure*.

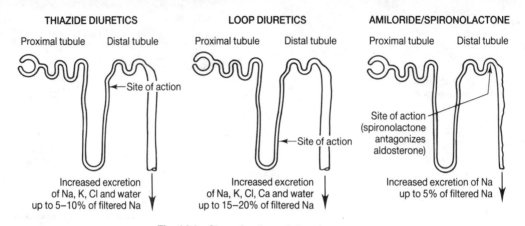

Fig. 14.1 Sites of actions of diuretics.

Renal function

The role of the kidney is to excrete the waste products of metabolism, drugs, etc., and maintain the correct amounts of water and electrolytes in the body by getting rid of any excesses which may be absorbed or produced by the body.

This is effected in two stages (Fig. 14.1).

1. At the glomeruli, water along with soluble substances is filtered from the blood. The volume of this filtration is about 100 litres of water per day and it contains glucose, electrolytes, urea and other substances.

2. In the renal tubules a selective reabsorption occurs. Glucose is normally completely reabsorbed. Water and electrolytes (including sodium, potassium, chloride and bicarbonate) are partially reabsorbed, whereas urea is almost entirely excreted. The exact amount of each substance finally excreted in the urine is controlled so that the composition of the body fluids remains constant.

DIURETIC DRUGS

All diuretic drugs produce their effect by decreasing reabsorption of water and electrolytes by the renal tubules and thus allowing more water and electrolytes to be excreted.

Water

It is common experience that in a normal person, increased ingestion of water results in an increased urine flow. When water is absorbed, it causes the plasma to become more dilute and this in turn decreases the release of antidiuretic hormone (ADH) by the posterior lobe of the pituitary gland. Less ADH reaches the kidney and this causes the tubules to reabsorb less water, so that more is excreted as the urine. In those with fluid retention, for example in heart failure, the normal response to water disappears and so it is no use as a diuretic in these circumstances.

OSMOTIC DIURETICS

Any substance which passes through the glomeruli and is not reabsorbed by the renal tubules will increase the concentration of the urine within the tubules. This prevents the reabsorption of salt and water from the tubule back into the blood and the water is then passed out and produces a diuresis. Osmotic diuretics are now little used in treating oedema.

Mannitol is sometimes used to lower raised intracranial pressure after a head injury or in a patient with a cerebral tumour. It is given intravenously as a 10% or 20% solution.

THIAZIDE DIURETICS

There are several diuretics in this group and although there are marginal differences in their actions, the general pattern of their effects is the same and they will be described together.

They are all absorbed from the intestinal tract and are therefore effective orally.

Their actions on the kidney are:

1. They interfere with the reabsorption of salt and water by the tubules, thus more fluid passes out of the tubules and causes a diuresis.
2. There is an increased excretion of potassium by the kidney.

Therapeutics:

1. *Cardiac failure*. The thiazides are used in treating the oedema of cardiac failure. They are usually given in the morning as the diuresis lasts throughout the day.
2. *Hypertension*. The thiazides have some blood pressure lowering action and may be used for this purpose, either alone or with other hypotensive drugs. For this purpose, small doses of thiazides are required, for example cyclopenthiazide 250 micrograms or bendrofluazide 2.5 mg once daily are adequate. Potassium supplements are not usually required.
3. *Cirrhosis of the liver with ascites*. The thiazides will produce a diuresis in this condition with reduction in the ascites and oedema. Care is required, however, as their use may be followed by mental changes with disorientation which it is believed is due to the potassium deficiency produced by these drugs.
4. *Nephrotic syndrome*. The thiazides can be used to treat the oedema found in this condition. Frequently, however, a more powerful diuretic will be required such as frusemide. Spironolactone (see below) can be given in addition to block the effect of aldosterone which may be produced in excess in this condition.

The following table gives some members of the group, with their relative strengths:

Preparation	Dose
Chlorothiazide	0.5–1g
Hydrochlorothiazide	25–100 mg
Hydroflumethiazide	50–100 mg
Bendrofluazide	2.5–10 mg
Cyclopenthiazide	0.25–1.0 mg
Polythiazide	0.5–4.0 mg

Chlorthalidone is very similar to the thiazides but it has a more prolonged action. The dose is 50–200 mg on alternate days.

Metolazone is a thiazide which generally has no advantage over others in the group but it will sometimes produce a diuresis when other thiazides have become ineffective or it may be combined with a loop diuretic, particularly in patients with impaired renal function. The dose is 5–10 mg daily.

LOOP DIURETICS

This group of diuretics is more powerful than the thiazides. It acts at a different site in the renal tubule (see Fig. 14.1) and interferes to a greater extent with the reabsorption of salt and water. Like the thiazides these diuretics also increase renal excretion of potassium.

Frusemide. Frusemide has a short duration of action; if given by mouth the diuresis lasts about 6 hours. It can also be given intravenously when there is an almost immediate massive diuresis which is finished in about 2 hours.

Therapeutics. Frusemide is particularly useful in:

1. Acute left ventricular failure with oedema of the lungs. In doses of 20–40 mg intravenously, frusemide rapidly clears the oedema.
2. Patients with congestive heart failure which is no longer responding to other diuretics. Frusemide is often effective when given orally in doses of 40–120 mg daily or more.
3. In oedema associated with the nephrotic syndrome especially if there is some degree of renal failure, oral frusemide is particularly useful. In these cases very large doses are sometimes used.
4. Large doses may be given when acute renal failure is developing to try and jolt the kidneys into resuming normal function.

Adverse effects of thiazide and loop diuretics

1. Hypokalaemia—this is due to increased potassium loss in the kidneys and is more marked

with high doses of diuretics. It is considered below.

2. Uric acid retention by the kidney, causing gout.

3. Decreasing glucose tolerance which may make control of diabetes more difficult and even lead to a diabetic-like state which, however, usually recovers when the drug is stopped. There may also be a temporary rise in plasma cholesterol concentration.

4. Sodium depletion—with large doses of loop diuretics, particularly when given intravenously, the patient's blood volume may be reduced rapidly causing hypotension and collapse. This can also occur with prolonged oral treatment.

5. A large and rapid diuresis can precipitate acute retention in those with prostatic enlargement.

Large doses of frusemide can cause transient deafness.

Interactions. Thiazide and loop diuretics can cause:

1. Lithium retention (see p. 128)
2. Renal damage when combined with gentamicin
3. Increase digoxin toxicity due to hypokalaemia.

NSAIAs and steroids reduce the efficacy of these diuretics.

Bumetanide. This powerful diuretic is similar to frusemide in its pharmacological action, although it is distinct chemically. It is given orally in doses of 1–4 mg daily and produces a rapid diuresis lasting about 3 hours. For an even more immediate effect it may be given intravenously. Its therapeutic uses and adverse effects are similar to those of frusemide.

DIURETICS AND POTASSIUM DEPLETION

Both the thiazides and loop diuretics cause loss of potassium through the kidney and if the plasma potassium is lowered excessively (< 3.0 mmol/litre) there is a risk of dangerous cardiac arrhythmias. This rarely occurs in patients on small doses of diuretic for hypertension or heart failure and it is adequate to check the plasma potassium level 1–2 months after the start of treatment. However, the following risk factors may require more careful monitoring and some form of potassium replacement:

1. Large doses of diuretics.
2. Poor diet—the elderly.
3. Concurrent use of digitalis—the toxicity of digitalis is increased by potassium deficiency.
4. Immediately following myocardial infarction—low plasma potassium is associated with an increased risk of dangerous arrhythmias.
5. Patients with cirrhosis of the liver are particularly sensitive to potassium depletion.
6. Concurrent use of steroids raises potassium loss.

In all these patients an attempt should be made to restore the body potassium levels. This may be achieved by:

1. **Potassium supplements**. These should be given in the form of potassium chloride. Unfortunately this substance is nauseating and can cause ulceration of the gut if given in tablet form. It is therefore formulated as *Effervescent potassium chloride tablets* (Sando-K) containing 12 mmol K or as *slow release potassium chloride tablets* (Slow-K) containing 8 mmol K.

Certain diuretics are made up as combined diuretic + potassium chloride, e.g. cyclopenthiazide + potassium chloride (Navidrex K), but are not recommended as they contain too little potassium to be useful.

2. **Potassium-sparing diuretics.** These substances have a diuretic action of their own, and if combined with a thiazide or loop diuretic prevent excessive loss of potassium.

POTASSIUM-SPARING DIURETICS

Triamterene. This drug increases the excretion of salt and water and reduces potassium excretion. It is thought that this is probably due to a direct action on the renal tubules and perhaps in addition, some anti-aldosterone activity.

Amiloride is similar but a little more powerful.

Therapeutics. Triamterene is usually combined with a thiazide diuretic to increase its efficacy and at the same time to prevent potassium loss. The dose is 200 mg daily if used alone. Amiloride can be used alone or in combination. The usual dose is 10–20 mg daily if used alone.

Adverse effects. Hyperkalaemia can occur in patients with impaired renal function and those taking ACE inhibitors or supplemental potassium.

Combinations. A thiazide or a loop diuretic can be combined with a potassium-sparing diuretic in one tablet to prevent potassium loss. Among the preparations available are:

- Co-amilozide—hydrochlorothiazide 50 mg + amiloride 5 mg per tablet
- Dyazide—hydrochlorothiazide 25 mg + triamterene 50 mg per tablet
- Co-amilofruse—frusemide 40 mg + amiloride 5 mg per tablet.

These preparations are effective and reduce potassium loss but it must be remembered that they have the adverse effects of both constituents and with co-amilozide both sodium depletion and potassium retention can occur, particularly in the elderly.

Spironolactone. Overproduction of aldosterone by the adrenal glands is a factor in maintaining oedema in a few patients with cardiac failure, and more frequently in cirrhosis of the liver and the nephrotic syndrome. The aldosterone causes increased retention of sodium and water by the kidneys.

Spironolactone blocks the action of aldosterone on the kidney and thus leads to less sodium and water retention and a diuresis. It will also cause some fall in blood pressure.

Therapeutics. Spironolactone is given orally in doses of 100 mg daily. It is usually reserved for those patients who have failed to respond to the usual diuretic drugs. It is more effective when combined with other diuretics.

It should not be used in the long term (e.g. in treating hypertension) as there is a remote risk of carcinogenicity.

Adverse effects appear rarely, but rashes and gynaecomastia have been reported.

Diuretics in cirrhosis of the liver

In such cases diuretics carry serious risks of hypokalaemia and hypotension leading to renal failure. It is best to start with spironolactone and then add a thiazide or loop diuretic cautiously a few days later. All drugs causing fluid retention (e.g. NSAIAs) should be avoided.

Diuretics in the elderly

For various reasons, not always sound, one in five people over 65 take diuretics and they are the commonest cause of adverse reactions in old people. These adverse effects are the same as those which occur in younger subjects but are more severe and may have serious consequences.

Most important is sodium depletion leading to a marked fall in blood pressure, particularly on standing, and causing faints, falls and confusion. As in other age groups disturbances of potassium and uric acid metabolism occur.

> **Nursing point**
>
> Swollen ankles in the elderly do not necessarily call for a diuretic—they may be due to sitting in a chair all day.
> If an old person taking diuretics develops diarrhoea and/or vomiting it is sometimes wise to stop the diuretic temporarily to prevent undue water and salt loss.

MISCELLANEOUS DIURETICS

Acetazolamide suppresses the activity of the enzyme carbonic anhydrase which is present in the renal tubule and the eye. In the kidney this prevents the reabsorption of sodium and water from the tubule and thus causes a diuresis. It is a poor diuretic as its effect is short-lived and is not now used for this purpose. In the eye,

---

Nursing point

The best way to monitor the efficiency of a diuretic is to weigh the patient regularly. Fluid balance charts are not always accurate but can be improved with the cooperation of the patient. Before leaving the hospital the timing of diuretic dosage must be tailored to the patient's daily programme. It is distressing to have a diuresis while stuck in your car in a traffic jam!

---

however, it reduces the formation of aqueous humour and is useful in lowering the intra-ocular pressure in glaucoma. For this purpose the initial dose is 500 mg orally or intravenously, then 250 mg 6 hourly (see p. 287). It will also help relieve mountain sickness which is due to salt and water retention.

DRUGS CHANGING THE REACTION OF URINE

Drugs making urine alkaline

Sodium citrate is the substance most commonly used to make the urine alkaline. It is usually given 2 or 4 hourly. The correct dose is that which keeps the urine alkaline, usually about 12 g daily. Sodium bicarbonate is often combined with sodium citrate and acts in a similar fashion.

Therapeutics. Occasionally urinary tract infections are treated by making the urine alkaline as this prevents the multiplication of certain bacteria. Some drugs are more rapidly eliminated by the kidney in an alkaline urine, particularly aspirin, and this may be useful in overdose.

FURTHER READING

Editorial 1988 Diuretics in the elderly, how safe? British Medical Journal 296: 1551
Editorial 1990 Thiazides in the 1990s. British Medical Journal 300: 168

Editorial 1991 Routine use of potassium sparing diuretics. Drug and Therapeutics Bulletin 29: 85
Odlind B O 1984 Site and mechanism of actions of diuretics. Acta Pharmacologica Toxicologica 54 Suppl. 1–5

15

Chemotherapeutic agents and antibiotics

Ever since it was realized that bacteria cause many diseases, man has been seeking a substance to kill the bacteria without harming the host.

The first advance was the preparation of neoarsphenamine, an organic compound containing arsenic, by Ehrlich and his co-workers. This would kill the bacterium *Treponema pallidum,* which caused syphilis, without untoward effects on the patient. Ehrlich hoped to eradicate the disease with a single injection but this proved inadequate and a long course was required.

In 1935 Domagk in Germany synthesized the first of the sulphonamide group of drugs and during the next 20 years several more were added. Before and during the Second World War the discoveries by Fleming, Florey and Chain led to the isolation of penicillin from the fungus *Penicillium notatum* and this was the first of the antibiotics. These are substances (produced by organisms) which either kill or inhibit the growth of bacteria, fungi or viruses. Since then a large number of antibiotics have been produced from various sources. Further, their structure has been modified in the laboratory to improve their efficacy and these drugs are known as semi-synthetic antibiotics.

Antibacterial drugs have revolutionized the treatment of infection and many diseases such as meningitis which previously were often fatal are now usually curable, but it must be realized that the battle against pathogenic bacteria is by no means over. Many organisms have become resistant to certain antibacterials and this requires a continuing search for new drugs and modification of those already in use. It also means that they should not be used unnecessarily.

It should be remembered that even with powerful antibacterial drugs the patient's natural resistance plays an important part in combating infection. The nurse will note that those with impaired immunity, due to prolonged illness, old age or perhaps the use of cytotoxic or immunosuppresive drugs, respond poorly to antibacterials and the infection is much harder to eradicate.

How antibacterial substances work

Drugs may interfere with bacteria in several ways. They may kill them (*bactericidal*) or prevent them multiplying (*bacteriostatic*)—in practice this distinction is not very important. It is essential that antibacterials, while eradicating the infection, do not damage the cells of the host. Figure 15.1 shows three ways in which they act.

Gram staining

In reading this chapter the nurse may be puzzled by the terms Gram-positive and Gram-negative when referring to bacteria. This indicates whether or not the bacteria take up a certain dye (Gram stain) and is a useful way to divide organisms into two groups:

Gram-positive	*Gram-negative*
Staphylococcus aureus	*Haemophilus (H.) influenzae*
Streptococcus pyogenes	*Neisseria (N.) gonorrhoea (Gonococcus)*
Streptococcus viridans	*Neisseria (N.) meningitidis (Meningococcus)*
Streptococcus pneumoniae (Pneumococcus)	*Escherichia (Esch.) coli*
	Proteus
	Pseudomonas
	Klebsiella

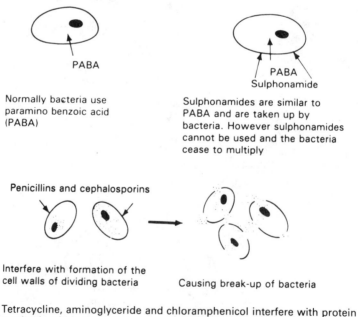

PABA

Normally bacteria use paramino benzoic acid (PABA)

PABA
Sulphonamide

Sulphonamides are similar to PABA and are taken up by bacteria. However sulphonamides cannot be used and the bacteria cease to multiply

Penicillins and cephalosporins

Interfere with formation of the cell walls of dividing bacteria

Causing break-up of bacteria

Tetracycline, aminoglyceride and chloramphenicol interfere with protein synthesis within the cell. In normal cells RNA is bound to ribosomes which are essential for protein synthesis. This group of antibiotics binds onto the ribosomes, excluding the RNA and preventing protein synthesis. Thus bacteria do not multiply.

Fig. 15.1   Some of the modes of action of antibacterial drugs.

Anaerobes

This term refers to a group of organisms with special requirements on culture and which may be responsible for various types of abdominal sepsis.

THE SULPHONAMIDES

This is one of the oldest groups of antibacterial agents. They differ to some extent in the range of organisms which they attack but most of their pharmacological properties are similar. In recent years they have been largely replaced and most have disappeared from use.

They are, with few exceptions, well and rapidly absorbed from the intestinal tract. They circulate widely in the body fluids and cross the meningeal barrier to enter the cerebrospinal fluid.

The sulphonamides circulate in the blood partially bound to the plasma proteins, and partially in the free state. Only that portion which is in the free state has antibacterial properties, or is capable of diffusing into the cerebrospinal fluid, or being excreted in the urine. After absorption the liver begins to acetylate the sulphonamides. The acetylated drugs together with unaltered sulphonamide are excreted in the urine. The acetylated sulphonamides are very poorly soluble and therefore there is danger that they will precipitate in the urine unless an adequate flow is maintained.

Most of the sulphonamides are effective against quite a wide range of bacteria, the most important of which are listed below.

Unfortunately certain of these bacteria have become resistant to the sulphonamides.

Organism	Disease
Strep. pneumoniae	Pneumonia
Strep. pyogenes	Tonsillitis, scarlet fever, septicaemia, etc.
Meningococcus	Meningococcal meningitis
Gonococcus	Gonorrhoea
Esch. Coli	Urinary infection
Various dysentery organisms	Dysentery

Table 15.1

Drug	Important features
Sulphadimidine	Well absorbed orally
Sulphasalazine	Used in ulcerative colitis. It is particularly useful for long-term maintenance treatment
Sulphacetamide	Non-irritant in solution and is used as eye drops
Silver sulphadiazine	Applied locally as a cream to prevent infection in severe burns

Table 15.1 gives a number of available sulphonamides.

Therapeutics. **Sulphadimidine** is still used in urinary infections provided that the infecting organism is susceptible. The dose is 2 g initially followed by 1 g 6 hourly. **Sulphasalazine** is given in doses of 0.5–1.0 g 6 hourly in the long-term treatment of ulcerative colitis and Crohn's disease. It is broken down in the colon to release sulphapyridine, an anti-bacterial agent, and 5-aminosalicyclic acid which has an anti-inflammatory action. The therapeutic effect is due to the 5-aminosalicyclic acid which is also available as a separate drug **mesalazine**. This is used when sulphasalazine causes side-effects. Sulphasalazine can also be used in rheumatoid arthritis (see p. 109).

Adverse effects:

1. *Nausea* can be troublesome and with sulphasalazine may be relieved by giving small and more frequent doses.
2. *Rashes* of various types, sometimes with fever.
3. *Blood dyscrasias.* Polyarteritis nodosa is a rare but dangerous complication.
4. *Sperm count* is reduced by sulphasalazine but recovers on stopping the drug.
5. *Precipitation in the urinary tract* causing obstruction. The patient should be given 2–3 litres of fluid daily to maintain a good urinary flow when on sulphadimidine.

Co-trimoxazole—trimethoprim and sulphamethoxazole (Bactrim-Septrin)

Sulphonamides affect bacteria by interfering with their use of para-aminobenzoic acid which is a precursor of folic acid which is ultimately essential in cell division. Trimethoprim also interferes with folic acid metabolism, at the phase when folic acid is changed to folinic acid to build up the cell nucleus. This requires the action of an enzyme and by combining with that enzyme, trimethoprim stops the reaction and the cell dies. The combination of a sulphonamide with trimethoprim is particularly effective in preventing bacterial cell division and is also bactericidal. Co-trimoxazole acts against the same organisms as listed under sulphonamides but can also be useful against *H. influenzae* and *salmonellae*.

Therapeutics. Each combined tablet of co-trimoxazole contains 80 mg of trimethoprim plus 400 mg of sulphamethoxazole, and the adult dosage is two tablets twice daily, although to prevent urinary tract infections one tablet daily or even less frequently is effective. Co-trimoxazole has been widely and successfully used in exacerbations of chronic bronchitis and in urinary infections. It also has a place in treating the more severe salmonella and other infections. Unfortunately, adverse effects (see below) may limit its use.

In large doses it is used to treat *pneumocystis* infection of the lung, a disease which occurs in patients whose immunity has been suppressed, often as a result of cancer chemotherapy or AIDS.

Adverse effects are largely those of the sulphonamides, namely nausea and vomiting, and occasionally blood disorders. More serious is the occasional development of the *Stevens–Johnson syndrome* with a bullous rash, mouth ulceration and fever which can be fatal.

Trimethoprim can also be used alone. At present it is largely used to treat urinary infection, the dose being 200 mg twice daily for an acute infection and for long-term use, 100 mg daily. It has less adverse effects than co-trimoxazole and has largely replaced it for urinary infections.

THE NITROFURANS

This group of chemotherapeutic agents has been investigated on and off for over 30 years. The only one now much used is nitrofurantoin.

Nitrofurantoin has quite a wide antibacterial spectrum and is considerably concentrated in the urine. It is used in the treatment of urinary tract infections, the oral dose is 100 mg four times daily. Nausea occurs sometimes but can be minimized by giving the drug after food. Other *adverse effects* include rashes and fever. It should not be used in renal failure as accumulation will occur.

THE QUINOLONES

This group of antibacterial drugs is increasingly important, several are available already and more will probably be introduced in the next few years. They interfere with an enzyme which is necessary for cell division of bacteria.

Ciprofloxacin acts against a wide range of organisms but is not very effective against some Gram-positive organisms, particularly pneumococci.

It is given orally in doses of 250–750 mg twice daily or by infusion. At present, its use should be confined to patients for whom older antibacterials are unsatisfactory, particularly for urinary infection and gonorrhoea. It is the preferred drug as a prophylactic for close contacts of meningococcal meningitis.

Adverse effects include gastrointestinal upsets and rashes. It should be avoided, if possible, in epileptics as it has a potential to cause fits, and in children it may cause damage to developing weight-bearing joints.

Interactions. It raises the blood levels of theophylline.

Enoxacin and Ofloxacin are similar to ciprofloxacin.

Norfloxacin is effective only in urinary tract infections because it is concentrated in the urine and is used when the infecting organism is resistant to the older antibacterials. The dose is 400 mg twice daily. For uncomplicated infection a 3-day course is adequate but prolonged treatment is required for severe or recurrent infections. It should be avoided in children and in pregnancy.

THE ANTIBIOTICS

β LACTAM GROUP

The β lactam antibiotics all contain the β lactam ring which is a chemical structure essential for their antibacterial activity. The group contains:

- The penicillins
- The cephalosporins
- Others.

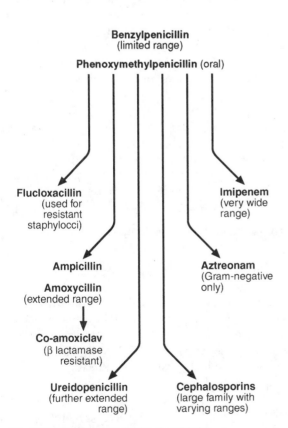

Fig. 15.2   The β lactam family of antibiotics.

PENICILLINS

The penicillins were the first of the antibiotics to be isolated. Over the years their structure has been modified repeatedly to deal with the problem of resistance to penicillin and to extend their antibacterial range. They are still probably the most widely used family of antibiotics.

Benzylpenicillin was the first penicillin to be used clinically. It is a white powder which is stable at room temperature for long periods provided it is kept sealed, but in solution it must be kept in a refrigerator and used within 5 days.

Benzylpenicillin is usually given by deep intramuscular injection which is painful and if a single dose of more than 1.8 g (3 mega units) is needed it should be given intravenously. It rapidly enters the blood stream and spreads through the body; it does not, however, cross into the cerebrospinal fluid in any great quantity, although this may be increased if the meninges are inflamed.

All penicillins are excreted by the kidneys partially through the glomeruli but the major part via the renal tubules. The excretion is rapid and blood levels have nearly fallen to zero 4 hours after injection.

If benzylpenicillin is given orally it is partially broken down by the gastric acid and is now rarely used by this route.

Benzylpenicillin is effective against a fairly wide range of organisms. The following are the most common:

Organisms	*Disease*
Streptococcus pyogenes	Tonsillitis, scarlet fever, septicaemia
Streptococcus viridans	Subacute bacterial endocarditis
*Staphylococcus aureus	Carbuncles, osteomyelitis, septicaemia, boils
Pneumococcus	Pneumonia
Gonococcus	Gonorrhoea
Meningococcus	Meningococcal meningitis

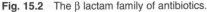

* Note that 90% of staphylococci found in hospital are now resistant to benzylpenicillin.

Treponema pallidum	Syphilis
Colstridium perfringens	Gangrene
Clostridium tetani	Tetanus
Actinomyces	Actinomycosis

Penicillins are bacteriostatic and in higher doses are bactericidal. When treating infection it is ideal to maintain the blood level of penicillin continually at bactericidal levels, and this requires 4-hourly injections. In milder infections, however, it is often adequate to give less frequent injections, for even when the blood levels of penicillin drop below bactericidal or bacteriostatic levels, the organism may take some time to recover and by that time the blood level of penicillin has risen again following a further injection.

Numerous attempts have been made to prolong the action of benzylpenicillin after injection by slowing down its release from the injection site. A successful method is to combine benzylpenicillin with procaine. The combination is called **procaine penicillin** and will maintain a satisfactory blood level for at least 12 hours. This preparation is, however, rather slow at producing a satisfactory blood level, so that if a rapid effect is required, benzylpenicillin should be given as well.

Triplopen is a mixture of benzylpenicillin, procaine penicillin and benethamine penicillin, the latter being very slowly released from the site of injection. It is given by deep intramuscular injection and because of its prolonged effect it is only needed every 2 or 3 days.

The action of penicillin can also be augmented and prolonged by slowing down its excretion. This can be done by giving *probenecid*, a drug which blocks the tubular secretion of penicillin, thus allowing the drug to accumulate in the body.

Certain organisms develop resistance to the action of penicillin. Organisms which were originally sensitive, appear to adapt themselves to the penicillin by producing a substance *penicillinase* which inactivates penicillin by attacking part of the penicillin molecule known as the β *lactam ring*. This structure is an essential part of penicillins and cephalosporins and the family of enzymes involved is sometimes known as the β *lactamases*. This is particularly so in the case of the staphylococcus and strains of this organism which are resistant to penicillin and other antibiotics are a serious clinical problem.

Other penicillins

1. There are a number of penicillins which are similar to benzylpenicillin but are effective by mouth. The example given below is not destroyed by the acid in the stomach and is fairly well absorbed from the intestinal tract. It maintains an adequate blood level for 6 hours and is therefore given four times daily.

Phenoxymethypenicillin—usual dose 250 mg four times daily.

Adequate absorption with a satisfactory therapeutic response usually occurs with oral penicillin but it is important that it is taken *30 minutes before a meal*. The patient must be carefully observed in case the drug is ineffective because of vomiting or inadequate absorption. Penicillin must then be given by injection.

2. The elucidation of the structure of the penicillin nucleus has made it possible to produce penicillins which are not broken down by penicillinase and are therefore effective against organisms (particularly the staphylococcus) which have become resistant to benzylpenicillin. In common use is:

Flucloxacillin—250–500 mg 6 hourly orally or by injection.

It is used almost exclusively for treating staphylococcal infections.

3. Broad spectrum penicillins. **Ampicillin** is an entirely new departure in that it is effective against a number of bacteria, including salmonellae, *Esch. coli*, shigellae and *Haemophilus influenzae* which are little affected by benzylpenicillin. It has proved particularly useful in chronic bronchitis, urinary infections and typhoid. The dose is 250–500 mg 6 hourly, by mouth. It can also be given by injection.

Amoxycillin is very similar to ampicillin but is better absorbed so a smaller dose is required. For this reason it is perhaps to be preferred to ampicillin. The dose is 250–500 mg 8 hourly. **Talampicillin** and **pivampicillin** both consist of ampicillin linked to another moiety. As they pass through the gut wall they are split and ampicillin is released. They, therefore, have no advantage over ampicillin except that they are rather better absorbed.

Some of the bacteria produce β lactamases which are capable of breaking down both ampicillin and amoxycillin together with other antibiotics. Antibiotics can be combined with a substance called **clavulanate** which prevents this breakdown and thus enables it to destroy β-lactamase-producing bacteria. The combined preparation of amoxycillin and clavulanate is called **Augmentin**.

4. There is a further group of extended spectrum penicillins (*ureido penicillins*) which have much the same antibacterial spectrum as ampicillin but are also effective against *Pseudomonas aeruginosa* and *Proteus morgani*. They are, however, inactivated by some β lactamases and are not therefore active against penicillin resistant staphylococci and in addition are not very effective against other Gram-positive organisms (e.g. *Strep. pneumoniae*). They are not absorbed from the gut and must be given by injection. They are reserved for serious infections with pseudomonas or when the causative organism is not known, in which case, due to deficiencies in their antibacterial spectrum they are usually combined with an aminoglycoside. They are very expensive. Some are shown in the Table 15.2.

As these drugs are excreted via the kidney the dose should be reduced in renal failure.

Mecillinam is the first of a new type of penicillin called the amidino-penicillins. It is effective against *Esch. coli* and salmonellae and has found some place in the treatment of urinary infections. Mecillinam can only be given by injection but **pivmecillinam** is well absorbed from the intestine. The usual dose is pivmecillinam 200 mg q.d.s. for urinary infections and 1.2–2.4 g daily for severe infections. Mecillinam is given i.m. or i.v. in doses of 400 mg 6 hourly.

Local applications. Penicillin can be applied as an ointment for treating infective conditions of the skin. It is effective but there is considerable risk of producing a sensitization rash, which may be worse than the original condition.

Eye drops. Penicillin may be used for conjunctival infection either as eye drops or ointment.

Adverse effects of penicillins

Considering the wide use of penicillin, it is remarkably free from toxic effects. Pain and rarely abscess formation may be seen at the site of injection. More commonly sensitization rashes occur either as a result of skin application or contact with the drug during or after systemic administration. The rash is often urticarial and is sometimes quite resistant to treatment. With ampicillin or amoxycillin the rash is sometimes erythematous and is particularly liable to occur if they are given to a patient with glandular fever or lymphoma. It may also appear after they have been stopped. Rarely penicillin causes an acute

Table 15.2

Drug	Dose	Special features
Azlocillin	15 g daily, given 8 hourly	The most effective agent against pseudomonas. Not quite so effective against other organisms
Mezlocillin	15–20 g daily, given 8 hourly	Reasonable broad spectrum action
Piperacillin	4 g every 6–8 h	Good all round activity
Ticarcillin	15–20 g daily given 4–8 hourly	Reasonable all round activity. Contains a lot of sodium so care is needed in heart failure

---

Nursing point

Always ask about previous drug reactions before giving a patient a penicillin, cephalosporin, or for that matter, any other drug.

Table 15.3 The older cephalosporins

Drug	Dose	Important features
Cephazolin	0.5–1.0 g 6 hourly	Some biliary excretion so used before surgery on the bile duct
Cephradine	0.5–1.0 g 12 hourly	Fairly β lactamase-stable

This group is being superseded.

anaphylactic reaction with collapse which can be fatal.

Other adverse effects include diarrhoea, and penicillins may reduce the efficacy of the contraceptive pill.

THE CEPHALOSPORINS

This is a large group of antibiotics which structurally bear some relationship to the penicillins in that they both contain a β *lactam ring*. They have a wide spectrum of antibacterial activity although there are differences in this respect between the older cephalosporins and the newer introductions. Most of them can only be given by injection.

Although they are efficient antibiotics they are rarely the drug of first choice as for many infections there are cheaper, effective substitutes. In the USA, however, they are more widely prescribed.

They can be divided into three groups:

1. The older cephalosporins
2. The recently introduced cephalosporins
3. Oral cephalosporins.

The older cephalosporins (Table 15.3)

These are active against:

- *Staphylococcus aureus* (including some strains resistant to penicillin)
- *Streptococcus pyogenes*
- *Streptococcus pneumoniae*
- *Esch. coli* (most strains)
- *Klebsiella* (most strains)
- *Proteus* (most strains)
- *H. influenzae* (variable)

Table 15.4 The newer cephalosporins

Drug	Dose	Important features
Cefuroxime	0.75–1.5 g 8 hourly	Good all round activity
Cephamandole	0.5–1.5 g 6 hourly	Effective against staphylococci
Cefoxitin	2 g 8 hourly	Active against *B. fragilis*
Cefotaxime	1–3 g 8 daily	Good all round activity against Gram -ve organisms
Ceftizoxime	2 g 8 hourly	Similar to cefotaxime
Ceftriaxone	1–4 g i.m. or i.v.	Once daily dosage
Ceftazidime	1–2 g 8 hourly	Useful in pseudomonal infection

They may be inactivated by β lactamases, and are excreted by the kidneys.

The newer cephalosporins

These are an improvement on the older members of the group. They are more β lactamase-stable and therefore effective against some resistant strains. In general they act against:

- *Streptococcus pyogenes*
- *Staphylococcus aureus*
- *H. influenzae*
- *Meningococcus*
- *Esch. coli*
- *Proteus.*

Some of them also have activity against pseudomonas and *B. fragilis*—important organisms in abdominal infection.

The very latest introductions do, however, show some falling off in their activity against certain Gram-positive organisms.

There are now so many of this group available that only a selection is shown in Table 15.4.

The main uses for these new cephalosporins:

1. To treat severe infection (septicaemias, etc.) when the causative organism is not known or other antibiotics are contraindicated.
2. Cefotaxime and ceftazidime penetrate well into the cerebrospinal fluid and are effective in neonatal and childhood meningitis.
3. Possibly in hepatobilary or abdominal sepsis.
4. Very rarely in resistant urinary infections.
5. Cefuroxime is effective in most chest infections even by Gram-positive organisms, i.e. pneumococci.

Most of this group are expensive.

Oral cephalosporins

Cefadroxil is given in doses of 500 mg 12 hourly and has a similar antibacterial range to the older cephalosporins. It can be used in urinary and respiratory infections.

Cefixime is similar but rather more effective against *H. influenzae*.

Although cefuroxime is ineffective if given orally a compound of it (*cefuroxime axetil*) is absorbed from the gastrointestinal tract and is now available.

Cross sensitivity to penicillin

Approximately 10% of patients who are allergic to penicillin will also be allergic to a cephalosporin. In general this excludes the use of cephalosporins in penicillin-sensitive patients although exception may be made in special circumstances.

OTHER β LACTAMS

Aztreonam has a relatively narrow spectrum of antibacterial action. It can be used against infections caused by *N. gonorrhoeae* and *H. influenzae* but is ineffective against the common Gram- positive organisms. It is given by injection, the dose being 1–2 g 8 hourly.

Imipenem has the widest antibacterial range of any antibiotic, including not only the usual Gram-positive and Gram-negative bacteria but also *pseudomonas* and *anaerobes*. The dose is 250 mg–1 g 8 hourly via an intravenous infusion, 500–750 mg 12 hourly by deep intramuscular injection. It is excreted via the kidney and is inactivated in the renal tubule by an enzyme; the urinary concentration is therefore very low. This can be prevented by combining it with *cilastatin* which inhibits the enzyme. At present its use is confined to patients in whom older antibiotics are contraindicated or ineffective.

Both these drugs can show cross sensitivity with penicillin.

THE AMINOGLYCOSIDES

This group of antibiotics interferes with protein synthesis in the bacteria and is bactericidal (i.e. they kill the bacteria rather than prevent them from multiplying). They have a fairly wide antibacterial range and one of them (streptomycin) is effective against the tubercle bacillus.

They have a number of common properties:

1. They are all given by injection if a systemic effect is required.
2. They are all excreted by the kidneys and accumulation occurs with impaired renal function.
3. They are all, to a greater or lesser degree, ototoxic and nephrotoxic.

Their antibacterial spectrum differs a little but they are generally active against a fair range of organisms.

Organism	*Disease*
Staphylococcus aureus	Septicaemia, abscesses, etc.
Strep. viridans	Endocarditis
H. influenzae	Pneumonia, meningitis
Brucella abortus	Abortus fever
Esch. coli	Renal and other infections
Proteus	Various infections,
Pseudomonas	largely abdominal
Klebsiella	Chest infection
*Tubercle bacillus	All forms of tuberculosis

*Streptomycin only.

Gentamicin

This antibiotic is widely used especially in treating severe infection by staphylococci and by various Gram-negative organisms. It is given intravenously or intramuscularly. Excretion, which is via the kidneys, is fairly rapid so that it is usually given three times daily.

It is important to maintain a correct blood level which should be measured twice weekly or more often if necessary. The peak level (half an hour after injection) should be between 5–10 mg/litre and the trough level (just before injection) should be below 2 mg/litre. The dose is adjusted to produce these levels. If the blood level is too low the antibiotic may not be effective, but if it is above 10 mg/1 for long, ototoxicity will result. It should be remembered that toxicity depends not only on the blood level but also upon the length of treatment.

The initial dose is usually 1 mg/kg body weight three times daily. This may be too little for severe infections when it is better to give 1.5 mg/kg/body weight. Elderly patients usually require reduced dosage.

Gentamicin is excreted via the kidneys and *accumulation and toxicity will occur if the drug is given to patients with impaired renal function.* In these circumstances lower dosage will be required and information is available which relates the dose necessary to the degree of impairment of renal function.

Interactions. Renal damage may occur if gentamicin is combined with frusemide or cephaloridine.

Gentamicin augments the action of curare-like neuromuscular blocking agents.

Nursing points

1. It is essential to monitor the blood levels of gentamicin etc. Renal function may deteriorate in the course of a serious illness and if impaired, accumulation and toxicity will occur.
2. Gentamicin reacts with many drugs in vitro, therefore it should be given as a bolus or separate injection.

Tobramycin, Amikacin and Netilmicin are very similar to gentamicin; however, they are sometimes effective against Gram-negative organisms which are resistant to gentamicin. They should only be used in this situation as they offer no other advantage. Side-effects are similar except that netilmicin is perhaps a little less toxic.

Spectinomycin has only one use, the treatment of gonorrheal infection due to organisms which have become resistant to penicillin. The dose is a single injection of 2 g in men and 4 g in women.

Adverse effects include rashes and vomiting.

Neomycin is an antibiotic which is bactericidal against a wide range of Gram-positive and Gram-negative organisms and against the tubercle bacillus. It is very poorly absorbed from the intestinal tract and because of toxicity is not given systemically. It is chiefly used to sterilize the gut in doses of 1 g 8 hourly for a day or two. It can also be applied locally as ear or eye drops.

Extensive local application to areas such as burns should be avoided as enough absorption can occur to cause ototoxicity.

Streptomycin

This antibiotic is derived from one of the actinomyces group of fungi.

Streptomycin is usually given by intramuscular injection. The maximum concentration in the blood is reached after about 1–2 hours and excretion is not completed for 24 hours or more. The drug is, therefore, rarely given more frequently than twice daily and often only once in 24 hours or even every other day. Following injection it spreads widely throughout the tissues but only low concentrations cross the meningeal barrier into the cerebrospinal fluid. Streptomycin is excreted in the urine. It is not absorbed after oral administration so this route is not used except for treating gut infections.

Resistance. The development of resistance to streptomycin is relatively common. It occurs rapidly with a sudden change in the bacteria rather than a gradual change as is the case with other antibiotics. This may be largely prevented by combining the streptomycin with some other chemotherapeutic agent or antibiotic to which the organism is sensitive; under such treatment the development of resistance is delayed or even prevented altogether.

Streptomycin in non-tuberculous infections

Streptomycin is now rarely used for the treatment of infections other than tuberculosis. It may be combined with tetracycline in the treatment of brucellosis.

Because it is poorly absorbed from the gut, large doses of streptomycin have been given by mouth for intestinal infections, 1 g three times daily being sufficient.

Streptomycin in tuberculosis

Streptomycin is very effective against the tubercle bacillus but resistant strains develop in about 6 weeks if it is used alone. This is prevented if it is combined with other antituberculous drugs. It is given by injection once daily, the dose being 1 g. In older patients this may be reduced to 0.75 g to decrease toxicity. In some regimes using drug combinations, streptomycin has been successful when given only twice a week. *Because it has to be injected and adverse effects can be troublesome it has now been largely replaced by other drugs.*

Adverse effects are not uncommon with streptomycin. The most important are those affecting the eighth nerve. The symptoms include high-pitched tinnitus and vertigo. This may be followed by varying degrees of deafness. The onset of these symptoms is related to the duration of treatment and the dosage of the drug employed.

Sensitization phenomena also occur with streptomycin. These may affect not only the patient but the person injecting the drug. Swelling of the eyelids is an early sign. Care should be taken when giving the drug to avoid contamination of the hands and face which may occur when the syringe is held at eye level

to measure the exact dose. The wearing of plastic gloves and a mask is advisable in those who handle large quantities of it. If hypersensitivity to it should occur, the subject can be desensitized.

Other drugs used in tuberculosis

Isoniazid. This drug is bacteriostatic and possibly bactericidal to tubercle bacilli. It is rapidly absorbed from the intestine and largely excreted by the kidneys. It diffuses widely through the body; it enters cells and it crosses the meningeal barrier to the cerebrospinal fluid in amounts adequate to inhibit the growth of the tubercle bacillus. The usual dose for an adult is 300 mg/day by mouth in divided doses.

Isoniazid is metabolized in the liver. It is possible to divide people into two groups, those who break isoniazid down rapidly and those who break it down slowly. As a result of this the rapidly inactivating group will have lower concentrations of the drug in the blood than the slow inactivators. In the dosage schemes used in the UK this is of no importance but in the Third World countries where the drug may be given less frequently to save cost, rapid inactivators are in danger of getting less than a full therapeutic effect from the drug.

Slow inactivators given large doses may develop nerve damage which can be prevented by giving *pyridoxine.*

Rifampicin. Rifampicin is effective against several Gram-positive and Gram-negative organisms and in particular against the tubercle bacillus. Its use is largely confined to tuberculosis but it can also be used in legionnaire's disease and to prevent infection in subjects who have had close contact with meningococcal meningitis. It is well absorbed orally, the dose being 450–600 mg once daily before breakfast. It is mainly excreted in the bile. It is useful in the treatment of tuberculosis but must be combined with other antituberculous drugs to prevent resistance developing.

Adverse effects are uncommon but it should not be used in patients with liver disease as it can cause changes in liver function. It may cause red discoloration of the urine and sputum and by increasing the rate of breakdown of oestrogen may reduce the effectiveness of oral contraceptives.

Ethambutol is usually satisfactory. It is given in doses of 15 mg/kg body weight. The most important side-effect is damage to the optic nerve leading to deterioration of visual acuity and colour vision. Correct dosage reduces this risk but vision should be tested before starting treatment and at 6-monthly intervals.

Pyrazinamide is powerful and effective with good penetration into tuberculous lesions and the CSF. Its use is somewhat limited by adverse effects but is justified, particularly in tuberculous meningitis, provided that the correct dose is given and the course lasts no longer than 2 months. During treatment liver function tests should be performed and alcohol avoided. The usual dose is 20–30 mg/kg/body weight daily by mouth.

Adverse effects include liver damage with jaundice, light sensitization (use a barrier cream) and attacks of gout.

Sodium aminosalicylate (PAS) inhibits the growth of tubercle bacilli. It is well absorbed after oral administration and diffuses widely with some penetration into the cerebrospinal fluid. The usual dose is 10–15 g a day in divided doses. It has an unpleasant taste and may cause vomiting and diarrhoea. Because of this it has now been superseded.

Treatment of tuberculosis

There are now a number of drugs which are effective against the tubercle bacillus. It is important, however, that:

1. At least two drugs are used at the same time to prevent the emergence of resistant organisms.
2. Treatment is continued for a long time to eradicate the infection completely. The choice of drugs is determined by the sensitivity of the infective tubercle bacillus. However, the regimes commonly used are:

Pulmonary tuberculosis

Rifampicin 10 mg/kg
Ethambutol 15 mg/kg   once daily before
Isoniazid 4–5 mg/kg   breakfast for 2 months
Pyrazinamide 20–30 mg/kg

followed by

Rifampicin
Isoniazid   for a further 4 months.

Genito-urinary tuberculosis

Isoniazid 300 mg daily for 4 months
Rifampicin 450 mg daily for 4 months
Pyrazinamide 20 mg/kg daily for 2 months

Tuberculous meningitis

Isoniazid 10 mg/kg
  + pyridoxine
Rifampicin 10 mg/kg   once daily for 8 weeks
Pyrazinamide 20–30 mg/kg

followed by

Isoniazid daily   for 10 months.
Rifampicin daily

Dexamethasone may be used early in treatment of meningitis to prevent exudates from becoming organized and causing blocks with obstruction to the flow of CSF.

Variation in the drugs used is due to their differing penetration of tissue, their effectiveness against dividing organisms and their ability to sterilize a lesion. The excellent penetration of isoniazid and pyrazinamide into the cerebrospinal fluid makes them particularly useful in meningeal tuberculosis. Resistance by the tubercle bacillus to one or other drug may require a change of regime.

Although the discovery of these drugs has revolutionized the treatment of tuberculosis, it must be realized that they form only part of the treatment. The basic measures of rest, good food and good nursing are as important as ever.

TETRACYCLINES

Following the discovery of penicillin and streptomycin a large-scale investigation was carried out into substances that were produced by various fungi.

Three important antibiotics which were discovered are known as the tetracyclines. They are very similar in chemical structure and toxic effects and are effective against the same wide range of organisms. They are: **chlortetracycline, oxytetracycline** and **tetracycline**.

The properties of these drugs are so similar that they may be considered together.

They are usually given orally and are quite well absorbed from the intestinal tract and 6-hourly dosage is satisfactory. Tetracycline hydrochloride may also be given by intravenous injection. It is, however, very irritating to the vein and is best given by continuous intravenous infusion.

After absorption the tetracyclines spread widely through the body. The penetration across the meningeal barrier into the cerebrospinal fluid is variable, being greatest in the case of tetracycline itself. The greater part of these drugs is excreted in the urine, the fate of the remainder is unknown.

The tetracyclines have a very wide antibacterial range which includes not only true bacteria but some of the larger viruses.

However, with some bacteria, resistant strains have emerged which limit their use. The main uses for the tetracyclines at present are:

Organism	Disease
H. influenzae	Bronchitis
Streptococcus pneumoniae	
Mycoplasma	Pneumonia
Chlamydia	Non-specific urethritis
Rickettsia	Typhus, Q fever etc.
Brucella abortus	Abortus fever

They are also used over long periods in the treatment of acne. Whether their efficacy in this condition is due to their antibacterial action or is due to some other factor is not known. They are usually given orally and their *absorption is reduced by* concurrent administration of iron and magnesium compounds and of calcium (including milk).

The dose for all three is 250 mg 6 hourly. Tetracycline can also be given intravenously, 500 mg being infused over 1 hour. Chlortetracycline is available as an ointment.

Demechlocycline is similar to the others in the group but rather smaller doses are required and its action is more prolonged. The dose is 150 mg four times daily.

Doxycycline is similar to the older tetracyclines but is excreted slowly so that only one dose is required daily. The other important difference is that, unlike tetracycline, it can be used when renal function is impaired (see below).

Adverse effects. A certain amount of nausea, vomiting and epigastric disturbance due to a direct irritant effect often follows administration of these drugs.

Because of their wide antibacterial spectrum the tetracyclines cause considerable changes in the bacterial flora both in the intestine and elsewhere. This often results in diarrhoea which usually recovers quickly when the drug is stopped. Occasionally, they may cause a serious enteritis due to the multiplication of a resistant organism, usually a staphylococcus. *Candida* is the other troublesome organism which may emerge in those receiving tetracyclines, causing 'thrush' in the mouth or vaginal candidiasis.

Tetracyclines damage and discolour developing teeth and should he avoided if possible from the fourth month of pregnancy until the child is 8 years old. Other toxic effects are rare but include skin rashes and other sensitization phenomena.

Tetracyclines (except doxycyline) should not be given when renal function is impaired as they cause an increased tissue breakdown with a subsequent rise of breakdown products in the blood, and exacerbation of the renal failure.

CHLORAMPHENICOL

Chloramphenicol is a broad spectrum antibiotic closely related in its action to the tetracyclines; it has, however, serious but rare toxic effects on the bone marrow which limit its use to those patients who cannot obtain benefit from any other form of treatment.

It is given by mouth and is rapidly absorbed from the intestine. It diffuses widely and crosses the meningeal barrier into the cerebrospinal fluid. It is excreted via the kidneys. Like the tetracyclines it is effective against a wide range of organisms with the important addition of *Salmonella typhi* and the *paratyphoid* group.

Therapeutics. Bone marrow toxicity limits its use and the chief indication for chloramphenicol in this country is meningitis due to *Haemophilus influenzae* and acute epiglottitis. It is also very effective in typhoid and paratyphoid fevers, though resistant strains are emerging and ciprofloxacin may be preferred. The dose for adults is 50 mg/kg daily, divided into 6-hourly doses. It is also commonly used in solution as eye and ear drops.

Adverse effects. The most serious toxic effects of chloramphenicol are on the bone marrow. Although they are rare (perhaps about 1 in 30 000 treatment courses), they are nearly always fatal when they occur. The commonest effect is aplastic anaemia, the other reported change being depression of white cells and platelets.

Toxic effects are more common after prolonged or repeated courses of chloramphenicol and their appearance may be delayed for up to 2 months after receiving the drug.

In the new-born, chloramphenicol is less rapidly broken down so that accumulation may occur producing the *'grey syndrome'* with circulatory collapse and shock.

THE MACROLIDES

Erythromycin

Erythromycin was first introduced in 1952. It is absorbed rather erratically after oral administration and diffuses widely but does not enter into the cerebrospinal fluid very well. It is bacteriostatic and acts against a wide range of organisms, including *Streptococcus pyogenes*, *Staphyloccus aureus*, *Mycoplasma pneumoniae* and *Legionella pneumophila* (causing legionnaires' disease). It is not, however, always effective against *H. influenzae*, a common cause of respiratory infection.

Resistance. Bacteria fairly readily become resistant to erythromycin, but do not show cross resistance to other antibiotics.

Therapeutics. Erythromycin has a similar range of activity to penicillin and is used instead of that drug in those who are sensitive to penicillin. It is used for various respiratory diseases including *Mycoplasma pneumoniae* and legionnaires' disease. The usual dosage is 2 g a day divided into 6-hourly doses. To reduce nausea it is best taken with food. Erythromycin can be given by injection as the preparation Erythrocin lactobionate.

Adverse effects are rare and include diarrhoea and vomiting and rarely jaundice, if injected.

Several new macrolides have been introduced.

Clarithromycin has a similar antibacterial spectrum to erythromycin but higher concentrations are found in the tissues and it has more effect against *H. influenzae*. Gastrointestinal upsets are less frequent. The dose is 250 mg twice daily.

Azithromycin appears to be similar but with a long half-life; one daily dose is adequate.

Table 15.5 The antibacterial activity of antibiotics and chemotherapeutic agents

Organism	Diseases	Co-trimoxazole	Benzyl-penincillin	Gentamicin	Ampicillin Amoxycillin	Others
Staphylococcus aureus	Purulent infection	+	++[†]	++	++[†]	Erthromycin ++ Flucloxacillin ++ Sodium fusidate ++
Streptococcus pyogenes	Tonsillitis Scarlet fever	++	++	0	++	Erythromycin ++
Streptococcus viridans	Infective endocarditis	+	++	+	++	Erythromycin ++
Streptococcus pneumoniae	Pneumonia	++	++	0	++	
Meningococcus	Meningitis	++	++	0	++	
Gonococcus	Gonorrhoea	++	++	++	++	Spectinomycin ++
Esch. Coli	Urinary tract infection	++	0	++	++	Co-trimoxazole ++ Nitrofurantoin ++
Shigella	Dysentery	+	0	+	++	Neomycin +
Salmonella typhus	Typhoid	+	0	+	++	Chloramphenicol ++
Haemophilus influenzae	Meningitis and pneumonia	+	0	+	++	Chloramphenicol ++
Treponema pallida	Syphilis	0	++	0	0	Erythromycin ++
Pseudomonas aeruginosa	Various infections, septicaemia	0	0	++	0	Ureido penicillins ++ some new Cephalosporins +
Chlamydia	Non-specific urethritis	0	0	0	++	Erythromycin ++ Tetracycline ++

Very effective ++   Sometimes effective +   Little or no action 0
[†] owing to resistance—flucloxacillin + +

The precise place of these new macrolides in treatment is still not settled but they appear to be an improvement on erythromycin. They are, however, considerably more expensive at present.

MISCELLANEOUS ANTIBIOTICS

Lincomycin and clindamycin are effective against many Gram-positive organisms and in addition clindamycin can be used to treat infections by anaerobic organisms particularly those which complicate bowel surgery. They are well absorbed when taken orally and appear to penetrate into bone. This makes them particularly useful for treating infection in bone. The dose of clindamycin is 150 mg four times daily.

Adverse effects are not common; diarrhoea may be a problem and rarely takes the form of a serious colitis (*pseudomembranous colitis*).

Polymixin is effective against a wide range of Gram-negative organisms. It is particularly useful applied locally for resistant infections by such organisms as pseudomonas, for example, otitis externa.

Sodium fusidate is effective against resistant *staphylococci*. Its main use is combined with other antibiotics in the treatment of severe staphylococcal infections. It is given orally in doses of 1–2 g daily and is relatively free of side-effects though high doses may cause jaundice which recovers when the drug is stopped.

Vancomycin is particularly useful in treating severe staphylococcal infections which are resistant to other antibiotics. It is given by slow intravenous infusion and the dose is controlled by measuring blood levels. It is ototoxic and nephrotoxic and is often given into a central vein as it can cause venous thrombosis.

Teicoplanin is similar but with considerably less adverse effects. The dose is 200–800 mg daily i.v. or i.m.

ANTIBIOTICS USED IN FUNGAL INFECTIONS

Nystatin. This antibiotic binds to the wall of the fungus causing it to leak. It is very poorly absorbed after oral administration and is therefore used to treat infections of the intestinal tract or is applied locally. It is particularly used in *Candida* infection. Oral infections respond to nystatin tablets (500 000 units) dissolved in the mouth four times daily but some patients find the taste intolerable and may prefer nystatin pastilles (100 000 units). It is very effective in treating vaginal candidiasis, one pessary being inserted daily for 14 days. Nystatin cream should be applied to the penis of the sexual partner over the same period.

Clotrimazole and miconazole are most effective if applied locally as pessaries in the treatment of vaginal candidiasis. Miconazole is available as a gel for treating oro-pharyngeal infection. Both can be applied to the skin as a 1% ointment for dermatophytoses.

Ketoconazole is largely used in severe candidiasis and other systemic fungal infections. It can be given orally and is well absorbed, the dose being 200–400 mg daily.

Adverse effects. The most important is jaundice when the drug must be stopped. Others include nausea, drowsiness and rarely, adrenal suppression.

Itraconazole is used in systemic candidiasis and dermatophyte infections. The dose is variable and the capsules should be taken immediately after food to ensure maximum absorption. It should not be used in liver disease.

Fluconazole is effective in candidiasis and serious adverse effects, particularly liver damage, have not been reported. For vaginal candidiasis a single oral dose of 150 mg is adequate and for oro-pharyngeal injection 50 mg daily for 7–14 days is required.

Griseofulvin is administered orally in the treatment of various fungal infections. It is used in most types of fungal infection of the skin, particularly in ringworm of the scalp. The dose is 250 mg twice daily by mouth and the drug may be continued for several weeks.

Adverse effects. Gastrointestinal upsets may occur when it is used and griseofulvin may enhance the action of alcohol taken at the same time as the drug.

Terbinafine is given orally for tinea infections. The dose is 250 mg daily for 2–4 weeks.

Amphotericin B. This is used in systemic infection with yeast-like organisms, namely systemic *candidiasis, cryptococcal meningitis* and *histoplasmosis*. It is given intravenously by infusion of 250 micrograms/kg over 6 hours. This frequently causes fever and nausea which can be reduced by giving 50 mg of hydrocortisone i.v. at the start of treatment. In addition, systemic treatment usually causes some renal damage. The dose is increased up to 1 mg/kg every other day. It is also available in lozenges containing 10 mg of amphotericin B which are given four times daily in the treatment of oral candidiasis.

Flucytosine is an antifungal agent which is effective against *Candida albicans* and *Cryptococcus*. It is given orally in doses of 200 mg/kg per day divided into four doses. It is excreted by the kidney and therefore reduced dosage may be required in patients with impaired renal function. Side-effects are rare but depression of the blood count has been reported.

CANDIDIASIS

This is common and troublesome problem. It can occur for no apparent reason but is particularly common in the ill, particularly those on broad spectrum antibiotics, those receiving drugs which suppress immunity (i.e. cytotoxics and steroids), AIDS sufferers, diabetics and infants. It may affect the mouth (thrush), the vagina or other mucous surfaces. Rarely, it enters the blood stream and becomes a systemic infection.

Treatment

Oral Candidiasis

Acute   Nystatin 500 000 unit tablets sucked 6 hourly or amphotericin B 10 mg tablets sucked 6 hourly.

Chronic   Fluconazole 50 mg daily or itraconazole 100 mg daily for up to 14 days.

Children   Miconazole gel.

Oesophageal, intestinal or systemic candidiasis

Fluconazole 50–400 mg daily.

Vaginal candidiasis

Fluconazole single oral dose of 150 mg or itraconazole 200 mg twice daily for 1 day Clotrimazole vaginal tablet 500 mg, one inserted at night as a single dose.

Nursing points

1. In oral candidiasis remove dentures (if any) during treatment. They should be soaked in 1% sodium hypochlorite overnight and rinsed before being worn again.

2. In vaginal candidiasis do not forget to treat the partner (if any) with a cream preparation.

Systemic fungal infections

These are an increasing problem because of the large number of immunocompromised subjects due to AIDS, cancer chemotherapy and other causes. Until fairly recently amphotericin B and flucytosine were the only drugs available but recent introductions including fluconazole and itraconazole are equally, and sometimes more, effective. The correct drug for a particular fungal infection is still being studied and the choice of treatment requires expert guidance.

TRICHOMONACIDES

Trichomonas vaginalis is a small mobile parasite which frequently causes vaginitis and occasionally urethritis in the male.

Metronidazole. Metronidazole given orally in doses of 200 mg three times daily for 1 week will eradicate trichomonas in about 90% of patients. It is relatively free of *adverse effects* but may cause nausea, headaches and skin rashes. *It interacts with alcohol producing headaches and flushing and with prolonged use can cause nerve damage.*

Metronidazole is also used in treating infections by anaerobic organisms such as bacteroides. Such infections frequently complicate abdominal operations involving the intestines. It may be used prophylactically before operation, a suppository containing 1 g being given 2 hours before operation and repeated 8 hourly until oral medication with 400 mg 8 hourly can be started. For established infection 400 mg 8 hourly is satisfactory or the drug can be given intravenously, the dose being 100 ml (500 mg of metronidazole) infused every 8 hours. It is highly effective in amoebiasis and giardiasis (see p. 226).

It is advised that metronidazole is not used in the first 3 months of pregnancy although there is no evidence that it causes fetal damage.

ANTIVIRAL AGENTS

Viruses cause a number of diseases and there is a continuous search for a cure. The difficulty in treating viral infections is that viruses live within the human cell and they are not very accessible and, being simple structures, are not easy to kill. Furthermore, a great deal of virus multiplication occurs before the patient develops symptoms.

Idoxuridine has been shown to be useful in acute dendritic ulcers of the eye caused by the virus of herpes simplex. It is applied to the eye as a 0.1% solution at frequent intervals. It may also be applied as a 5% solution (Herpid) to the rash of herpes zoster (shingles) to promote healing.

Note: *Herpid must not be applied to the eyes.*

Acyclovir. This agent is effective against the herpes viruses. It enters the infected cells where it is changed into a powerful antiviral agent.

Therapeutics.

1. It can be applied as a 3% ointment five times

daily to treat ulceration of the cornea due to herpes simplex virus and should be continued for 3 days after healing.

2. Given orally in doses of 200 mg five times daily for 5 days it accelerates the healing of genital herpes. Very severe attacks may require parenteral treatment.

3. A 5% cream of acyclovir is only effective in labial herpes if used in the prodromal period when there is only a local burning sensation.

4. In generalized herpes simplex infection in the immunosuppressed or in herpes meningo-encephalitis it is given by intravenous infusion, 5 mg/kg over 1 hour, every 8 hours. This may cause an apparent deterioration of renal function which should be monitored. Patients with impaired renal function will require smaller doses.

5. Acyclovir is not usually needed in herpes zoster (shingles) but if the ophthalmic branch of the trigeminal nerve is involved, this may be followed by prolonged neuralgia and damage to the eye and acyclovir 800 mg five times daily should be given for 7 days. It should be started within 48 hours of the onset of symptoms.

Adverse effects include rashes, nausea and vomiting.

Amantadine (see also p. 151) has some action against the influenza virus. 100 mg twice daily for 5 days may prevent an attack in those at risk.

Ganciclovir is used specifically for the treatment of serious infections by the cytomegalovirus. The disease is usually mild except in the immunosuppressed (e.g. AIDS) and as a risk to the fetus in pregnancy. It is given by intravenous infusion.

The most serious *adverse effect* is suppression of the white cell count and of the platelets, which usually recover when the drug is stopped.

THE INTERFERONS

This is a family of protein-like substances produced by various cells in the body in response to viral infections. They have the ability to act on cells and increase their resistance to viral infections and may also modify the immune response. In addition they control the growth and differentiation of certain cells.

Interferons can now be produced synthetically and have been used in both neoplastic and infective disease in man. Their main success has been in treating leukaemias particularly the hairy-celled types, and to a lesser degree in some other forms of cancer. In the control of viral infections their usefulness is limited. They are given by injection which may cause an influenza-like illness.

BACTERIAL RESISTANCE

With the increasing use of antibiotics some organisms have produced resistant strains, especially common with some organisms (for example staphylococci and *Esch. coli*). Certain antibiotics seem particularly liable to produce resistant strains.

Resistance may be produced in several ways. In any population of bacteria there may be a few organisms which are resistant to an antibiotic and when all the sensitive organisms have been killed off, the resistant ones are left to flourish and multiply. These resistant organisms have often been produced by mutations (changes in their nuclear make-up). It has also been shown that certain Gram-negative bacteria can transmit resistance to each other, and even to different types of bacteria. It follows therefore that wherever antibiotics are widely used (as in hospitals) resistant strains will appear. In order to reduce resistance to a minimum certain precautions should be taken.

1. Antibiotics should only be used when really necessary.

2. Antibiotics should be given in adequate doses.

3. The use of antibiotics prophylactically is generally to be deplored as it breeds resistant strains. There are exceptions to this rule, i.e. the use of penicillin to prevent tonsillitis in patients who have had rheumatic fever and to prevent endocarditis when those with damaged heart valves

have dental treatment or before certain operations.

4. In certain circumstances, i.e. the treatment of tuberculosis, the use of several antibiotics together may prevent resistant strains developing.

ANTIBACTERIALS IN THE TREATMENT OF SOME COMMON INFECTIONS

Tonsillitis

Minor sore throats are usually viral and do not require antibiotic treatment but streptococcal throat infection should be treated with phenoxymethylpenicillin 250 mg four times daily. If vomiting is a problem, benzylpenicillin should be given by injection. This drug is also used in smaller doses over long periods to prevent throat infection in those who have had rheumatic fever and thus decrease the chance of recurrence.

Bronchitis

A mild attack of acute bronchitis in an otherwise healthy adult does not usually require antibiotic treatment and is frequently due to a viral infection. A severe attack or an acute exacerbation of chronic bronchitis is best treated with co-trimoxazole 2 tablets 12 hourly or amoxycillin 250 mg three times daily as the infection in these circumstances may be due to *Haemophilus influenzae*, *Streptococcus pneumoniae* or *Moraxella catarrhalis*.

Pneumonia

The problem with pneumonia is that it may be caused by various bacteria with different antibiotic sensitivities. The following table is a guide but is by no means definitive.

Type of pneumonia	Usual organism	Antibiotic
Lobar	*Pneumococcus*	Benzylpenicillin 600 mg i.v. or i.m. 6 hourly
Severe in previously healthy	*Pneumococcus* *Staphylococcus*	Ampicillin 600 mg i.v. +
cause unknown	*Legionella* *Mycoplasma*	Erythromycin 500 mg i.v. both 6 hourly
Bronchopneumonia often in chronic bronchitis	*Pneumococcus* *H. influenzae*	Amoxycillin 500 mg orally 8 hourly
Postinfluenzal	*Staphylococcus* (often)	Ampicillin 500 mg i.v. + Flucloxacillin 500 mg i.v. 6 hourly. If staph. proved, add sodium fusidate 500 mg i.v. 8 hourly
Primary atypical	*Mycoplasma*	Erythromycin 500 mg 6 hourly
Legionnaires' disease	*Legionella*	Erythromycin up to 1.0 g 6 hourly + rifampicin 600 mg i.v. daily
Aspiration pneumonia (postoperative)	Mouth organisms	Ampicillin 500 mg i.v. 6 hourly + metronidazole 400 mg 8 hourly

Sputum and blood cultures may help the *correct choice of antibiotic when results are available.*

Urinary infections

Urinary infections are usually due to *Esch. coli* and respond satisfactorily to trimethoprim 200 mg 12 hourly for 5 days. Another approach which has proved useful is to give two doses of amoxycillin (3 g per dose) at 12 hourly intervals.

In some areas the organism has become resistant to these antibacterials and norfloxacin 400 mg twice daily or ciprofloxacin should be used. In serious infections gentamicin can be added to the regime.

It is sometimes necessary to use antibacterials prophylactically, particularly in children. Trimethoprim 100 mg or less at night or on alternate days is usually adequate.

Meningitis

Meningitis may be caused by a variety of organisms and its treatment is complicated because certain antibiotics penetrate poorly into the cerebrospinal fluid. Drugs which penetrate poorly have been given intrathecally.

Good penetration

Sulphonamides
 (particularly
 sulphadiazine)
Chloramphenicol
Tetracycline
The newer cephalosporins

Poor penetration

Penicillin
Streptomycin

Meningococcal meningitis

This should be treated with benzylpenicillin 2 mega units (1.2 g) intramuscularly, every 4 hours. A certain amount of penicillin will pass through the inflamed meninges and this is adequate. Alternatively cefotaxime or ceftriaxone are equally effective.

Prevention. Close contacts of patients with meningococcal meningitis should be given rifampicin 10 mg/kg twice daily for 2 days for children, or ciprofloxacin 500 mg single dose for adults.

Meningitis in neonates

This is usually due to Gram-negative organisms and is treated either with gentamicin and ampicillin or with a new cephalosporin such as ceftriaxone or cefotaxime.

Streptococcus pneumoniae meningitis

This does not usually respond so well as meningococcal infection. The usual treatment is with benzylpenicillin 20 mega units i.v. daily; however, resistant strains may make it preferable to start treatment with cefotaxime.

Haemophilus influenzae meningitis

This is treated with chloramphenicol 1 g i.v. followed by 500 mg 6 hourly i.v. or orally. Alternatively cefotaxime 100–200 mg/kg/day in divided doses (for children) is equally effective.

Infective endocarditis

This is an infection of damaged heart valves usually with the *Streptococcus viridans*. Because the organisms are buried in the thick vegetation on the valves they are difficult to reach and kill with antibiotics, so that prolonged treatment with high doses is needed. If the organism is sensitive to penicillin, benzylpenicillin 1.2 g i.v. 4 hourly plus gentamicin is given for 2 weeks followed by amoxycillin 500 mg 8 hourly for a further 2 weeks. If the organism is less sensitive, benzylpenicillin and gentamicin should be continued for 4 weeks. Other organisms may require other regimes and the management should be worked out with a microbiologist.

If a 'butterfly' needle is used to give the antibiotics intravenously, it is necessary to change the site of the cannula regularly or local infection will occur.

Prevention. The trauma of dental treatment often releases micro-organisms into the blood. If the patient has damaged heart valves, the organism settles on the valve and sets up infection. This can be prevented by giving an antibiotic to cover dental treatment. A single oral dose of 3 g of amoxycillin given 1 hour before treatment is easy to give and most satisfactory. For children from 5–10 years the dose is 1.5 g and for those under 5 years is 750 mg. For people who are sensitive to penicillin, erythromycin 1.5 g orally 1 hour before treatment followed by 500 mg 6 hours later or clindamycin 600 mg can be used.

Staphylococcal infections

These cover a wide range including simple boils and carbuncles, and extending to severe and sometimes fatal septicaemias, pneumonias and osteomyelitis. Mild infections usually respond to phenoxymethylpenicillin, but the severe infections are often due to organisms which have become resistant to penicillin. In these circumstances flucloxacillin 250–500 mg four times daily by mouth or by injection is given. Other useful antibiotics in staphylococcal infections are gentamicin, erythromycin, clindamycin, sodium fusidate and vancomycin or teicoplanin. One or other of these is often combined with flucloxacillin.

Staphylococcus epidermidis which lives on the skin and was considered unlikely to cause infection is now emerging as a danger in the immuno-suppressed and patients with artificial heart valves. Careful choice of the correct antibiotic is required and vancomycin may be needed.

Intestinal infections

Intestinal infections can be caused by various organisms, the common ones in this country being *salmonellae* and *shigellae*. Although these organisms are sensitive to a number of antibiotics it has been found that their use does not hasten recovery and may lead to an increased number of chronic carriers of these infections. Antibiotic treatment is not indicated, therefore, except in the dangerous systemic infection by *Salmonella typhi* (typhoid or paratyphoid fever) which is treated with ciprofloxacin or chloramphenicol.

Septicaemias

Septicaemias are becoming common particularly in ill and/or immunosuppressed patients. Various bacteria may be implicated and initial treatment aims at a wide antibacterial effect until the nature of the infection becomes clear as a result of blood cultures. Gentamicin combined with flucloxacillin and metronidazole is frequently used but there are many other possibilities.

Gram-negative septicaemia in particular affects those who have undergone extensive surgery or have depressed immunity. It is a very dangerous infection leading rapidly to organ failure. It should be treated as early as possible with a combination of antibiotics. In addition, *Centoxin (HA-1A)* which neutralizes the toxin produced by Gram-negative organisms, can be given and this reduces mortality. It is infused intravenously over 30 minutes. The main problem is expense—at the time of writing a single dose costs £2200; therefore, it is important that strict criteria are laid down for its use.

Listeriosis which is rare but particularly attacks pregnant women and immunosuppressed subjects responds to amoxycillin. Gentamicin should be added in seriously ill patients.

Acquired immunodeficiency syndrome (AIDS)

This is caused by the human immunodeficiency virus (HIV). Following infection with the virus there is a latent period, often lasting several years before AIDS develops. Whether all those infected with the virus will ultimately develop AIDS is not known.

The virus enters and destroys the T (helper) cells which are necessary for the immune response, thus the patient becomes susceptible to infections which are eventually fatal.

Anti-infective treatment can therefore be:

1. To interfere with the HIV virus itself
2. To treat the complicating infections.

There is as yet no agent which can eradicate the virus; the difficulty is that it lives within the host cell and uses the processes in that cell to reproduce itself.

Zidovudine delays or arrests the replication of the HI virus and, thus, the progress of the disease but its effects are temporary. It is used to treat patients with HIV infection who have developed symptoms and has been shown to enhance well-being and to prolong life. It does not, however, cure the disease. It does not prevent the development of AIDS if given to asymptomatic patients with HIV infection.

Adverse effects include bone marrow suppression, nausea, headache and muscle pains. Toxicity is increased by concurrent paracetamol.

Complications of HIV infection

Pneumocystis carinii pneumonia is common and is treated by high-dose co-trimoxazole or by intravenous *pentamidine*.

Relapse can be prevented by long-term treatment with co-trimoxazole, inhaled pentamidine or dapsone.

Patients with AIDS are also susceptible to various fungal and viral injections and to tuberculosis.

PREVENTION OF SURGICAL SEPSIS

Antibacterial agents are now commonly given before operations to prevent postoperative sepsis. Opinions differ as to the best drugs to use but the following are popular. Prophylaxis is most effective if antibiotics are given within 2 hours before surgery.

Acute appendicitis	Metronidazole suppository inserted 2 hours before surgery and repeated 8 hourly until oral treatment is possible. Continue for 48 hours + cefuroxime at induction and for 48 hours.
Large bowel surgery	Metronidazole as above + cefuroxime at induction followed by doses at 8 and 16 hours.
Biliary surgery	Not required in elective surgery, otherwise, cefuroxime as above with premedication and then 8 hourly for 48 hours.
Amputation of ischaemic limb	Metronidazole as above + flucloxacillin 500 mg i.v. with premedication and 8 hourly for 48 hours.
Hip replacement	Ampicillin + flucloxacillin as above for 48 hours.

Practical points in the administration of antibiotics

1. Oral penicillins and tetracyclines should be given 30 minutes before meals to facilitate absorption. Erythromycin, sodium fusidate and metronidazole should be given with or after food to minimize nausea.

2. In general, intravenous antibiotics should be given as a bolus. A few, e.g. piperacillin, are given as short-term infusions. If long-term infusions are used, remember that some antibiotics are unstable in certain solutions and rapidly lose their potency. Among the most important are:

Benzylpenicillin, Ampicillin	Lose activity in dextrose solutions.
Gentamicin	Unstable in solution and inactivated if combined with penicillins.

Do not as a rule mix drugs in an infusion bottle and if this is necessary, check their compatibilities with the pharmacist.

3. When making up solutions for injection avoid contamination of hands etc. due to the risk of contact dermatitis. Hands should be washed after as well as before giving injections and in certain circumstances gloves may be worn.

4. When patients are taking antibiotics at home, compliance must be assured by full explanation of its importance.

FURTHER READING

Angel J 1992 The modern management of pulmonary tuberculosis. Prescribers Journal 32: 144
Classen D et al 1992 The timing of the prophylactic administration of antibiotics and the risk of surgical wound infection. New England Journal of Medicine 326: 281
Editorial 1987 Ciprofloxacin—an important new antibiotic. Drug and Therapeutics Bulletin 25: 69
Editorial 1988 Zidovudine and other drugs against HIV.

Drug and Therapeutics Bulletin 26: 101
Editorial 1990 The penicillins today. British Medical Journal 300: 1289
Editorial 1991 More macrolides. British Medical Journal 303: 594
Editorial 1993 Zidovudine, now or later? Lancet 329: 351
Finch R 1988 Antibacterial chemotherapy: Medicine International 52: 2146
Finch R 1989 Bacterial meningitis. Prescribers Journal 29: 2
Infection Today 1988 Lancet Ltd, London

16

Sera, vaccines and the antihistamines

SERA AND VACCINES

THE IMMUNE REACTION

The human body is continually subjected to the risk of infection by microorganisms (bacteria, viruses, fungi) or to damage by toxins produced by bacteria. These are known collectively as antigens.

The cells that recognize and react to antigens are called lymphocytes. They are distributed throughout the body in blood, lymph and lymphoid tissues (spleen, lymph nodes, tonsils and adenoids). All lymphocytes originate in the bone marrow, but there are two main groups, the B and T cells which mature differently and help to defend the body against foreign antigens in different ways (Fig. 16.1).

Humoral immunity

Humoral immunity is a property of the B lymphocytes which mature in the spleen and lymph nodes after they leave the bone marrow. B lymphocytes are specific for particular antigens and the body can produce hundreds, possibly thousands of types of B lymphocytes each able to respond to a different microorganism. When an antigen gains access to the tissues the B lymphocytes become activated, dividing many times to form a clone of identical plasma cells. The plasma cells release proteins called immunoglobulins, also known as antibodies. Antibodies circulate in the blood and combine with antigens to neutralize their effects and destroy them. Once the

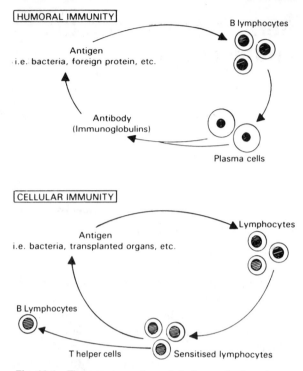

Fig. 16.1 The sequence of events in the production of humoral and cellular immunity.

antigens have been removed most of the plasma cells disappear but a few persist as memory cells. If a second exposure occurs the memory cells multiply rapidly and release antibodies even more swiftly than during the first exposure. This establishment of 'memory' by the B lymphocytes forms the basis of active immunization against bacteria and the harmful toxins they produce (see below).

Cell-mediated immunity

Cell-mediated immunity is a property of the T lymphocytes which mature in the thymus gland before they enter the circulation. T lymphocytes do not produce antibodies but are an essential component of the immune respond as B lymphocytes require them to function properly. Some T lymphocytes (T helper cells) appear to play an important role 'switching on' the immune response when antigens invade, while others 'switch off' the immune response when the body

no longer requires it. Cell-mediated immunity is especially important in the rejection of foreign materials such as transplanted organs, and in chronic infections like tuberculosis. People whose cell-mediated immunity is impaired by HIV infection, which destroys the T helper cells, become very prone to fungal and protozoal infections which T lymphocytes usually keep in check.

ACTIVE IMMUNIZATION

The principle of this method is to promote the production by the patient of antibodies or sensitized lymphocytes to certain bacteria or toxins produced by bacteria, before infection occurs. If the patient then becomes infected, the antibodies are quickly produced and are capable of rapidly dealing with the infecting organism or its toxin and thus preventing or minimizing the disease.

Antibodies are usually produced by injecting into the patient killed or modified bacteria which, although harmless, are still capable of producing antibodies. These bacteria are known as a vaccine. Two good examples of this method are the production of immunity to typhoid by injection of dead typhoid bacilli and the widespread immunization against poliomyelitis by the Sabin vaccine which is a live virus which has been rendered harmless.

Similarly, bacterial toxins may be modified to produce toxoids which are no longer harmful, but capable of acting as antigens. They are then injected and protect against future damage from the particular toxin. Good examples of toxoids are the various diphtheria toxoids which produce immunity to the very dangerous toxin produced by the diphtheria organism.

Following injection of the antigen, whether vaccine or toxoid, there is usually an interval of a few days before antibodies appear; these may then persist for varying periods from a few months up to many years. It is often the practice to give two or more injections of the antigen to produce a higher level of immunity.

Active immunization is used in the prevention of the following diseases: measles; mumps; rubella; diphtheria; whooping cough; tetanus; typhoid; typhus; yellow fever; cholera; tuberculosis; smallpox; poliomyelitis; hepatitis A and B; influenza; meningitis; rabies.

As can be seen from the foregoing paragraph, active immunization may take several weeks before enough antibodies are produced to be effective. This is quite satisfactory as a prophylactic measure, but is not much good to treat established disease. Under these conditions passive immunization is used.

PASSIVE IMMUNIZATION

In this method of immunization the appropriate antibody against the invading organism or toxin is injected. This antibody is produced on a large scale by injecting an antigen, either vaccine or toxoid, into an animal until a high blood level of antibody is obtained. Some of the animal's blood is then removed and the antibody extracted and stored until it is required. Following injection of antibody, immunity will last about 2 weeks.

This method suffers from the disadvantage that it is not possible to completely purify the antibodies produced and there is therefore a risk of a hypersensitivity reaction. Certain types of antibody can be obtained from human blood, either after the subject has been actively immunized or has suffered a particular infection. These antibodies contained in human immunoglobulin are safer and rarely produce a serious reaction although there may be discomfort at the injection site. Common examples are diphtheria antitoxin which is obtained from horse serum and antitetanus immunoglobulin injection from human blood.

ADMINISTRATION OF SERUM

Antitoxin raised in animals, often called *antiserum*, carries a real risk of a hypersensitivity reaction. This is particularly liable to occur in patients who have had previous serum injections or who suffer from allergic disorders (e.g. asthma). It is due to the antibody in the serum reacting with antigens already present in the patient, releasing histamine and other substances. If possible, antibodies obtained from the blood of immune humans should be used. They are called immunoglobins and reactions are much less likely to occur. Serum reactions take two forms.

Immediate or anaphylactic reaction. Within a few minutes of injection the patient collapses with difficulty in breathing, low blood pressure and sometimes, widespread urticaria. Rarely it can be fatal.

Serum sickness occurs about a week after injection of serum. The patient is pyrexial with a rash and arthritis. It clears up in a few days.

Nursing point
Sera and vaccines should be kept in a refrigerator at 2–8°C otherwise they may become inactive.

Precautions when injecting serum

Ask the patient:

- Have you had serum before?
- Have you had asthma or eczema?

If both answers are negative, give 0.1 ml of serum subcutaneously and if there is no reaction in 30 minutes the rest may be given and the patient kept under observation for a further 30 minutes.

If the patient has had serum previously or suffers from allergic disorders it is best to use 0.1 ml of a 1:10 dilution of serum for the test dose. These precautions may well be unnecessary if human immunoglobin is used but are mandatory for animal-raised serum.

The management of anaphylaxis and serum sickness are considered on page 265.

Whenever serum is injected by any route a syringe of 1:1000 adrenaline, an antihistamine and hydrocortisone hemisuccinate should be ready at hand in case of immediate reaction.

ANTISERA

Diphtheria antitoxin is an antiserum raised in animals and there is a real risk of a hypersensitivity reaction.

Dose: Prophylactic —500–2000 units
intramuscularly.
Therapeutic —Not less than 10 000 units
intramuscularly or
intravenously.

Tetanus antitoxin is an immunoglobin prepared from human sources, with little or no risk
of a hypersensitivity reaction. Following injury:

Immunized patients require a booster dose of
vaccine to stimulate immunity. Extensive and
dirty wounds may need a local infusion of tetanus immunoglobin plus antibiotic cover.

Non-immunized patients require 500 units of
tetanus immunoglobin and a course of tetanus
vaccine should be started. These should not be
given in the same syringe nor into the same site.
This should be combined with antibiotic cover.

VACCINES

Adsorbed diphtheria vaccine (BP) is prepared by adsorbing toxoid onto aluminium
phosphate:

Dose: Adult: Primary —0.5 ml, three
immunization doses at monthly
intervals.
Reinforcement —0.5 ml, one dose.
Child: Dose as instructed.

Adsorbed tetanus vaccine (BP). Dose: Three
doses of 0.5 ml i.m. at intervals of 6 weeks. In
addition to single vaccines, combined vaccines
stimulating immunity to diphtheria, whooping
cough and tetanus are available and are frequently used for immunizing infants.

Hib is a vaccine against *Haemophilus influenzae
type b*. Three doses are given at monthly intervals
in the first year of life.

**Diphtheria, tetanus and pertussis vaccine
(BP)** is given in doses of 0.5 ml i.m. For initial
immunization three injections are given at intervals (see Table 16.1).

Brain damage may occur occasionally after the
administration of pertussis vaccine; the frequency is difficult to assess but is probably less
than 1: 80 000. There is also, of course, the risk

Table 16.1

Age	Vaccine	Note
During first year of life	Triple (diphtheria tetanus and pertussis) + polio + Hib	First dose at 2 months 3 doses at 4-weekly intervals
During second year of life	MMR	
At school entry	Diphtheria, tetanus + polio MMR (if not previously given)	
At 10–14 years	BCG	If tuberculin test is negative
	Rubella	Girls only
On leaving school	Tetanus + polio	

Smallpox vaccination is not now given as a routine unless
the subject is going to a country which still requires a
certificate of vaccination despite the elimination of the
disease!

attached to getting whooping cough particularly
in infancy. Whether pertussis vaccine should be
given and to whom is outside the scope of this
book but the dilemma serves to underline the fact
that no active drug is entirely safe and that
possible benefits have to be weighed against
risks.

Subjects at risk from tetanus should receive a
booster dose of toxoid every 5 years.

Smallpox vaccine contains the living virus of
vaccinia and produces antibodies against smallpox. Dose 0.2 ml by scarification.

Typhoid, paratyphoid A and B vaccine (TAB).
Dose 0.5 ml subcutaneously, followed by either
0.5 ml subcutaneously or 0.1 ml intradermally, 28
days later.

Bacillus Calmette–Guérin vaccine. A suspension of living bacilli which will produce
tuberculosis antibodies. Dose 0.1 ml by intracu-
taneous injection.

Poliomyelitis vaccine may be either inactivated poliomyelitis viruses type 1, 2 and 3 (Salk
vaccine) or attenuated live virus (Sabin vac-

cine)—the latter is to be preferred as it avoids injections, provides a more prolonged immunity and by producing antibodies in the intestine it prevents the spread of infection.

The dose is three drops on a lump of sugar.

Rubella vaccine should be offered to seronegative women of childbearing age. It is important to exclude pregnancy when giving the vaccine and to avoid it for 3 months thereafter. The dose is 0.5 ml by subcutaneous injection.

Measles, mumps and rubella vaccine (MMR). This combined vaccine should be given as a single dose of 0.5 ml by intramuscular or deep subcutaneous injection to children aged 1–2 years and 4–5 before starting school. It occasionally produces malaise, fever, a rash and parotid swelling about 1 week after injection. Meningitis due to the mumps component occurs in about 1 in 1 000 000 doses.

Influenza vaccine. The 'flu' viruses are changing continually so the WHO recommends which strains of virus should be included in the vaccine for a particular year. The vaccine only protects about 70% of subjects for about 1 year and its use is confined to those at special risk, e.g. the elderly, those with heart, lung or renal disease and diabetics.

Immunization against viral hepatitis

1. Hepatitis A. This virus is spread by poor hygiene, and infection is usually due to contaminated food and water. A vaccine is now available and is given at 4-weekly intervals with a booster dose after 6 months. It appears to be very effective in preventing hepatitis A but the duration of protection is not yet known. There may be local soreness at the site of injection.

Alternatively, normal human immunoglobin given by intramuscular injection confers passive immunity for up to 2 months.

2. Hepatitis B. This viral infection is of particular importance to the nurse as it can be spread by infected body fluids (blood or saliva) and strict regulations should be enforced when nursing patients with this type of hepatitis. The problem is complicated as some people are symptom-free carriers of the virus, particularly those who frequently receive blood products (i.e. in dialysis units etc.).

A vaccine prepared from the surface antigen of the virus is available (H-B-Vax). Three injections of 1 ml i.m. are given—the first and second, 1 month apart and the third after 6 months. Immunity persists for at least 2 years. Passive immunization is also possible using a special serum containing large amounts of antibody against the hepatitis B virus.

Nursing point

A doctor may delegate the responsibility of immunization to a nurse provided that:

1. The nurse is willing to be accountable for the work.
2. The nurse has received training in the subject.
3. The nurse has been trained in the diagnosis and treatment of anaphylaxis.

Anaphylaxis is very rare with active immunization but treatment should be immediately available (see above).

Contraindications to immunization

1. Acute illness.
2. Live vaccines should not be given to those who have reduced immunity due to:
   a) High doses of steroids or cytotoxic drugs
   b) Active lymphomas including Hodgkin's disease.
3. Pregnancy. Rarely the risk of infection outweighs this precaution.

In case of doubt the nurse is referred to *Immunization against infectious disease*, HMSO 1992.

DRUGS WHICH BLOCK THE IMMUNE REACTION

THE ANTIHISTAMINES

The histamine released following an antigen–antibody reaction is responsible with other factors, for a variety of clinical syndromes. These include anaphylactic shock, serum sickness, hay fever and urticaria. A series of drugs have been produced which block this action of histamine and thus relieve or partially relieve some of these conditions. It is believed that these drugs prevent the stimulation of H_1 receptors by histamine and must be carefully distinguished from H_2 receptor blockers (see p. 79) which interfere with an entirely different action of histamine.

The antihistamine drugs are usually given orally and are well absorbed from the intestinal tract.

In addition to their antihistamine properties some of these drugs enter the central nervous system and have sedating and anti-emetic effects. Some also have anticholinergic effects such as dry mouth and urinary retention.

Therapeutics

Nonsedating antihistamines are used mainly for hay fever and other allergic reactions.

Terfenadine in doses of 60 mg once or twice daily is useful and is rarely sedating. It should not be used in patients with liver disease or be combined with erythromycin as it occasionally causes cardiac arrhythmias.

Certizirine 10 mg daily acts similarly.

Astemizole has a very long duration of action. The usual dose is 10 mg once daily. It has been reported as rarely causing cardiac arrhythmias in overdose or when combined with erythromycin. None of these drugs potentiates the sedative action of alcohol.

Sedating antihistamines are used for various allergic reactions but also for non-allergic itching and as anti-emetics and sedatives.

Chlorpheniramine can be given orally or slowly intravenously, the oral dose being 4.0 mg two or three times daily.

Clemastine, cyproheptadine and **triprolidine** are similar. **Trimeprazine** is very sedative and is used for this purpose. **Promethazine** is a useful anti-emetic which can be used in pregnancy.

The wide range of antihistamines is useful as patients vary in their response to treatment and it may be necessary to try several before finding the most suitable one.

Adverse effects. Except for drowsiness, already mentioned, toxic effects are rare.

The drugs should be kept out of the reach of children as they may mistake them for sweets and overdosage produces dangerous results.

Antihistamines are also available for local application to bites and stings. This is not recommended as they are not particularly effective and can cause local reactions.

Sodium cromoglycate

This compound prevents the release of substances from mast cells, which constrict the bronchi and produce an attack of asthma. It is given by inhalation in a 'Spincap' capsule, either as 20 mg of sodium cromoglycate alone or combined with 0.1 mg of isoprenaline. Usually one capsule is inhaled night and morning and at 4–6 hourly intervals—this dosage can be reduced.

Sodium cromoglycate is thus used to prevent asthma rather than treat the established attack. It is particularly effective in the allergic type of asthma occurring in young people.

It is available as a 2% solution as eye or nasal drops and as a nasal spray. Drops are instilled four to six times daily. It can also be given orally in doses of 200 mg four times daily before meals for treating various intestinal disorders.

Adrenaline (see p. 28)

Although not specifically blocking any of the substances which mediate the immune response, adrenaline is very effective in acute anaphylaxis as it reverses bronchospasm and vasodilatation. The usual dose is 0.5 ml of 1:1000 solution i.m.

Hay fever

This is a common complaint caused by an allergic response to pollen, with the release of histamine in the nose and eyes. It is therefore most severe in late spring and early summer. A similar allergic rhinitis may occur at any time of year or be more or less continuous.

Treatment can be systemic or local. Systemic oral antihistamines are useful and a non-sedative preparation is the first choice. Several are available without a doctor's prescription, e.g. terfenadine (Seldane) or astemizole (Pollen-eze). If this fails a nasal spray containing a steroid (beclomethasone or budesonide) can be added to the regime. Alternatively, sodium cromoglycate nasal spray can be used on a regular basis. Local applications have the advantage of avoiding systemic side-effects but may cause local stinging.

The associated conjunctival inflammation requires eye wash solution or local sodium cromoglycate. In severe intractable cases systemic steroids may be necessary for a short period.

IMMUNOSUPPRESSION

Under certain circumstances it is believed that the antibody-producing system becomes deranged and produces antibodies against various body tissues. Diseases which arise in this way are called 'autoimmune' and may include some types of nephritis, systemic lupus erythematosus, polyarteritis nodosa and possibly rheumatoid arthritis. If the antibody system can be suppressed there is reason to hope that the disease process can be controlled. This can be achieved to a certain degree by steroids (see p. 163) but often incompletely and more recently various cytotoxic drugs which are active against antibody-forming cells have proved useful. Those most frequently used are **azathioprine** or **cyclophosphamide;** the dose has to be carefully adjusted to avoid leucopenia. Such drugs are also used for the same reason to prevent rejection of transplanted organs by sensitized lymphocytes.

Cyclosporin A. The greatest problem in organ transplant is rejection of the graft by the immune system of the recipient. This is largely mediated by the lymphocytes and most drugs which have been used to prevent rejection (see above) suppress all aspects of immunity and also interfere with the formation of polymorphs and platelets. Cyclosporin A affects the T lymphocytes which are particularly concerned with graft rejection and is thus very useful in transplant surgery and is being tried cautiously in various auto-immune diseases.

It is however a difficult drug to use. It can be given orally or intravenously and is used to cover the organ or bone marrow transplant and then continued orally at a lower maintenance dose to prevent rejection. Estimation of blood levels may be required to control dosage.

Adverse effects include disturbances of renal and hepatic function, nausea and vomiting and tremor. There is also the possibility of the development of cancer as a delayed complication.

Interactions with other drugs may increase absorption and alter the metabolism of cyclosporin in the liver. Combination with aminoglycosides (e.g. gentamicin) or NSAIAs can be nephrotoxic.

FURTHER READING

Editorial 1992 Treating anaphylaxis with sympathomimetic drugs. British Medical Journal 305: 1107
HMSO 1992 Immunization against infectious disease. HMSO, London

Lockhead Y J 1991 Failure to immunise children under five years. Journal of Advanced Nursing 16: 130
Wood S F 1988 Choosing an antihistamine. Prescribers Journal 28: 21

17

Drugs used in the treatment of tropical and imported disease and anthelmintics

Tropical diseases, like their background, are inclined to be dramatic and florid. The majority are infective or due to dietary deficiency and in former times and even to some degree today, great epidemics have caused widespread disease with a very high death rate. During the last 50 years the causative organisms of nearly all these diseases have been discovered and drugs have been devised which are capable of dealing with them. The problem of treating tropical disease is further complicated by the primitive conditions which prevail in many parts of the tropics and the lack of proper medical and nursing facilities. However, in spite of these difficulties, immense progress has been made in this sphere. In recent years, air travel has brought tropical diseases much nearer home for it is possible to catch malaria in Central Africa and not be taken ill till after arrival in London. Some knowledge of these complaints is therefore necessary even if the nurse does not intend to carry on her profession in tropical countries.

The consideration of tropical disease will be carried out under headings of the disease rather than the drug.

TRAVELLERS' DIARRHOEA

A holiday in tropical or subtropical countries is often interrupted by an attack of diarrhoea, colic and vomiting which although rarely severe, interferes with a few days' pleasure. It is believed that there is usually an infective cause and the organism often implicated is an unusual variant of *Esch. coli*. Prevention should include care over drinking water and washing uncooked foods such as fruit and vegetables in chlorinated water. The prophylactic use of antibiotics is not recommended except for those at special risk (e.g. bowel disease) or if for social or business reasons diarrhoea must be avoided. In these cases *trimethoprim* 200 mg daily or *doxycycline* 100 mg daily are satisfactory. For the developed attack, fluid replacement with added glucose and electrolytes (e.g. Dioralyte or a similar preparation) is important. Symptoms can be improved with *codeine* or *loperamide* and in severe cases trimethoprim 200 mg twice daily should be given.

AMOEBIC DYSENTERY

Amoebic dysentery is an infection of the lower bowel with an organism called the *Entamoeba histolytica* and is characterized by chronic diarrhoea. Sometimes the infection spreads outside the bowel, particularly to the liver where it causes an abscess.

The chief drugs used in this infection are:

Metronidazole is now the first choice in treating amoebic infection of the bowel and abscess of the liver. It is given in doses of 800 mg three times daily, and a 5–day course is often sufficient (see also p. 211). At this dose level, vomiting can be troublesome. Metronidazole can be combined with **diloxanide furoate** which is active against organisms in the bowel lumen but not in the tissues. The dose is 500 mg three times daily for 10 days and the combination appears to be even more efficient at eradicating the infection.

Chloroquine (see also p. 229) is concentrated in the liver and is effective against the amoeba in that site. It is no use in the treatment of intestinal infection. The dose is 300 mg twice daily for 4 days followed by 300 mg daily for 2 weeks.

BACILLARY DYSENTERY

This may be caused by a variety of organisms of the *Shigella* group. In mild cases symptomatic treatment only is required and there is no evidence that antibiotics produce a more rapid cure.

In severe cases the organism should be cultured and its sensitivity to antibiotics defined. If there is no time for culture, treatment may be started with trimethoprim 200 mg twice daily. Ciprofloxacin is used if trimethoprim resistance is a problem. Fluid and electrolyte replacement is important.

CHOLERA

Cholera is due to an organism, the *cholera vibrio* which invades the intestine, producing severe and copious diarrhoea and vomiting. This leads to intense dehydration and sodium and potassium deficiency and is often fatal. The most important part of treatment is to replace the lost water and salts orally or by intravenous infusion.

The cholera vibrio is sensitive to tetracycline, and it can be used to eradicate the infection and to shorten the course of the illness.

In the Third World where this disease reaches epidemic proportions, large scale intravenous infusion may be difficult. An important advance has been the discovery that if glucose is added to the electrolyte replacement solution and given orally, water and electrolytes are well absorbed and i.v. infusion is less often required. The oral replacement solution contains:

Sodium chloride 3.5 g
Sodium bicarbonate 2.5 g
Potassium chloride 1.5 g
Glucose 20 g
Made up to 1 litre.

The volume given is titrated against the loss in the stools and by vomiting.

LEPROSY

Leprosy is a disease of great antiquity and is referred to in the Bible. It is caused by the *Mycobacterium leprae;* these bacteria cause chronic infection of the skin, visceral nerves and other parts of the body. Leprosy has long resisted treatment, but in recent years the introduction of new drugs has made the outlook more hopeful.

The *Mycobacterium leprae* can become resistant to the drugs used in treatment; therefore at least two antibacterials should be given together to prevent this. Three drugs are used in leprosy at present:

Dapsone is widely used. It is given orally, usually over long periods. The dose is 50–100 mg daily.

Adverse effects are uncommon but include headaches, cyanosis, anaemia and blood dyscrasias.

Clofazimine is useful in treating leprosy and is combined with other agents. It is given orally over long periods. Side-effects are rare but it may cause pigmentation of the skin.

Rifampicin (see p. 205) is also effective against the *Mycobacterium leprae,* although resistance may develop.

Treatment of leprosy

In patients with florid infection (*multibacillary*) treatment is:

> Rifampicin 600 mg once a month
> Clofazimine 50 mg daily with a 300 mg dose once a month
> Dapsone 100 mg daily.

The course should be continued for a minimum of 2 years. With a less florid infection (*paucibacillary*) treatment is:

> Rifampicin 600 mg once monthly
> Dapsone 100 mg daily.

The course is continued for 6 months.

MALARIA

Malaria has been known for thousands of years and is one of the most widespread diseases which attack mankind.

Although it is largely confined to tropical and subtropical zones, air travel has led to its increased frequency in this country. Malaria is caused by a small organism called a plasmodium. There are three varieties of plasmodia which produce the commonly found varieties of human malaria. They are:

- *Plasmodium vivax*—causing benign tertian malaria.
- *Plasmodium malariae*—causing quartan malaria.
- *Plasmodium falciparum*—causing malignant tertian malaria.

These plasmodia are injected into the human victim by the mosquito. They are carried to the liver where they go through a stage of division known as the exo-erythrocyte stage. After a short period some plasmodia enter the red cells of the blood stream. Here they divide in a simple asexual fashion to form more plasmodia which rupture the red cells and then re-enter further red cells: the breaking up of the red cells corresponds with the rise of temperature with rigor and later sweating which is so characteristic of the disease.

Other plasmodia which have entered the red cells form male and female gametes which may then be sucked out when a mosquito bite occurs and continue the cycle in the infected mosquito. The cycle is shown graphically in Figure 17.1. The drugs which are effective in treating malaria may be divided into two groups:

1. Those which act on the asexual stage of the malarial parasite in the blood.

> Quinine
> Chloroquine
> Proguanil
> Halofantrine
> Mefloquine
> Pyrimethamine.

2. Those which act on the exo-erythrocyte stage in the liver and the gametocytes.

> Primaquine.

Quinine. Quinine is described first, because it was the first effective remedy.

It is one of the alkaloids obtained from the bark of the cinchona tree and has been known to be effective against 'fever' for several hundred years.

For some years it was largely replaced by newer antimalarials but is now proving useful in

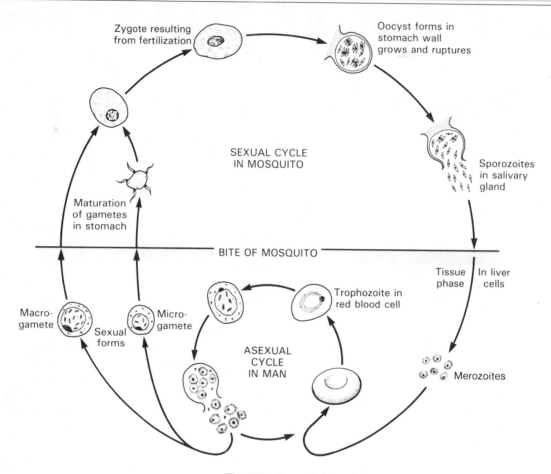

Fig. 17.1 The malarial cycle.

infections due to parasites which are resistant to other drugs.

Quinine is given either orally or intravenously. It is well absorbed from the intestine.

It suppresses the multiplication of the plasmodia in the blood stream and relieves the symptoms of malaria in about 4 days. It does not, however, have any effect on the gametes or exo-erythrocyte stages of the malarial life cycle and thus symptoms may recur when quinine is stopped.

Quinine has a number of other actions. It has a depressing action on the heart similar to that of quinidine; it is also said to cause contraction of the uterus and should, therefore, be avoided in pregnancy.

Adverse effects are quite common with quinine—the syndrome produced being known as cinchonism. This may occur with large doses but some people are hypersensitive to the drug and develop toxic effects after small amounts; the chief symptoms are vertigo, tinnitus, deafness and visual disturbances. There is some evidence that *blackwater fever*, in which there is widespread but unexplained breaking down of red cells, is connected with the taking of quinine.

Therapeutics. The usual therapeutic dose of quinine sulphate for treating malaria is 600 mg (540 mg base) three times a day.

If quinine is given intravenously, which is occasionally required in fulminating malignant tertian malaria, it should be given as quinine hydrochloride, 10 mg/kg dissolved in 500 ml of saline and given by slow intravenous infusion and repeated 8 hourly.

Chloroquine is a most useful drug to treat malaria but resistant strains of *P. falciparum* are common.

It can be given orally, intramuscularly or intravenously. It is rapidly absorbed and is stored in various organs of the body, part being destroyed and part excreted in the urine.

It is effective against the asexual forms of the plasmodia in the blood stream, but has no effect on the gametes or on the exo-erythrocyte stages. Strains of malaria which are resistant to chloroquine have appeared in South-east Asia and South America and Central and East Africa.

Adverse effects are rare and include nausea and headaches, and as it may cause fetal damage it should not be used in pregnancy.

Therapeutics. In an acute attack of malaria, adults should receive 600 mg of chloroquine base followed by 300 mg after 6 hours, then 300 mg daily. Prophylaxis against malaria is obtained by taking 300 mg of chloroquine base weekly.

Mefloquine is effective against chloroquine-resistant *P. falciparum* and is used in those parts of the world where this is common. It is excreted very slowly so a single dose of 25 mg/kg is used.

It can also be used prophylactically in doses of 250 mg once weekly and no longer than 3 weeks should be spent in an endemic area.

Adverse effects. Nausea and giddiness are rather common and it should not be given in pregnancy.

Halofantrine is also used to treat resistant infections with *P. falciparum*. It is given in doses of 500 mg 6-hourly for 1 day. Absorption is rather irregular but can be improved by giving it with fatty foods.

Adverse effects. Cardiac arrhythmias—avoid in heart disease.

Proguanil. Proguanil is given by mouth. It is rapidly absorbed but disappears rather rapidly from the blood stream.

It is effective against the blood stream asexual phase of the plasmodia and also has some action against the gametocytes and against the exo-erythrocyte stage of *P. falciparum*.

It is, however, rather slower at relieving the acute attack of malaria than chloroquine and furthermore resistant strains of plasmodia have been encountered. Toxicity is very low.

Therapeutics. Proguanil is very slow in its antimalarial action and it is therefore largely used as a suppressant. The usual dose for this purpose is 100–200 mg daily.

Pyrimethamine. Pyrimethamine is effective against the asexual blood stream phase of the malarial parasite but it is too slow to be used in treating an acute attack. Owing to the emergence of resistant strains it is now only used in combination, e.g.

> Pyrimethamine + dapsone—Maloprim
> Pyrimethamine + sulfadoxine—Fansidar.

It can be seen that all the drugs so far described with the possible partial exception of proguanil, while effectively suppressing the asexual blood stream phase of the malaria organism and relieving acute symptoms are ineffective against the exoerythrocyte stage in the liver and against the gametocytes.

This is particularly important when it is caused by *P. vivax* or *P. malariae* as a relapse may occur on stopping treatment. In these types of malaria the initial treatment should be followed by a drug which acts against the parasites in the exo-erythocyte stage.

Primaquine. Primaquine is effective against the exo-erythrocyte stage and against the gametocytes. It is not free from toxic effects and may produce nausea and vomiting.

It is not used alone in the treatment of the acute malarial attack but may be combined with chloroquine, the dose being 15 mg daily for 2 weeks when it is particularly valuable in eradicating benign tertian malaria. Relapses will not occur unless there is reinfection.

Before starting treatment it is important to test the patient for G6PD deficiency, an inherited disorder of the red blood cells which results in severe haemolysis with primaquine and some other drugs.

The treatment of malaria

It is impossible to give precise instruction as to the best drug or drugs in the treatment of malaria as this is not yet settled and may also vary with different forms of malaria infection.

It must be realized that there are three possible ways in which malaria may be attacked by drugs.

Suppressive. Regular administration of a drug to prevent clinical manifestation of the disease.

The best drug for this purpose varies in different parts of the world. This is because the widespread use of antimalarials has led to the development of resistant strains of *P. Falciparum* particularly in South-east Asia but also South America and parts of Africa. At the time of writing the following may be recommended, but it is wise to obtain up-to-date advice before travelling, from the Malaria Reference Laboratory (071 388 9600).

North Africa	Proguanil 200 mg daily
Sub-Saharan Africa	Proguanil 200 mg daily + Chloroquine 300 mg weekly or Mefloquine 250 mg weekly
South-east Asia, Central and South America	Proguanil 200 mg daily + Chloroquine 300 mg weekly or Mefloquine 250 mg weekly
Oceania	Maloprim 1 tablet daily + Chloroquine 300 mg weekly

The chosen drug must be started 1 week before entering the malarial area and *continued for 1 month after leaving it.*

In addition, precautions should be taken against mosquito bites including the use of nets at night.

Treatment of established disease. The really dangerous type of malaria is that due to *P.*

falciparum which may prove fatal unless treated rapidly. Strains from some parts of the world are resistant to one or more antimalarial drugs so it is necessary to discover whether the patient acquired the infection in an area where resistance, particularly to chloroquine, exists and to treat accordingly.

P. falciparum	Chloroquine base 600 mg orally followed by 300 mg after 6 hours, then 300 mg daily for 3 days. In severe infections, 200–300 mg of chloroquine can be given i.v. in 250 ml of saline.
P. falciparum (chloroquine resistant or cerebral malaria)	Quinine 600 mg 8 hourly for 5 days followed by Fansidar*, a single dose of 3 tablets. In severely ill patients quinine can be given by i.v. infusion. This is a potentially dangerous procedure. A loading dose of 20 mg/kg of the salt[†] is infused over 4 hours. A dose of 10 mg/kg is then repeated at 8-hourly intervals. If it is impossible to monitor the infusion, quinine salts can be given, well diluted, intramuscularly. Oral treatment with quinine is continued when the patient can swallow. This is followed by Fansidar as above.
P. vivax or *P. malariae*	Chloroquine as above followed by primaquine base 15 mg daily orally for 14 days to eliminate exo-erythrocyte forms.

LEISHMANIASIS (KALA-AZAR)

There are several varieties of kala-azar caused by closely related organisms. These organisms may invade the spleen, liver, lymph glands and bone marrow producing a generalized disease with

---

*Fansidar is a combination of pyrimethamine and sulfadoxine. Its long-term use is not recommended as it can cause a severe and unpleasant rash (Stevens–Johnson syndrome).
[†]This dose is correct provided quinine sulphate hydrochloride or dihydrochloride is used.

constitutional symptoms or produce a local ulcerative lesion.

The most useful drugs for treating leishmaniasis are those which contain antimony. They are believed to interfere with enzymes within the parasite.

Sodium stibogluconate given as an initial dose of 5 mg/kg body weight followed by daily doses of 10 mg/kg body weight for 20 days is usually adequate. The drug, being irritant, should be given by slow intravenous injection. Sometimes it may be necessary to repeat courses at intervals of 2 weeks.

Adverse effects include irritation at the site of injection, muscle aches and cardiotoxicity with arrhythmias.

The patient usually responds within 2 weeks and should be restored to full health within 2 months.

SCHISTOSOMIASIS

This disease is caused by flukes which inhabit the veins of the bladder and the lower bowel leading to haematuria and rectal bleeding.

Praziquantel has now emerged as the most useful drug in schistosomiasis. It is effective against all types of the disease and unlike drugs formerly used, it appears free from serious adverse effects. A single dose of 40 mg/kg is adequate for *S. mansoni* and *S. haematobium* and three doses of 20 mg/kg for *S. japanica*. The cure rate is around 80%.

ANTHELMINTICS

Anthelmintics are drugs which are used to treat worm infestations. Although such infestations, with the possible exception of threadworms, are not common in this country they may occur in immigrants, being endemic in some regions of the world and are of great medical and economic importance.

The anthelmintics are a diverse group of sub-stances with widely differing properties and they will be described under the headings of the type of infestation they are used to treat.

THREADWORMS (*Enterobius vermicularis*)

These worms appear like short lengths of thread. They live in the caecal region and the females migrate to the anus where they lay eggs and provoke intense itching. The resulting scratching leads to the hands becoming contaminated with eggs which may then be transferred to food and thus further infestation occurs.

General cleanliness and scrubbing of the nails before meals is important in treating this condition.

It must be remembered that the whole family of an infected patient must be examined for infestation as it is common to find several members of a family harbouring worms and reinfection will occur unless the worms are eradicated from the whole family.

Piperazine. This is effective in treating threadworm infections, and is not liable to produce side-effects.

The dose for infants up to 2 years is 50–75 mg/kg once daily. For adults the dose is 2 g once daily. This should be given for a week followed by a week's rest and then a further week's treatment.

Adverse effects are rare but it should not be used in epileptics, in pregnancy or in patients with peptic ulcers. It may cause gastrointestinal upsets and rashes.

Mebendazole as a single dose of 100 mg is effective. It should not be given to children under 2 years or in pregnancy and, rarely, it causes nausea and diarrhoea. A second dose can be given after 3 weeks.

Pyrantel paralyses the worms and is effective as a single dose of 10 mg/kg.

WHIPWORMS

This worm is common in the tropics and infects

children predominantly. Infestation may be asymptomatic but it can cause diarrhoea.

Mebendazole in doses of 100 mg twice daily for 3 days is the only effective remedy.

STRONGYLOIDES STERCORALIS

This worm which is common in the tropics lives in the intestines. The larvae can penetrate the anal skin and thus reinfect the host so infection can last for a long time. Usually they only cause mild intestinal symptoms but if the patient is immunosuppressed (i.e. given large doses of steroids or has AIDS) widespread penetration of the bowel occurs which may be fatal.

Thiabendazole in doses of 25 mg/kg twice daily for 3 days is effective but side-effects of nausea and drowsiness are common.

TAPEWORMS

There are two common types of tapeworm. They are *Taenia solium* and *Taenia saginata*. Both these worms inhabit the small intestine of man where they may reach several feet in length. They consist of a head which is embedded in the wall of the intestine and a body consisting of a large number of segments. These segments containing eggs are shed and pass out in the faeces.

The eggs may then infect the animal host which is the pig in the case of *Taenia solium* and bullock in the case of *Taenia saginata*. In the animal's gastrointestinal tract the larval form is released and migrates via the blood stream throughout the carcase where it remains until the animal is killed, the meat is eaten by man and reinfection occurs.

There are several drugs which can be used to treat tapeworms, the most effective being:

Niclosamide. This is effective against tapeworm. No preparation is required. In the morning 1 g of the drug is chewed and swallowed on an empty stomach. After 1 hour the dose is repeated. This is followed 3 hours later by a saline purge. In *Taenia solium* infestation a more powerful purge should be used as it is important

to clear all the ova from the gut. Treatment may be preceded by metoclopramide to minimize the risk of vomiting.

The drug appears very free of side-effects and acts by actually killing the worm.

ROUNDWORMS (*Ascaris lumbricoides*)

The roundworm is similar to a pale-coloured earthworm. It lives in the small intestine and its eggs are passed out in the faeces. If reinfection occurs, the larval forms are liberated in the gastrointestinal tract and pass via the blood stream to the lungs. They then migrate up the trachea to the pharynx and are swallowed, thus completing the cycle.

There are several drugs used in the treatment of roundworms.

Piperazine. This is useful in treating roundworms. It paralyses the muscle of the worm which is passed alive per rectum. A single dose of 75 mg/kg body weight (maximum dose 4 g) is effective. Alternatively, one Pripsen sachet (containing 4 g of piperazine + 15.3 mg of sennosides) may be used, the purgative helping to clear the bowel of worms.

Pyrantel as a single dose of 10 mg/kg is also effective.

HOOKWORM

The hookworm, although not seen in this country, is extremely common in the tropical and subtropical countries in both the Old and New World.

This worm lives in the small intestine of man, the fertilized eggs are passed out in the faeces and develop into larvae in the soil. The larvae penetrate the skin and pass via the blood stream to the lung. Here they enter the bronchial tree and migrate to the intestinal tract via the trachea.

Severe infestation can cause iron deficiency anaemia.

Mebendazole in doses of 100 mg twice daily for 3 days is effective. It should not be used in pregnancy or for children under 2 years old.

FILARIASIS

The parasitic worms *Loa Loa*, which cause subcutaneous swellings, and *Wuchereria bancrofti*, another filarial parasite which causes elephantiasis, may be eradicated by **diethylcarbamazine**. The initial dose is 50 mg a day and this should be increased to 150 mg three times daily and continued for 3 weeks.

FURTHER READING

Chemoprophylaxis and treatment of malaria 1988. New England Journal of Medicine 319: 1538

Editorial 1988 Imported diseases: a symposium. Prescribers Journal 28: 69

Editorial 1993 Prophylaxis against malaria for travellers from the UK. British Medical Journal 306: 1247

Lockwood D N J, Parvol G 1994 Recent advances in tropical medicine. British Medical Journal 308: 1559

White N J 1992 Antimalarial pharmacokinetics and treatment regimes. British Journal of Clinical Pharmacology 34: 1

18

The vitamins

Vitamins are substances which are present in certain foods but which man cannot manufacture for himself and are necessary for the proper functioning of animal tissues. Deficiency of vitamins in the diet leads to a number of diseases which are specific for each particular vitamin. Many of the vitamins exert their action by taking part in the complex chemical reactions which occur within the cell.

It is important to realize that provided a sufficiency of vitamins is taken, which should be provided by a good mixed diet, there is no advantage to be gained by taking further large doses of the various vitamins; in fact the taking of excessive amounts of certain vitamins may even be harmful. At present there is no firm evidence that extra vitamins protect against cancer and heart disease to any appreciable extent and reports that supplementary vitamins given to children increase their IQ should be treated with scepticism until confirmed.

The vitamins may now be considered in detail.

Vitamin A (retinol)

Vitamin A is a fat-soluble, oily liquid. It is present in diary products such as milk, butter and cream and in fish liver oils.

Beta carotene, a substance which is closely allied to vitamin A and can be converted to vitamin A by the body, is found in carrots, green vegetables and liver.

The absorption of vitamin A is helped by the presence of fat and bile salts in the intestine.

Vitamin A is concerned with maintaining the health of the epithelium. Deficiency leads to keratinization of the epithelium of the nose and respiratory passage and to changes in the conjunctiva and in the cornea which may lead to blindness.

Vitamin A is also concerned with the mechanism of dark adaptation by the retina and deficiency leads to night blindness.

Therapeutics. Vitamin A should be given in cases of deficiency causing night blindness or epithelial changes.

Minimum human requirements. Adult 2250 IU daily.

Therapeutic dose. 50 000 IU.

Toxicity. Overdosage with vitamin A can produce liver damage and hair loss.

Pregnant women are advised to avoid vitamin A supplements as there is some evidence that excessive intake is associated with fetal defects.

Vitamin B1 (thiamine)

Vitamin B1 is a white crystalline solid, soluble in water. It is obtained from wheat germ, yeast, egg yolk, liver and some vegetables.

Vitamin B1 is essential for certain stages in carbohydrate metabolism. Deficiency of this vitamin leads to a condition known as **beri beri**. This deficiency may not only result from an inadequate intake of vitamin B1, but may also occur in disturbances of metabolism in which requirements of vitamin B1 are higher than normal, a good example being chronic alcoholism. Beri beri is characterized by heart failure and polyneuritis.

Therapeutics. Beri beri responds rapidly to vitamin B1. Severe cases will require up to 100 mg daily by i.m. injection, in milder cases oral administration is satisfactory.

Vitamin B1 is also used in the polyneuritis of chronic alcoholism and in Wernicke's encephalopathy which is also usually due to excess alcohol.

Minimum human requirements. Adult 2 mg daily.

Therapeutic dose. 50 mg orally or i.v. daily.

Vitamin B2 (riboflavin)

This vitamin is found in vegetables, yeast and liver. It is concerned in intracellular metabolism. Deficiency in man causes cracking and fissures at the corner of the mouth. Vitamin B2 may be given in doses of 2 mg daily.

Nicotinic acid

Nicotinic acid is found in yeast, dairy products and liver. Deficiency of nicotinic acid leads to a condition known as **pellagra** which may occur in alcoholism and renal failure as well as with deficient diets. This disease is characterized by the 3 Ds, diarrhoea, dermatitis, and dementia. It may be relieved by nicotinic acid. It is worthwhile remembering that nicotinic acid is also a vasodilator. If it is taken in large doses flushing and tingling of the face may occur.

Although deficiency of vitamins in the B group have been discussed separately, it is common to find that deficiencies are often mixed and in treating patients who show evidence of vitamin B deficiencies it is worth giving all the vitamins of the group.

Pyridoxine is concerned with protein metabolism. It is sometimes used in the treatment of vomiting of pregnancy or following radiation. It can be used to prevent the polyneuritis which rarely complicates the use of high dose isoniazid in doses of 10–20 mg daily (p. 205).

Vitamin B 12 (cyanocobalamin) (see p. 240)

Vitamin C (ascorbic acid)

Vitamin C is a crystalline solid, soluble in water. It is found in fresh fruits, particularly citrus fruit, blackcurrants, tomatoes and green vegetables. It is important to remember that vitamin C is relatively unstable and it is destroyed by boiling especially in an alkaline solution. Thus green vegetables should be eaten raw if required for their vitamin C content.

Vitamin C is necessary for the formation and maintenance of a cement-like substance between cells and deficiency leads to a condition known as scurvy. Requirements are increased with prolonged exercise and illness.

Scurvy has been recognized for hundreds of years. It was particularly liable to attack mariners who in the days of sailing ships were away from land for long periods and were thus deprived of fresh food and vegetables. Infants and children are also susceptible, for although breast milk contains about 6 mg of vitamin C per 100 ml, cow's milk contains considerably less.

Scurvy is rarely seen in England at the present time, although it is occasionally found in people who for medical reasons, or more often supposed medical reasons, have been living on a very restricted diet such as bread and weak tea.

Scurvy is characterized by a tendency to bleed due to increased capillary fragility. Haemorrhages occur into the skin and mucous membranes; sponginess and haemorrhage around the gums may be found in those with teeth. Bleeding also occurs under the periosteum of bones and into joints producing great pain and tenderness; the patient is anaemic. If vitamin C is not given the disease will prove fatal.

Therapeutics. Scurvy is cured by giving vitamin C, the dose for adults being 150 mg daily. The bleeding is arrested and the anaemia which is not entirely secondary to haemorrhage, is relieved. Vitamin C is also used in a number of other conditions where it is of doubtful value; it does appear, however, to be useful in promoting the healing of wounds in those who, although showing no evidence of scurvy, have a mild degree of deficiency.

Very high doses of vitamin C are sometimes taken to prevent colds and other forms of ill health. The efficacy of this medication is not proven but it does not seem to do any harm.

Minimum human requirements:

- Children 100 mg daily
- Adults 30 mg daily
- Pregnancy 200 mg daily
- Lactation 150 mg daily.

Therapeutic dose. 500 mg daily.

Parentrovite contains high doses of B and C vitamins and is given intravenously or intramuscularly. Rarely it can cause a severe allergic reaction and infusion should be over at least 10 minutes.

Vitamin D (cholecalciferol) (Fig. 18.1)

This fat-soluble vitamin is found in fish liver oils and dairy produce and is also formed in the skin on exposure to sunlight. It is essentially concerned with calcium metabolism and bone formation. After absorption it is modified in the liver to form *25-hydroxycholecalciferol*, and undergoes further change in the kidney to form *1–25-hydroxycholecalciferol*. This substance is highly active in facilitating calcium absorption from the gut and the laying down of calcium and phosphate during bone formation. A deficiency in vitamin D leads to inadequate calcification of the bones resulting in their becoming soft and easily deformed. This condition when it occurs in children is known as **rickets** and these children with their bowed legs and deformed chests were a familiar sight in former times; with the arrival of cheap milk, cod liver oil and Infant Welfare

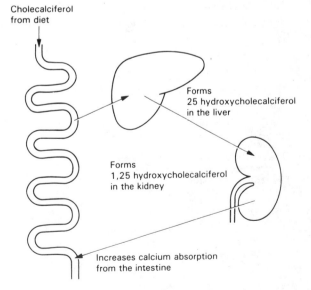

Fig. 18.1 The changes undergone by cholecalciferol (vitamin D) in the body.

Centres it has now become rare, although there has been a reappearance of the disease in coloured immigrants to this country. In adults, prolonged deprivation of vitamin D gives rise to a condition similar to rickets but it is very rarely seen in this country although certain groups, e.g. the elderly, Asians and vegetarians, are at some risk.

Vitamin D deficiency can also result from poor absorption from the intestine as in coeliac disease and from resistance to the action of vitamin D which is found in renal failure leading to stunting in children (*renal rickets*).

Therapeutics. 5000 IU of vitamin D daily is adequate for the treatment of rickets. In coeliac disease doses of vitamin D up to 50 000 units daily may be required at first but these requirements diminish as the disease is controlled by diet. In chronic renal failure large doses of vitamin D or alfacalcidol are used.

Overdose with vitamin D is dangerous and leads to deposition of calcium in the kidneys and other organs.

Minimum human requirements:

- Young children 600 IU daily.
- Adults 400 IU daily.
- Pregnancy and lactation 1000 IU daily.

Alfacalcidol (1-alpha-hydroxycholecalciferol) is closely related to vitamin D and is used in treating various disorders in which there is a resistance to the action of vitamin D. The usual dose is 1 microgram daily.

Vitamin K (phytomenadione)

Vitamin K is a precursor of prothrombin which is essential for the coagulation of blood.

Vitamin K is fat soluble and requires bile salts for proper absorption from the intestine. It is also synthesized in the gut by bacteria. After absorption it is used by the liver for the synthesis of prothrombin.

Deficiency in vitamin K will lead to bleeding and may result from insufficient uptake due to various intestinal diseases or to deficient utilization following liver disease or anticoagulant drugs. It is given to the new-born to prevent haemorrhage due to prothrombin deficiency. This arises because the bacterial flora of the gut at birth does not synthesize vitamin K. Recently, there has been some evidence that injection of vitamin K at birth may predispose to childhood cancer but not if it is given orally. At the time of writing the situation is not clear.

It can be given by injection as **phytomendadione** or orally as **menadiol sodium diphosphate.**

Nursing point
Nurses should be aware of the importance of a good diet but should be on their guard against fads.

FURTHER READING

Editorial 1992 Vitamin K and childhood cancer. British Medical Journal 305: 326
Gregory J et al 1990 Dietary and nutritional survey of British adults. HMSO, London
Ministry of Agriculture, Fisheries and Food 1991 Dietary supplements and health foods. Report of the Working Group. MAFF Publications, London
Smith S 1985 How drugs act No 7 Vitamins. Nursing Times 81(3): 35

19

Drugs used in the treatment of anaemia

IRON DEFICIENCY ANAEMIA

Iron is an essential constituent of haemoglobin which is contained in the erythrocytes (red cells) of the blood. Haemoglobin is concerned with the transport of oxygen from the lungs to the tissues. When the red cells break down the iron is retained by the body and built up again into further haemoglobin molecules. There is very little iron held in storage depots, the major portion being constantly in use. A little iron, probably about 2 mg a day or less, is lost by desquamation of cells by the skin and gut, but the chief drain of iron from the body occurs in the various forms of blood loss, either menstruation or parturition or due to chronic bleeding usually from the gastrointestinal tract. In pregnancy the growing fetus requires a certain amount of iron and during lactation iron is lost in the mother's milk.

It can be seen, therefore, that although the average diet which supplies about 25 mg of iron a day is sufficient for most people, if there is any prolonged iron loss, a deficiency will occur. This leads to failure to produce enough haemoglobin with resulting anaemia.

Iron, when taken by mouth, is converted into the ferrous form in the stomach. It is absorbed from the upper part of the small intestine, forming a loose compound with a protein in the intestinal wall which is called *ferritin*; in this form it is transported across to the blood stream where it forms a compound with another protein and with carbon dioxide and is carried to the bone marrow for the synthesis of haemoglobin. The absorption of iron is carefully regulated so that just enough is absorbed to make good any deficiency.

Iron deficiency anaemia is sometimes associated with deficient secretion of hydrochloric acid by the stomach and this leads to a failure of release of ferrous iron from the diet.

If a deficiency of iron occurs, less haemoglobin is synthesized and the amount of haemoglobin in the erythrocytes decreases.

Iron is given to correct a deficiency. It is usually given orally. The rise in blood haemoglobin level should be at least 0.7 g/litre per week and *treatment should be continued for 4 months after the blood haemoglobin level has returned to normal in order to replace depleted iron stores.*

It is also given during pregnancy when the iron requirements increase (see under folic acid, p. 241).

Ferrous sulphate

Ferrous salts are rapidly changed to ferric salts in the air and thus ferrous salts are given as coated tablets. Ferrous sulphate tablets are a satisfactory way of giving iron to most people. The dosage is about 200 mg, three times a day. In sensitive individuals ferrous sulphate may cause gastric discomfort and nausea or diarrhoea or sometimes constipation.

Ferrous sulphate tablets are usually coated with sugar; *children are therefore very liable to take them and fatal poisoning by ferrous sulphate is not uncommon.* Like all drugs they should therefore always be kept in a position of safety.

Ferrous gluconate is another ferrous salt. It is less irritating to the stomach than most ferrous salts. The dose is 300 mg three times daily.

Ferrous glycine sulphate is a complex of ferrous sulphate and the aminoacid glycine. It is perhaps less liable to cause gastrointestinal disturbances and is useful in sensitive individuals.

Liquid preparations are also available. **Sodium ironedetate (Sytron)** and a **polysaccharide–iron complex (Niferex)** are satisfactory and do not stain the teeth. Although slow release iron preparations are used they may be less effective as iron

absorption takes place in the upper small intestine but these preparations release it lower down the gut.

Iron can also be given by intravenous or intramuscular injection in those who are not absorbing iron satisfactorily. *Before injecting iron, oral iron should be stopped for at least 72 hours as this appears to reduce the chances of a reaction after injection.* The compounds used are:

Iron-dextran. This is a complex of iron and dextran. It can be given by deep intramuscular injection or intravenously. If given intramuscularly care must be taken to displace the skin prior to injection so that the needle track is sealed off, as leakage into the skin will cause a disfiguring stain. Reactions may occur and it is wise to start with a test dose of 0.5 ml. The dose thereafter is 1–2 ml and each ml contains 50 mg of iron.

It can be given into alternate buttocks daily or at longer intervals.

Adverse effects include anaphylaxis with collapse, rashes, joint pains and fever.

Iron-sorbitol citrate is an iron preparation for intramuscular injection. It is rapidly absorbed from the injection site. It contains 50 mg of iron per ml of solution. Side-effects appear slight but shock-like reactions can occur and care must be taken when giving the injection.

DRUGS USED IN TREATING OTHER ANAEMIAS

Cobalamins (vitamin B12). There are several factors required for the proper maturation of the red cells. The best known of these is vitamin B12. A deficiency in this vitamin leads to a failure in production of erythrocytes. There is, therefore, a decrease in the number of circulating erythrocytes and those which do manage to mature appear abnormal, being large and irregular in shape and size. Primitive red cells may also appear in the blood.

Besides the change in the blood, deficiency in cobalamin leads to glossitis and degenerative changes in the nervous system. The syndrome produced by cyanocobalamin deficiency is known as *pernicious* or *Addison's anaemia.* This deficiency is believed to be due to a failure to absorb cobalamin from the intestine. In the normal person, a factor (*the intrinsic factor*) is produced by the stomach and is necessary for the absorption of cobalamin in the intestine. In patients with pernicious anaemia there is a lack of this gastric factor and cobalamin cannot therefore be absorbed (Fig. 19.1).

Treatment is to give cobalamin by injection. There are two cobalamins available, **hydroxocobalamin,** which is stable and which is highly bound by the plasma proteins so that it is excreted slowly and thus its action is prolonged, and **cyanocobalamin**, which is effective but more rapidly excreted.

Therapeutics. Treatment is started with hydroxocobalamin 1 mg three times weekly and then reduced to 1 mg every 6–8 weeks when a satisfactory remission has been produced. Maintenance doses of cyanocobalamin, however, should be given every 3–4 weeks.

The lesions in the nervous system also respond to cobalamin, but it may be many months before the full effect of treatment is seen.

Occasionally, vegans may develop vitamin B12 deficiency due to a shortage in the diet. To prevent this 1 mg of hydroxycobalamin can be added weekly to their diet.

Folic acid. Folic acid is obtained from animal and vegetable sources and is also synthesized by bacteria. It is necessary for the maturation of red cells, and deficiency will produce changes in the blood similar to those found in pernicious anaemia.

The common causes of deficiency in this country are:

1. Malabsorption syndromes such as coeliac disease.
2. Pregnancy. Some women fail to absorb folic acid in the later months of pregnancy and thus become anaemic. In addition, folic acid taken during pregnancy reduces the incidence of *neural tube defects*. Iron deficiency is also common in pregnancy and it is usual to give both folic acid and iron supplements at this time.

Therapeutics. Folic acid can be given orally in doses of 10–15 mg daily. If the anaemia is severe the first dose should be given intramuscularly. Tablets containing both iron and folic acid are available for use in pregnancy. 'Pregaday' contains ferrous fumarate equivalent to 100 mg of ferrous iron plus folic acid 350 micrograms, the dose being one tablet daily. *It is important not to treat pernicious anaemia with folic acid for, although it will improve the anaemia, it will worsen the neurological complications of pernicious anaemia.*

Erythropoietin deficiency

Erythropoietin is a hormone manufactured by the kidney, which is necessary for erythrocyte formation. If the kidneys fail, the level of erythropoietin in the blood falls with resulting anaemia.

Epoetin is a genetically engineered analogue of erythropoietin and two forms, alpha and beta, are available commercially. They are essentially the same. In patients with renal failure and anaemia epoetin is given weekly by subcutaneous or intravenous injection until a satisfactory haemoglobin level is produced. Treatment then continues with weekly maintenance doses.

Adverse effects. Hypertension is quite common and may be severe. The blood pressure should be measured every week in the initial stages of treatment and then at 6-weekly intervals. Thrombosis and 'flu'-like symptoms occasionally occur.

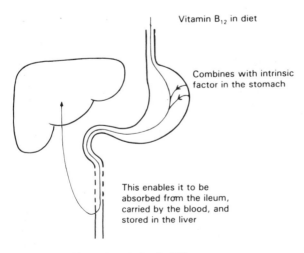

Vitamin B$_{12}$ in diet

Combines with intrinsic factor in the stomach

This enables it to be absorbed from the ileum, carried by the blood, and stored in the liver

Fig. 19.1 Absorption of vitamin B12.

Patient education

Severe hypertension requires immediate treatment.
Patients or relatives should be told to report
headaches or confusion at once.

FURTHER READING

Hibbard B M, Horn E 1988 Iron and folate supplements
during pregnancy. British Medical Journal 297: 1324
Kong C H, Brown S M 1991 Recombinant human
erythropoietin in the management of anaemia. ERSO
Professional Nurse 6(11): 650

20

Drugs used in the treatment of malignant disease

Although a great deal has been discovered about normal cell function and cell division, after many years of research it is still not known why malignant cells behave as they do. The pattern of their behaviour is familiar. Instead of differentiating in an orderly fashion to take their place in the formation of some organ, they multiply in a haphazard way showing little if any attempt at differentiation and, further, instead of remaining in their organ of origin they invade neighbouring structures. Cell emboli from new growths are swept in the blood or lymphatic circulation to distant parts of the body, take root and set up further tumours known as secondary deposits or metastases.

CELL DIVISION AND CYTOTOXIC DRUGS

The cells of the body vary enormously in appearance and function but have some characteristics which are common to all types of cell. With very few exceptions (e.g. erythrocytes), cells consist of a nucleus surrounded by cytoplasm. The most vital component of the nucleus is deoxyribonucleic acid (DNA), which consists of two chains of molecules arranged rather like a spiral staircase. DNA is very important because it contains the code which determines the type of protein that is made by the cell and thus ultimately how the cell functions.

One of the important components of the cell cytoplasm is ribonucleic acid (RNA). This substance receives instructions from the DNA in the

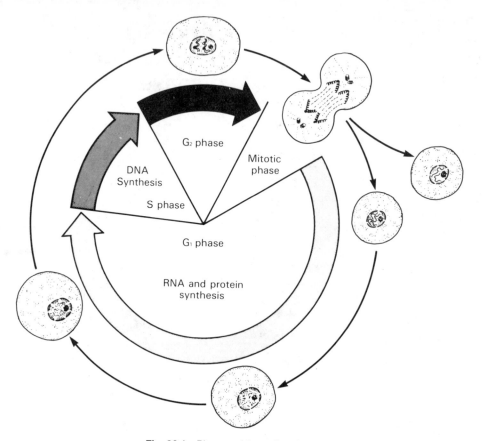

Fig. 20.1 Phases of the cell cycle.

cell nucleus and is actually responsible for the manufacture of protein.

Most cytotoxic drugs interfere with DNA or RNA, and thus they have a profound effect on cells and their functions. Unfortunately, these actions are not confined to the malignant cells but affect normal cells as well.

Some cells in the body divide frequently to replace those which have become worn out, particularly the cells of the bone marrow, the lymphatic system and the lining of the intestinal tract and are particularly sensitive to the action of cytotoxic drugs.

During its life the cell passes through a series of changes, and cell division itself is a complicated process. The newly formed cell enters the G_1 stage, which is a period of protein synthesis and intense metabolic activity. This may last for a variable time, from a few hours to many years.

Many cells remain in this phase throughout the life of the organism, but some undergo division and enter the S phase. This phase is short and is concerned with DNA and RNA synthesis so that the DNA strands may split when cell division occurs. It is a period of great metabolic activity. The G_2 phase which follows is a short period of consolidation before cell division occurs. In the mitotic phase the DNA spiral splits longitudinally so that each daughter cell has its full complement of DNA, which is exactly the same as that in the parent cell (Fig. 20.1).

Some cytotoxic drugs will affect cells at any phase in their life cycle; others will only act at a single phase of the cell cycle, usually when the cell is dividing, and are called *phase specific*. It follows therefore that when using phase specific drugs repeated dosage is necessary if maximum effect is to be achieved.

A proportion of the cells in a cancer are in a resting phase, sometimes called the G_0 phase, when they are not dividing. This is important because in this stage they are very resistant to chemotherapy.

The aim of treatment of neoplastic disease with drugs is to find a drug which will kill the neoplastic cells while leaving the normal cells of the body unharmed. However, the metabolic process of the neoplastic cells is so very similar or perhaps even the same as that of normal cells that so far it has been impossible to reach this ideal. Nearly all drugs which have so far been discovered, although having a marked toxic effect on neoplastic cells, have some adverse effect on the normal cells of the body especially those of the bone marrow. The best that can be done is to give the cytotoxic drug or drugs at repeated intervals so arranged that the recovery of normal cells can occur but little recovery of cancer cells is possible. It *may* then be possible to progressively reduce the number of malignant cells without unduly reducing the normal ones until ultimately all the malignant cells are eradicated (Fig. 20.2).

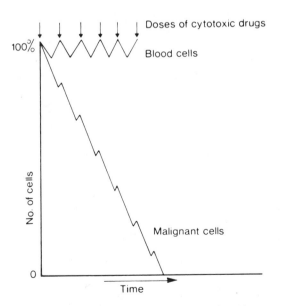

Fig. 20.2 Progressive reduction in the number of malignant cells produced by repeated doses of a cytotoxic drug, with recovery of the normal blood cells. An ideal therapeutic response.

There are several types of drug used in the treatment of neoplastic disease.

ALKYLATING AGENTS

These are chemically very active substances which combine with the DNA in the cell nucleus and thus damage or kill the cell. Unfortunately, although these substances have a marked effect on certain types of malignant cells, they also damage normal cells, particularly those of the bone marrow and gastrointestinal tract which have a high rate of division.

There are a number of alkylating agents now available.

Mustine (nitrogen mustard) is related to mustard gas and is used in the treatment of neoplastic diseases of the lympho-reticular system such as Hodgkin's disease and with less success in certain carcinomas such as those of the ovary and bronchus.

Therapeutics. Nitrogen mustard is given by intravenous injection and as it is very irritant it is common practice to set up an intravenous drip of saline and inject nitrogen mustard into the drip tubing and flush it through the vein with saline.

Adverse effects. Most patients experience nausea and vomiting for some hours after treatment. Bone marrow suppression is an ever present risk, usually affecting the white cells and platelets.

Mustine may also be injected into malignant effusions and may either slow down or prevent their formation.

Cyclophosphamide was developed in an attempt to improve the therapeutic effectiveness of this type of drug. Cyclophosphamide itself is non-toxic, but in the liver it is split by enzymes which release cytotoxic metabolites. It can be given orally or intravenously, either daily or weekly and is frequently combined with other cytotoxic agents. The dose varies between 100 mg and 1 g or more according to the regime being used. The therapeutic effect is usually delayed for a week or more.

Adverse effects include depression of the bone marrow and loss of hair. A metabolite is excreted in the urine which can cause a severe cystitis. This may be avoided by giving a high fluid intake (4 litres a day) or combining it with mesna (see below).

Ifosfamide is closely related to cyclophosphamide from which it differs slightly in efficacy. It is less likely to depress the blood count than cyclophosphamide but is more likely to damage the kidneys and bladder. To prevent this adverse effect it is combined with a drug called **mesna** which neutralizes ifosfamide in the kidneys and bladder and thus prevents toxicity.

Chlorambucil is a useful drug of the mustine group. It is effective by mouth and although depression of the bone marrow can occur, vomiting is unusual.

Therapeutics. Chlorambucil is given orally and a usual course of treatment is to give 10 mg daily for 14 days in every month. It can be used on an outpatient basis but the patient should attend monthly for blood counts. It is effective against the same disorders as mustine and is probably the drug of choice in chronic lymphatic leukaemia.

Busulphan is particularly used in chronic myeloid leukaemia where it has a selective depressing action on the abnormal white cells. Excessive dosage will produce dangerous depression of normal white cells and platelets.

Therapeutics. Busulphan is usually given in doses of 2–4 mg daily. Treatment is continued over weeks or months and is modified by the response of the patient.

Adverse effects. In addition to bone marrow depression it can cause pigmentation and fibrosis of the lungs.

Melphalan is used particularly in multiple myelomatosis. The usual dose is 10 mg daily for a week, which may be repeated if the blood count is satisfactory. Melphalan is a powerful depressant of white cells and platelets.

Lomustine (CCNU) is similar in many ways to the alkylating agents and though its mode of action is different it is effective against the same types of cancer. It is given orally as a single dose and should not be repeated for 4 or preferably 6 weeks as depression of white cells and platelets may be delayed. Nausea and sometimes vomiting is common for about 12 hours after dosage.

ANTIMETABOLITES

These agents resemble substances used by the cells for their metabolic processes. They thus become incorporated in the cells and because they cannot be metabolized normally they cause the cell to die.

Malignant cells often have a very rapid metabolic turnover and thus incorporate antimetabolites more rapidly than normal cells. It is thus possible to kill the majority of malignant cells without interfering too drastically with normal cells. Excessive dosage will inhibit normal cell production, particularly in the bone marrow.

Methotrexate. This is similar in structure to folic acid and it blocks one of the chemical processes necessary for the production of cell nuclear material from folic acid. Methotrexate can be given orally, intravenously or intrathecally but large doses are not well absorbed from the intestine and must be given by injection. Dosage schedules depend on the type of cancer being treated. It is excreted via the kidney and it is essential that renal function is measured before starting treatment. With impaired function the dose is reduced.

In certain types of malignant disease, a very large and potentially lethal dose of methotrexate is given; then after 24 hours, the action of the drug is reversed by giving folinic acid. It is extremely important that this is carried out precisely. This method is known as *folinic acid rescue*.

Adverse effects. In addition to bone marrow suppression methotrexate can cause liver damage and mouth ulceration.

6-Mercaptopurine is closely related chemically to adenine and hypoxanthine, two substances used in the formation of the cell nucleus.

It is believed that 6-mercaptopurine replaces these substances in the nucleus of cells and thereby prevents their further division. It is used in combination with other drugs in the treatment of acute leukaemia, a disease where the bone marrow is rapidly overgrown by very malignant white cells.

6-Mercaptopurine can also be used in chronic myeloid leukaemia.

Therapeutics. The dosage of 6-mercaptopurine is 2.5 mg/kg body weight/day by mouth and the course of treatment is determined by the response of the patient. Excessive or prolonged treatment will produce depression of normal white cells.

5-Fluorouracil is another antimetabolite which is used with some benefit in a wide variety of tumours including those of the gastrointestinal tract. It is given by intravenous infusion; the dose lies between 250 mg and 1 g, depending on circumstances. It produces leucopenia and in particular ulceration of the mouth.

Cytarabine is a drug which interferes with the nuclear function in the malignant cell and is used in acute leukaemia. It can cause bone marrow depression.

VINCA ALKALOIDS

Vinblastine is an extract of periwinkle. It is believed to act at the stage of cell division (mitosis) and is therefore phase specific. Vinblastine is useful as part of a cytotoxic drug regime in treating certain lymphomas and is given in a single weekly injection of 6 mg/m^2. It can cause a leucopenia which is, however, usually short-lived.

Vincristine which is related to vinblastine is also given intravenously usually at weekly intervals. The dose is between 1–2 mg/m^2 i.v. It is used as an initial drug in acute leukaemia to induce a remission and is also useful in lymphomas and other cancers. It is less likely to cause leucopenia but may also damage peripheral and autonomic nerves producing constipation with abdominal distention and tingling and numbness in the limbs.

MISCELLANEOUS DRUGS

Doxorubicin (Adriamycin). This cytotoxic drug is an antibiotic; it has a fairly wide antitumour range. It is given by intravenous injection, every 3 weeks, usually in combination with other cytotoxic drugs. It is believed to interfere with DNA and RNA function.

Adverse effects. It can depress bone marrow and this occurs about 2 weeks after treatment, rather later than with most cytotoxic drugs. It is toxic to heart muscle and this requires regular ECG monitoring. Toxicity is dose related and the total cumulative dose of the drug should not exceed 500 mg/m^2. Other effects are nausea, vomiting and hair loss.

Procarbazine is also used in the lymphomas in doses of 50–150 mg daily. Nausea is less likely if the drug is given after meals and it may have to be combined with an anti-emetic. If alcohol is taken at the same time as the drug it may produce a reddish flush.

Dacarbazine (DTIC) is largely used in treating Hodgkin's disease and melanomas. It has to be given intravenously and is highly irritant so it must be injected *very* slowly into a fast running drip. It also causes considerable vomiting.

Bleomycin is another antibiotic with relatively weak anticancer effects. However, unlike all the drugs already discussed, it does not depress the bone marrow. It is usually injected at weekly intervals, and injection may be followed by a spike of fever. Prolonged use (usually more than a total cumulative dose of 200 units) leads to lung fibrosis.

Etoposide is related to podophyllin, an extract of mandrake which can be applied locally in the treatment of warts. Its action is to prevent cell division.

Etoposide can be given orally or intravenously and is usually used in combination in the treatment of a wide range of malignancies.

Adverse effects include bone marrow depression and vomiting in a small number of patients.

Cisplatin is based on the metal platinum. It is effective in a number of cancers but has found a particular use in regimes designed to treat cancer of the testicle and has proved very successful.

Therapeutics. Cisplatin is given intravenously and usually in combination with other anticancer agents. The dose is 50 mg/m^2 or more, given intravenously at 3–4 week intervals. Certain precautions must be observed:

1. A diuresis is essential when the drug is given or it will damage the kidneys.
2. Hearing should be tested regularly as it damages the inner ear.
3. Vomiting is usually very troublesome.

It follows, therefore, that this drug should only be given by those who are aware of the complications which can occur.

Carboplatin is similar and is used in ovarian carcinoma. It is not, however, so nephrotoxic as cisplatin.

Mitozantrone is given as a single injection at 3-weekly intervals. It is used in a variety of cancers. The incidence of adverse effects is relatively low and it is useful in controlling the disease, particularly on an outpatient basis.

COMBINATION THERAPY

In most forms of malignant disease which can be treated successfully by drugs, better results with less toxicity are achieved if several cytotoxic agents are combined in the course of treatment. Most regimes consist of repeated courses given at intervals of 1–2 weeks and extending over 6–12 months or even longer. This enables the malignant cells to be attacked at different stages in their cell cycle; also careful timing enables the normal cells of the body to recover while the malignant cells remain suppressed. Treatment can often be carried out on an outpatient basis, or with the patient remaining in hospital overnight when he receives the drugs. As an example of a

treatment which has been used for widespread Hodgkin's disease, the MOPP regime is shown below:

Mustine 6 mg/m^2 body surface, i.v., on days 1 and 8.
Vinblastine 10 mg i.v., on days 1 and 8.
Procarbazine 100 mg, orally on days 1 to 15.
Prednisolone 40 mg daily, orally, days 1 to 15.

After a rest period of 1 month the course is repeated until six courses have been given. Courses are sometimes then repeated every 3 months for 1 year and every 4 months for the next year.

Many combination regimes are now being used in the treatment of various types of cancer. Among the malignant diseases which can nearly always be improved and quite often cured are:

- Acute lymphoblastic leukaemia
- Hodgkin's disease
- Non-Hodgkin lymphomas
- Testicular cancer
- Ovarian cancer
- Childhood cancers
- Chorionepithelioma.

Chemotherapy may be combined with other types of treatment such as surgery or radiotherapy and the management of a patient is often an integral operation. Although a great deal of cancer will continue to be treated in general hospitals there is much to be said for the more complicated regimes being carried out in special oncology units.

In terms of nursing organization it requires frequent short-term admissions or special outpatient facilities and careful checks on the general health of the patient and the blood count.

Special training is now available for nurses who wish to work in the field of cancer treatment.

ADJUVANT THERAPY

It is common experience that, although a malignant growth appears to have been totally removed, a recurrence may occur somewhere else in the body at a later date. This must mean that at the time of operation there was already a

Table 20.1 Storage and preparation of cytotoxic drugs

Drug	Storage	Diluent	Stability in solution*	Administration
Mustine	Refrigerate	Water for injection	Unstable, use immediately	i.v.
Cyclophosphamide	Cool place	Water for injection	Stable for 2 h	i.v. or oral
Chlorambucil	Room temp	—	—	oral
Melphalan	Room temp	—	—	oral
Vinblastine	Refrigerate	Saline	Stable in fridge for 48 hours	i.v.
Procarbazine	Room temp	—	—	oral
5-Fluorouracil	Refrigerate	Water for injection	—	i.v.
	Room temp	—	—	oral
Methotrexate	Room temp	Water for injection	Stable in fridge for 24 h	i.v.
	Room temp	Saline	—	i.v. and intrathecal[†]
				oral
Adriamycin	Room temp	Water for injection	Unstable	i.v.
Lomustine	Room temp	—	—	oral
Bleomycin	Room temp	Saline	Unstable	i.v. or i.m.
Dacarbazine	Refrigerate and protect from light	Water for injection	Use within 8 h	i.v.
Cisplatin	Room temp	Water and diluted in 2 l of saline	20 h at room temp	i.v. infusion

* Although some cytotoxic drugs can be used for periods after the solutions have been prepared, it is wise to discard all unused remnants at the end of a treatment session owing to the risk of bacterial contamination.
[†]Special preparation required for intrathecal injection, must be free of irritant preservatives.

seedling deposit, and the object of adjuvant therapy is to give cytotoxic drugs after operation even if there is no evidence of spread to eradicate hidden small deposits which are particularly susceptible to drug treatment. There is now a considerable body of evidence that in early breast cancer, adjuvant therapy results in an improved prognosis as judged by a 10-year follow up. Premenopausal women do best with chemotherapy but it is confined to those with a relatively poor prognosis as treatment carries with it quite serious adverse effects. In postmenopausal women simple hormone treatment with tamoxifen (see p. 253) is adequate.

Palliative chemotherapy

In some types of advanced cancer, chemotherapy can relieve symptoms and prolong life but is not curative. Most regimes have some side-effects and before embarking on palliative chemotherapy it is very important to weigh possible benefits against disadvantages. This will require a compassionate discussion with the patient and ascertaining the views of relatives, nursing staff and others who are involved. As with all chronic diseases much supportive care will be necessary, and generally, such treatment should be given in specialist oncology units.

It is impossible to discuss the palliation of all the cancers in which this treatment is an option but the group includes:

- Carcinoma of the breast
- Small cell carcinoma of the lung
- Carcinoma of the ovary and cervix
- Colorectal carcinoma
- Carcinoma of the bladder
- Head and neck cancer
- Various lymphomas
- Malignant melanoma.

If the nurse requires further information, the subject is discussed by R D Rubens et al (1992) British Medical Journal 304: 35.

SOME PRACTICAL POINTS
Preparation of solutions (Table 20.1)

The preparation of solutions of cytotoxic drugs for injection should only be carried out by:

1. Medical staff
2. Pharmacists
3. Nurses who hold a certificate of competence.

Some of these substances are very irritant and, in addition, can be highly dangerous if absorbed. The following precautions should be observed:

1. Wear plastic gloves and a plastic apron when making up solutions or crushing tablets. If any of the drug splashes onto the skin it should be washed off immediately. Some of the drugs are irritant and there is always the risk of an allergic reaction.
2. Avoid getting any of the drug into the eyes and wear protective spectacles. If the drug comes into contact with the eyes, they should be washed out with water and further advice should be sought.
3. Care should be taken to avoid absorbing the drug either systemically or by inhalation. Hands should be washed after preparing a drug (even when gloves are worn). The drugs should be prepared in a designated area, well away from food, crockery, etc. and not at the bedside. Ideally, they should be handled under an extraction fan. Although at present there is no evidence that those who handle cytotoxic drugs are more liable to suffer long-term ill-effects, there are certainly no grounds for complacency and every care must be taken.
4. Made-up solutions should only be used during the session for which they are prepared.
5. Pregnant staff should not prepare cytotoxic solutions.
6. If spillage occurs, it should be mopped up with absorbent paper which must be disposed of properly and the whole area washed down thoroughly.

Administration of cytotoxic drugs

In view of the possible danger when giving cytotoxics the following authorization should be applied:

a. Oral—no special restriction
b. i.m. or i.v. infusion—nurses holding a certificate of competence

c. Intravenous bolus—oncology nurse, specialist or medical staff
d. Intrathecal or intra-arterial—medical staff.

Never use the brachial vein for vesicant drugs. Use a no. 23 butterfly or a Venflon 21 or 22 for intravenous administration.

Vesicant drugs should be given into a fast running infusion over at least 5 minutes.

Extravasation of cytotoxic drugs on injection

Even if great care is taken, some leaking of the injected drug may occur around the vein and this can cause problems.

Vesicant drugs carry a high risk of severe tissue necrosis if they extravasate.

Vesicant drugs:

Dactinomycin	Mustine
Daunorubicin	Plicamycin
Doxorubicin	Vinblastine
Epirubicin	Vincristine
Mitomycin	Vindesine

Bleomycin and ifosfamide are irritant drugs which cause pain but do not lead to tissue damage. For bleomycin and ifosfamide, 1% lignocaine is adequate to relieve the pain but for vesicants the following full extravasation procedure should be carried out:

a. Leave the needle in situ and flood the area with saline.
b. Inject 100 mg of hydrocortisone through the needle.
c. Continue flushing and infiltrate the periphery with 100 mg of hydrocortisone.
d. The area should be flooded with at least 100 ml of saline which should then be gently massaged away.
e. The needle can now be removed.
f. Record the episode in the patient's notes.
g. Consult an expert.
h. Inspect the area after 24 hours and as often as necessary thereafter.

Policies may vary in different units and local policies and procedures should be available and strictly followed.

Occasionally, necrosis occurs despite all the measures and skin grafting may be required.

Vomiting with cytotoxic drugs

Many cytotoxic drugs cause the patient to vomit a few hours after administration.

Severe	Moderate	Mild
Cisplatin	Cytarabine	Bleomycin
Cyclophos-phamide (high dose)	Etoposide	Busulphan
Dacarbazine	Procarbazine	Chlorambucin
Daunorubicin	Vinblastine	Fluorouracil
Doxorubicin		Melphalan
Lomustine		Mercaptopurine
Mustine		Methorexate
Plicamycin		Vincristine
Streptozocin		

There is as yet no complete remedy for this troublesome side-effect. A variety of regimes may be tried in an attempt to mitigate the symptoms and patients vary in their preference. It is usual to give cytotoxic drugs in the late evening so that the patient may sleep as much as possible through the period of nausea.

For mildly or moderately emetic cytotoxics prochlorperazine, domperidone or low-dose metoclopramide can be used.

Combinations are often more effective and:

Lorazepam 2 mg orally +
Haloperidol 3 mg orally +
Dexamethasone 10 mg i.v., is particularly useful.

It is believed that the most severely emetic drugs (e.g. cisplatin) stimulate the $5HT_3$ receptors in the gastrointestinal tract and brain stem. *Ondansteron*, a $5HT_3$ antagonist, 8 mg i.v. followed by 8 mg orally twice daily for 2 days is the most effective anti-emetic for this type of cytotoxic drug.

Some patients, particularly towards the end of their course of treatment, become anxious and tensed up before treatment and may indeed vomit before receiving their drugs. This is a difficult problem. Diazepam (5 mg) an hour before coming to hospital may be tried and sometimes psychiatric support with a desensitization programme helps.

Care of the mouth

Mouth ulceration may occur with many cytotoxic regimes. This is partially due to the direct effect of the drugs on the mucous membrane of the mouth and also the general suppression of immunity, particularly of the white blood cells, encourages infection. This unpleasant complication can be minimized.

1. Before starting treatment, the patient should be seen by a dentist or dental hygienist and have any infections treated.
2. If the white count drops or the mouth becomes sore, the patient should have nystatin pastilles (for candida) 6 hourly and Corsodyl mouth washes twice daily.
3. If ulceration develops, the pain can be relieved by Difflam Oral Rinse which contains benzydamine, a local anaesthetic. The mouth is rinsed out every 3 hours with the undiluted solution. Lignocaine gel can also be applied to the painful area.

Infection

Patients who are being treated with cytotoxic drugs are liable to develop infection because their immunity is suppressed by the drugs. In addition to those caused by the usual bacteria, infections may be due to fungi, viruses and even organisms which do not normally cause disease in healthy people. Attempts have been made to diminish the risk of infection by isolating the patients but this is difficult and, if strictly implemented, very expensive. In most cases it appears to be sufficient to avoid obvious sources of infection. Those caring for these people should always watch for signs of infection and the patients should be told to report any suspicious symptoms. Immunosuppressed patients often respond poorly to antibacterial treatment and the infecting organism may be obscure, so a combination of antibiotics is often used.

Long-term risks of the use of cytotoxic drugs

Most cytotoxic drugs interfere in some way or other with the structure of the cell nucleus and this can have serious long-term implications.

1. Second malignancy. These drugs may induce changes in normal cells so that they ultimately become malignant. This means that although the original cancer is eradicated, a different malignancy may develop at a later date. Second malignancies are more common after certain cytotoxic drugs and if drugs are combined with radiotherapy. It is necessary to get this risk in perspective as the chance of dying from the initial cancer, if untreated, is much greater than that of developing a further cancer. Some information is now available as to the risk of second malignancies with various cytotoxic drugs and the situation is becoming increasingly well defined. This risk will be one factor to be considered when choosing a suitable regime.

2. Many cytotoxic drugs damage the gonads. In men permanent sterility may result, in women amenorrhoea is common but periods usually return after stopping treatment. It is now possible to store a man's sperm before treatment in case gonadal function is permanently suppressed.

3. If pregnancy is avoided for 6 months from the end of treatment, there does not seem to be an increased risk of an abnormal infant being born.

The role of the nurse in cancer chemotherapy

The establishment of units specializing in oncology has enabled nurses to receive advanced training which is of direct benefit to patients and their families. A multidisciplinary approach is important in the treatment of cancer and the team will consist of nurses, doctors, pharmacists and social workers. In most centres part of the work will be concerned with therapeutic trials and this will require ancillary staff.

The management of malignant disease may be by chemotherapy alone or may involve surgery or radiotherapy. In this book only the problems of chemotherapy are considered. In addition to technical knowledge the nurse will have a most important role in patient support. The distress and fear of having cancer is enough to shake the stoutest heart and, indeed, chemotherapy is usually prolonged and often unpleasant.

In the initial assessment nurses should try to establish what patients know about malignant disease and their beliefs, if any, about treatment. They will appeal to the nurses for information and this provides an opportunity to dispel myths and at the same time explain what treatment will entail. Patient education is multipronged and can take the form of booklets, videos, question and answer sessions and group discussions so that sufferers can gain support from others in similar circumstances. Patients usually attend oncology units at regular intervals for treatment and follow-up so it is possible for the nursing staff to build up a supportive relationship with those who know and trust them.

A good deal of research is in progress by oncology units to mitigate the unpleasantness of chemotherapy and one of the key areas being examined is the use of self-help measures at home.

HORMONES IN MALIGNANT DISEASE

Various hormones will produce a temporary remission in malignant disease. Their mode of action is not clear but it is believed that certain malignant tumours are in part dependent on hormones. By removing these hormones (i.e. by removing the endocrine glands where they originate) or by suppressing them by giving other hormones, the stimulus to growth is removed from the malignant. cells and they regress.

Examples of such forms of treatment are the orchidectomy or the administration of oestrogen or gonadotrophin releasing hormone (*goserelin*) in patients with carcinoma of the prostate, and adrenalectomy or the administration of oestrogen or testosterone to patients with carcinoma of the breast.

Tamoxifen competes with oestrogens for receptors in the malignant cells. In some way which is not understood this causes regression of the tumour in carcinoma of the breast. It is given in doses of 20 mg orally daily for metastatic disease in both pre- and postmenopausal women and is also used in the adjuvant treatment of postmenopausal women.

Adverse effects are mild and include occasional nausea, oedema, flushing and bone pain.

Interactions. Increases the anticoagulant effect of warfarin.

Aminoglutethimide inhibits steroid synthesis in the adrenals and also suppresses oestrogen and androgen production in the peripheral tissues. For this reason it is used in the treatment of advanced breast cancer. It can also be used to control the overproduction of adrenal steroid hormones in Cushing's disease.

FURTHER READING

Banks C 1991 Alleviating anticipatory vomiting. Nursing Times 87 (16): 42

Byrne J et al 1987 Effects of treatment on fertility in long-term survivors of childhood or adolescent cancer. New England Journal of Medicine 317: 1315

Freeman E 1990 Making sense of cancer chemotherapy. Nursing times 86 (31): 45

Gibbs J 1991 Handling cytotoxic drugs. Nursing times 87 (11): 54

Holmes S 1990 Cancer chemotherapy. Lisa Sainsbury Foundation, Austin Cornish, London

Kaye S B 1988 Prevention of vomiting due to cytotoxic drugs. Prescribers Journal 28: 144

Richardson A 1992 The Royal Marsden Hospital manual of core care plans for cancer nursing. Scutari Press, London

Stuard N S A, Blackledge G R P 1989 Side effects of cytotoxic chemotherapy. Prescribers Journal 28: 155

Swerdlow A J et al 1992 Risk of primary cancer after Hodgkin's disease. British Medical Journal 304: 1137

Williams C J 1985 Handling cytotoxics. British Medical Journal 291: 1299

Department of Health 1988 Policy for safe handling of cytotoxic drugs. Health Management System and Personal Division, WHC (88) 65, HMSO, London

21

Drugs at the extremes of age

Most facts about drugs are obtained from observations on adults. However, age may modify the way drugs are handled by the body and also the way the body reacts to the actions of drugs. In recent years, increasing interest has led to studies of drugs given at the extremes of age.

DRUGS IN PREGNANCY

Drugs can affect the fetus either by interfering with some important function in the mother which indirectly damages the fetus or by passing across the placenta and acting directly on it. *Most drugs cross the placenta.*

The fetus may be damaged at three stages of pregnancy.

1. Implantation (5–15 days). Drug toxicity at this stage usually results in abortion.
2. Embryo stage (15–55 days). During this period it is changing from a group of cells into a recognizable human being. The embryo is particularly susceptible to drug toxicity at this time which leads to fetal malformation such as occurs with thalidomide.
3. Fetogenic stage (55 days–birth). As the fetus continues to grow and develop drug damage becomes less likely but it is still possible.

In this country about 30% of women take some drug during pregnancy, though only 10% take one in the first trimester when the fetus is most vulnerable to damage. Those most commonly taken are mild analgesics and antibiotics.

It is important to discover which drugs can

produce fetal damage and which are safe to use. This is difficult for two reasons;

1. Fetal abnormalities can occur for various reasons even when no drugs are taken.

About 2% of babies have some abnormality at birth but only about 5% of these are believed to be drug-related.

2. If the drug only rarely causes an abnormality, thousands of pregnant women need to be studied before a connection between a certain drug and fetal damage can be confirmed. Experiments with pregnant animals have only a limited value.

At present drugs can be divided into three groups:

A. Drugs known to produce fetal abnormalities

Thalidomide
Folic acid antagonists
Tetracyclines
Androgens
Warfarin (during the first 4 months of pregnancy)
Diethylstilboestrol
Etretinate
Lithium
Some anticonvulsants

B. Drugs suspected of producing fetal abnormalities

Oral hypoglycaemic agents
Various cytotoxic drugs
Anorexics (amphetamines)
ACE inhibitors

A number of other drugs which are under suspicion or for which information is not available.

C. Drugs which probably do not harm the fetus (see British National Formulary, Appendix 4)

Simple analgesics	— Paracetamol for minor pain.
	— NSAIAs can be used if really necessary and ibuprofen, being mild

and short-acting, is preferred.

Powerful analgesics	— Opioids can be used (but see below).
Drugs for dyspepsia	— Antacids.
Drugs for constipation	— Bulk purges.
Drugs for nausea	— Avoid if possible and treat by modifying diet.
	— Promethazine if necessary.
Antibacterials	— Penicillins, cephalosporins, erythromycin stearate.
	— Trimethoprim should be avoided in the first 3 months of pregnancy if possible.
Antimalarials	— Chloroquine (low dose) proguanil.
Antiasthmatics	— β_2 agonists, inhaled steroids, short courses of systemic steroids if really necessary.
Centrally-acting drugs	— Benzodiazepines (but see below).
	— Neuroleptics and tricyclic antidepressants probably safe.
	— Antiepileptics—see page 150.
Hay fever	— Topical preparations.
	— Antihistamines (chlorpheniramine, terfenadine).

Further information can be obtained from: *Prescribing in Pregnancy*, P. C. Rubin (ed) 1986 British Medical Journal or from a drug information unit.

When treating pregnant women some general rules should be observed:

1. Avoid giving drugs if possible, especially in the first 3 months of pregnancy.
2. Give drugs at lowest effective dose for as short a time as possible.
3. Avoid recently introduced drugs if possible.
4. Drugs on lists A and B should be avoided if

possible. The problem arises when there is no satisfactory substitute and treatment is vital. This is a matter of risk to the fetus against risk to the mother (and often therefore, the fetus as well).

5. *Ethanol.* Alcohol taken by the mother during pregnancy can damage the fetus, resulting in an infant with a small head, facial abnormalities and of low intelligence. Although it may well be better to avoid alcohol altogether in pregnancy, there is no evidence that one glass of wine, or its equivalent, daily causes any harm.

Pregnancy and dosage

Pregnancy causes a number of changes in the way the drug is handled by the body. The volume of water in the body is increased so that the concentration of a given dose will be decreased, though this may be offset by a fall in protein binding which leaves more free active drug in the blood.

Liver enzymes increase so that some drugs are broken down more rapidly and renal excretion may also be enhanced. Where dosage is not critical this does not matter, but for a few drugs (e.g. anticonvulsants and theophylline) adjustment of the dose may be necessary.

DRUGS IN THE NEW-BORN

During the hours of labour drugs may be given to the mother and some of these can pass via the placenta to the neonate. Among those which are important are:

Analgesics and hypnotics. Morphine and similar drugs affect the fetus and may lead to difficulties in starting breathing immediately after birth.

Excessive dosing of the mother with barbiturates and benzodiazepines leads to accumulation of these drugs in the fetus and after birth the infant will be floppy with depressed breathing and failure to suck.

β **blockers** pass to the fetus and produce a slow pulse rate.

Kernicterus and drugs. Certain drugs given to the mother late in pregnancy or to the infant in the first few days of life bind onto the plasma protein and displace bilirubin from the binding sites. This can be dangerous because too much uncombined bilirubin in the blood causes brain damage. Drugs that have been implicated are:

Sulphonamides
Tolbutamide
Aspirin.

Chloramphenicol. The new-born are not able to break down drugs as effectively as older children or adults thus accumulation may occur after repeated dosing. With chloramphenicol this can be dangerous as accumulation of the drug produces the 'grey syndrome' which is due to collapse of the circulation.

Oxygen. Treating a new-born infant with a high concentration of oxygen is known to cause blindness due to retrolental fibroplasia.

BREAST FEEDING AND DRUGS

Most drugs will pass into the breast milk but usually at very low and innocuous concentrations. However, this is not inevitable and a few drugs being taken by the mother can be a hazard to the baby. Generally, drugs should be avoided by nursing mothers, but if a drug is essential the baby should feed just before the mother takes her dose when blood levels will be low.

Certain drugs should not be used by nursing mothers and if unavoidable, will require transfer to bottle feeding.

For further information there is a comprehensive list of safe and unsafe drugs in the British National Formulary, Appendix 5.

DOSAGE OF DRUGS IN CHILDREN

Children should not be regarded as small adults when prescribing for them particularly in the first few months of life. They differ in:

1. Body composition.
2. Elimination of drugs.

In the first few weeks of life the breakdown of drugs by the liver is reduced but thereafter, because of the relatively large size of a child's liver, the rate of breakdown is greater, weight for weight, than in the adult. This discrepancy progressively disappears until adulthood.

Renal excretion is similarly reduced in the first few weeks of life but reaches normal levels by about 6 weeks. It follows therefore that except for the first few weeks of life, weight-related doses of most drugs are higher in children than in adults.

This means that dosage has to be carefully considered for each individual drug. Young children find it difficult to swallow tablets so liquid preparations are preferable. However, they should not be mixed in the feeding bottle as milk may interfere with drug absorption. Older children respond to drugs more like adults but, even here, there may be differences.

There is no completely satisfactory way of calculating the correct dose of a drug for children. In practice three methods may be used:

1. Dose = Adult dose $\times \dfrac{\text{Patient's weight in kg}}{70}$

2. Dose = Adult dose $\times \dfrac{\text{Patient's body surface area (metres}^2)}{1.7}$

3. Age	Wt in kg	% of adult dose
New-born	3.5	12.5
4 months	6.5	20
1 year	10	25
3 years	15	33
7 years	23	50

·*Note*: This assumes that the child is 'average'.

The first is most satisfactory in deciding the initial loading dose but the second, which takes into account the rate of breakdown of the drug, is to be preferred for maintenance dosage. Both methods are only approximate and with certain drugs the dose in adults and children differs considerably.

DRUGS IN THE ELDERLY

Old people are responsible for about one-third of the expenditure on drugs by the National Health Service. It is therefore important to know whether the action of drugs is modified by old age and how advancing years may alter the handling of drugs by the body.

1. Drug absorption. At present there is little evidence that the absorption of drugs after oral administration changes with age, provided there is no disease of the gastrointestinal tract.

2. Drug distribution. After absorption drugs are carried round the body in the blood. They are to a greater or lesser extent bound to the plasma proteins, particularly albumin. Old people have less albumin in the blood so, of certain drugs less is protein bound and more is free in the blood and tissue fluids and can therefore produce a greater pharmacological effect.

3. Drug metabolism (breakdown). Many drugs are broken down by enzymes in the liver, but with advancing age these enzymes become less active and, in addition, the blood supply to the liver decreases. The result is a slower breakdown of drugs with a tendency for accumulation to occur and signs of overdosage to develop. Those implicated include:

Lignocaine	Tricyclic antidepressants
Propranolol	Caffeine

4. Drug excretion. Drugs are also excreted via the kidney. Old age, sometimes associated with kidney disease, leads to a decline in renal function, so that by the age of 80 years renal function is only half that at age 40. This again may cause drug accumulation and the most important drugs in this case are:

Digoxin	Aminoglycosides
Propranolol	

5. Organ sensitivity. This is more difficult to assess but there is evidence that certain systems become more sensitive to drug action with advancing years. Brain function is easily disturbed in old people so that hypnotics can easily produce confusion and excessive drowsiness.

6. Compliance. Complicated drug regimes may be impossible for old people to follow so they either give up taking their drugs or take the wrong doses at the wrong times, sometimes with disastrous results.

7. **Adverse reactions** to a drug are two or three times more common in the elderly than in younger adults and there are several reasons for this:

a. Elderly patients often need several drugs at the same time and there is a close relationship between the number of drugs taken and the incidence of adverse reactions.

b. For reasons given above the elimination of drugs may be impaired in the elderly so that they are exposed to higher concentrations unless the dose is suitably adjusted.

c. Elderly patients are often severely ill and this may interfere with elimination.

d. Drugs which are associated with adverse reactions such as digoxin, diuretics, NSAIAs, hypotensives and various centrally-acting agents are often prescribed for the elderly.

This does not mean that diseases should not be treated in old people but drugs must be prescribed with care.

All these considerations have made it necessary to observe certain general principles when using drugs for the elderly:

1. A full **drug history** is important as the patient may have experienced an adverse effect from a drug in the past. Medication already being taken may raise the possibility of an interaction. It will also enable the nurse to assess the patient's ability to manage the regime alone or whether help may be needed from relatives.

2. Keep the regime simple and use as few drugs as possible.

3. Prescribe the smallest effective dose and if possible, use drugs which are short acting.

4. Do not continue to use a drug for longer than necessary.

5. If an old person's condition deteriorates remember that a drug may be responsible.

6. Certain formulations such as elixirs may be easier than tablets for an old person to take, particularly if the tablets are very large or very small.

7. Clear and simple instruction should be given to the patient and the container must be clearly labelled. Various types of calendar packs are available but it is important to ensure that the patient can use them.

Specific therapeutic problems

Sleep. Elderly people generally require rather less sleep and broken sleep during the night is quite common. They do not usually require a hypnotic but should avoid sleeping in the day and take more exercise. Alcohol, taken in the evening, may induce sleep but often leads to waking in the night because its hypnotic effect wears off rapidly. If, however, the patient is used to a little alcohol before sleep it is usually best not to interfere. Various disorders can cause sleeplessness and they should be sought and treated if possible:

Pain	Depression
Urinary frequency	Heart failure
Constipation	Dementia

The main dangers of hypnotic drugs for old people are:

1. They may cause mental confusion during the night.

2. They may have hangover effects into the next day.

Old people appear very sensitive to most centrally-acting drugs. Those most commonly used for insomnia are the *benzodiazepines*.

Temazepam 5–15 mg is short acting and to be preferred.

Despite their safety these drugs can produce excessive drowsiness, confusion and ataxia and the smallest possible dose must be used.

Triclofos is related to chloral. The usual dose is 10–20 ml (1–2 g) of the elixir. It is particularly useful in the restless and the disorientated.

Tranquillizers. Agitation with restlessness is common in old people especially if they are demented. This can be controlled by phenothiazines, such as *thioridazine* 25–50 mg, but with all phenothiazines remember postural hypotension, Parkinson-like symptoms and akathisia (restlessness and anxiety).

Depression. Tricyclic antidepressants are useful but postural hypotension, urinary retention and dry mouth can all be troublesome. Avoid in glaucoma.

Parkinson's disease. (See p. 150.) Small doses of *levodopa*, combined with a dopa decarboxylase inhibitor, are useful. In the elderly postural hypotension can be a problem. Anticholinergic drugs often cause troublesome side-effects, i.e. urinary retention and glaucoma and constipation should be avoided.

Hypertension. There is now considerable evidence that treating hypertension in older subjects is worthwhile and it is possible to reduce cardiovascular complications in this group. The cardiovascular systems of old people do not adapt to change so well as in youth therefore a gentle approach is needed. A low dose thiazide diuretic (bendrofluazide 2.5 mg daily) is often enough but if this fails a small dose of a β blocker can be added. The use of ACE inhibitors and calcium blockers is still under review. The blood pressure should be taken standing and lying as the elderly may have a large postural fall.

Chronic heart failure is increasingly common and is usually, but not always, due to coronary artery disease. Treatment is along the same lines as in younger patients (see p. 46) but certain problems are more liable to arise in older people:

Diuretics — Sodium deficiency may develop causing postural hypotension and fainting on standing.
— With loop diuretics, the rapid diuresis can cause acute retension in men with enlarged prostates.
— With large doses, potassium deficiency occasionally occurs, requiring potassium supplements or the addition of a potassium-sparing diuretic.

ACE inhibitors — Hypotension, particularly with the first dose and in those already on diuretics.
— Developing renal failure.

Digoxin — Toxicity due to reduced renal elimination. Low doses should be given.

Oral hypoglycaemic agents. Diabetes in old people can be treated with these drugs. Tolbutamide or glipizide are to be preferred as they are rather short-acting and the risks of hypoglycaemia are less.

Epilepsy which is usually due to cerebrovascular disease is not uncommon in the elderly. The most useful drugs are carbamazepine, sodium valproate and phenytoin. The same problems arise as in younger patients (see p. 147). The initial dose should be small and adverse effects are more easily provoked, mainly because of slower elimination. It is also important to remember that interference with cognitive function, which occurs with many centrally-acting drugs, is more marked in old people.

Antibiotics. There is no particular contraindication to antibiotics in the elderly as long as care is taken with aminoglycosides as reduced renal function can lead to high blood levels and toxic effects.

FURTHER READING

Cargill J 1992 Medication compliance in elderly people: interfering variables and interventions. Journal of Advanced Nursing 17: 422

Conn V C 1991 Older adults: factors that predict the use of over-the-counter medication. Journal of Advanced Nursing 16: 1190

Curnock D A 1985 Prescribing for the newborn baby. Prescribers Journal 25: 62

Glasper A, Oliver R W 1984 A simple guide to infant drug calculations. Nursing 2nd Series 22: 649

Grant E, Golightly P 1992 Drugs in breast feeding. Prescribers Journal 32: 90

Montamat S C et al 1989 Management of drug therapy in the elderly. New England Journal of Medicine 321: 303

Rubin P C 1986 Drugs in Pregnancy. British Medical Association, London

Rylance G (ed) 1987 Drugs for children. WHO, Geneva

Rylance G 1988 Prescribing for infants and children. British Medical Journal 296: 984

Report of Working Group 1991 Cardiological intervention in elderly patients. Journal of the Royal College of Physicians, London

22

Adverse reactions to drugs. Testing of drugs

TYPES OF ADVERSE REACTIONS

During the last few years, adverse reactions to drugs have become increasingly common. They are responsible for about 2% of acute admissions to hospital and occur in 10–20% of hospital inpatients. This is probably due to the enormous increase in the range and number of drugs now in use. It is particularly important for the nurse to be aware of the possibility of drug reactions as she may be the first to realize that something is wrong, and so the drug can be stopped before too much damage is done.

The classification of adverse reactions to drugs has been simplified by Professors Rawlins and Thompson of the University of Newcastle. They have suggested that reactions can be divided into:

Type A reactions which are due to the normal pharmacological actions of the drug which for various reasons are greater than would normally be expected. They are therefore predictable.

Type B reactions which are totally unrelated to the drug's normal pharmacological action. They are therefore unpredictable and not related to the dose of the drug.

Type A reactions

They can be due to:

1. Excessive absorption

This is uncommon.

2. Decreased elimination

This is due to slower breakdown or poor excretion by the kidneys. This in turn leads to accumulation of the drug in the body and adverse effects.

Examples:

- Slow breaking down of morphine by the liver in patients with liver damage causing undue sedation and even coma.
- Poor elimination of gentamicin by the kidneys in renal failure causing accumulation of the antibiotic and damage to the ears.

3. Undue sensitivity of organs

Undue sensitivity to the action of a drug.

Examples:

- The increased sensitivity of the heart to digoxin leading to toxicity in patients with potassium deficiency.
- The respiratory centre of patients with chronic lung disease may be unduly sensitive to opioids, so that normal therapeutic doses cause symptoms of overdose.

This type of reaction is usually related to the dose of the drug and can be relieved if a lower dose is given or the drug is stopped for a time.

Type B reactions

These are bizarre and unexpected reactions and are not dose related. In many cases the reason for and mechanism of this type of adverse reaction is not known: for example, chloramphenicol causes severe depression of the bone marrow in about 1:30 000 treatment courses. It is therefore very difficult to relate the adverse effect to the drug when it occurs in such a small proportion of patients.

Among the known causes of type B reactions are:

1. Genetic factors

A tendency to certain reactions of this type is related to the genetic make-up of the individual.

Example:

- Subjects of tissue type HL-A D3 are more likely to suffer from gold toxicity.

Genetic factors may make the drug act in a completely abnormal way.

Example:

- Primaquine, an antimalarial agent causes breakdown of red cells in about 10% of American negroes. This has been shown to be due to an enzyme deficiency in the red cell.

A similar deficiency is responsible for favism, in which red cells break down as a result of eating certain beans.

2. Environmental factors

These have been little studied but it is possible that in certain individuals diet, tobacco or alcohol consumption and other, as yet unknown, factors may influence the response to a drug.

3. Allergic reactions (See also p. 217)

Allergy plays an important part in unexpected drug reactions although here the mechanism is partially understood.

This type of reaction implies that the patient has been exposed to the drug on some previous occasion. This exposure has resulted in the production of an antibody against the drug. Antibodies are proteins which are formed in the body as the result of the introduction of some foreign substance (antigen). They often serve a useful purpose, for example antibodies formed against bacteria combine with and destroy the bacteria. Several different types of antibodies are produced in response to drugs. Sometimes these antibodies combine with a drug in such a way as to cause damage to tissue and so produce the symptoms of an allergic reaction. Four types are described:

Type I—The antibody (produced in response to a drug) may become attached to the surface of certain cells called mast cells which are scattered throughout the body. If the drug is given on a second occasion the drug (antigen) and antibody combine on the surface of the mast cells which are destroyed, liberating substances such as histamine which cause an acute anaphylactic reaction (see below).

Type II—The antibody may become attached to the surface of red cells. On second exposure to the drug, the combination occurs on the surface of the red cells which are destroyed, producing a haemolytic anaemia.

Type III—Antigens and antibodies may combine in the blood stream to form immune complexes. They may penetrate various organs where they are deposited together with a further substance called complement which is present in the blood. The antigen/antibody/complement combination stimulates inflammation which may affect the skin, kidneys and other organs.

Type IV—Drugs acting as antigens may sensitize lymphocytes which, on further contact with the antigen, will cause tissue damage. This type of reaction usually causes rashes.

Although the exact mechanism of all allergic reactions is not understood, some form of drug/antibody combination is always involved.

Allergic reactions cause a number of clinical disorders:

Acute anaphylaxis (see also p. 119) may follow the injection of foreign serum and also occurs with penicillin and various other drugs. The onset is rapid with chest pain, pallor, collapse and low blood pressure occurring soon after the patient has been given the drug. This type of reaction is sometimes fatal.

Treatment. Acute anaphylaxis should be avoided if possible. *Patients must always be questioned about previous reactions before they are given a drug and particular care is required with sufferers from certain allergic disorders (asthma, hay fever and infantile eczema) as they are more prone to anaphylactic reactions.*

The treatment depends on the severity of the reaction; if severe it consists of:

1. Adrenaline 1:1000 solution 0.6 ml (600 micrograms) intramuscularly
2. Hydrocortisone hemisuccinate 100 mg intravenously, and repeated as required
3. Chlorpheniramine 10 mg intravenously
4. Sometimes cardiopulmonary resuscitation and oxygen may be required
5. *The nurse should never leave the patient alone.*

Serum sickness develops about a week after the serum or drug has been administered. There is usually an urticarial rash with stiffness and swelling of joints, sometimes a mild nephritis and lymph node enlargement. Spontaneous recovery is usual but calamine lotion applied to the rash, and oral chlorpheniramine 4 mg t.d.s. together with prednisolone 10 mg t.d.s. for a few days in more severe cases will relieve the symptoms and speed recovery.

Rashes may occur as a result of drug allergy, but not all rashes which occur when drugs are given are due to allergy. A good example of a non-allergic drug rash is the typical erythmatous rash which often occurs when ampicillin is taken.

Other allergies have been implicated as the cause of various other disorders including depression of the bone marrow leading to leucopenia, thrombocytopenia and anaemia, haemolysis (breakdown) of red cells, jaundice and renal damage. These drug reactions are not always caused by allergic mechanisms and in

---

Nursing point

Adverse reactions cannot be eliminated entirely but they can be minimized by:

1. Taking a *drug history* to discover whether patients are already taking medicines and whether they have had adverse effects from a drug or drugs in the past.
2. Reducing prescribing to a reasonable minimum.
3. Remembering that certain patients (i.e. the elderly, those with liver or renal disease) may not handle drugs in the usual way and dose modifications may be required.
4. Always remembering that some unexpected change in a patient's condition may be due to an adverse drug reaction.

many cases the exact way in which a drug damages the tissues and organs is not known.

DRUG INTERACTIONS

If the prescription sheet of a patient in hospital is examined it will probably show that he is receiving at least half a dozen separate drugs. This treatment with multiple drugs which has become a feature of medical practice, has brought with it the danger that certain drugs may interact, occasionally with disastrous consequences. Dangerous interactions are particularly liable to occur:

1. In seriously ill patients because they will probably be taking several drugs at the same time
2. In the elderly because they may be very sensitive to relatively small changes in the blood concentration of certain drugs
3. When there is only a small difference between the toxic and therapeutic dose of the drug.

Interaction may occur before the drugs enter the body. Intravenous infusions are commonly used, particularly in very ill patients, and a veritable cocktail of drugs may be mixed in the infusion bottle. Some of these drugs may be incompatible in solution and precipitation or modification may occur. It is therefore very important that when drugs are given via a drip infusion, they should wherever possible be given as a bolus injected into the plastic tubing and flushed into the patient. If drugs have to be mixed in the infusion bottle, the advice of the pharmacist or doctor should be sought.

After administration of drugs, interactions can occur at numerous sites:

1. In the intestine
2. In the blood
3. At the site of action of the drug
4. At the sites of elimination of the drugs
   a. Liver
   b. Kidney

The intestine

Most drugs are absorbed by diffusion through the gut wall. If a drug which is well absorbed becomes attached to a drug which is poorly absorbed, the well absorbed drug will be held in the intestine and absorption will be decreased. For example, if tetracycline and iron are given together the tetracycline is held in the intestine by the iron which is poorly absorbed.

The blood

Many drugs are transported partially attached to the plasma proteins and partially free in the blood. Only the free drugs have any pharmacological action. If two drugs (A and B) of this type are given together they may compete for sites of attachment to the carrier plasma protein. Drug A may be displaced from the carrier sites by drug B so that there is more drug A free, and thus drug A has an increased pharmacological action. For example, the anticoagulant warfarin is largely carried by the plasma proteins. If an oral hypoglycaemic agent is given to a patient taking warfarin, the warfarin is pushed off the carrier protein, more free warfarin is available, resulting in increased pharmacological action and bleeding.

Drugs which will displace others from the plasma protein include NSAIAs, sulphonamides, and tolbutamide.

At site of action

Drugs may antagonize or augment each other at their site of action, for example, the effect of a drug depressing the nervous system (e.g. a benzodiazepine) will be enhanced by another depressant (e.g. alcohol).

There may be antagonism at the receptors, for example, β agonists (e.g. salbutamol) and β blockers (e.g. propranolol) compete for receptors in the walls of the bronchi and thus produce bronchodilatation or bronchoconstriction depending on the circumstances.

At sites of elimination

Many drugs are broken down in the liver where enzymes can be modified by drugs in two ways:

1. They can be made more active (*enzyme induction*) so that other drugs are broken down more rapidly and their effect decreased. Phenytoin and rifampicin are both powerful enzyme inducers.

2. They can suppress enzyme activity. The antibiotic chloramphenicol is an enzyme suppressor.

One of the most important enzymes which breaks down drugs and also some naturally occurring substances such as adrenaline and noradrenaline, is monoamine oxidase. It is possible to inhibit this enzyme with drugs called monoamine oxidase inhibitors (MAO) which are used in treating depression (see p. 128). If patients on monoamine oxidase inhibitors are given certain drugs or even foods containing amines, these substances will accumulate in the body and cause an abrupt and serious rise in blood pressure.

Such drugs are:	*Such foods are:*
Adrenaline	Cheese
Noradrenaline	Broad beans
Amphetamine	Marmite and Bovril

In addition the effects of some drugs are potentiated, particularly those of:

Pethidine
Barbiturates
Anaesthetics.

Drugs may also be excreted via the kidney and in many cases they are passed through the renal tubular cell into the urine. At this site competition can occur. Perhaps the best known examples are probenecid and penicillin, both of which are excreted via the renal tubular cells. Probenecid blocks the excretion of penicillin and this fact is used when very high levels of penicillin are required. Similarly, thiazide diuretics block the renal excretion of lithium and small increases in blood levels of lithium lead to severe and dangerous toxicity.

Important interactions

The number of drug reactions which have been described is now very large and many of them are of little or no clinical importance. In general those interactions which are important occur when the dose of a drug is critical and a small change in the blood concentration or the patient's sensitivity to the drug results in toxicity, or conversely, a lack of therapeutic effect. It is quite impossible for the nurse or doctor to remember them all but most of the important ones concern:

ACE inhibitors	Lithium
Anticoagulants	Oral contraceptives
β Blockers	Phenytoin
Cimetidine	Rifampicin
Digoxin	Theophylline
Hypoglycaemic agents.	

When these drugs are being given to a patient the possibility of interactions must be remembered if further drugs are added to the treatment regime. In outpatient prescribing it should be remembered that the patient may be taking over-the-counter drugs.

Nursing point

Charts are now available which show the more important interactions and it would be sensible to display such a chart in every ward and outpatients' department.

Many patients would not consider alcohol as a drug but nevertheless it can cause serious interactions and should therefore be avoided when certain drugs are taken.

Disulfiram	These drugs interfere
Griseofulvin	with the metabolism of
Procarbazine	alcohol causing flushing,
Metronidazole	headaches, sweating and
Chloropropamide	nausea.
Hypnotics and sedatives	Potentiated by alcohol.
Warfarin	Anticoagulant action enhanced with acute

overdose of alcohol. Chronic overdose may reduce effect by increasing the rate of breakdown.

Monoamine oxidase inhibitors — Hypertensive crisis, particularly with Chianti.

Metformin — Risk of lactic acidosis.

Aspirin — Increased risk of gastric bleeding. This risk is small and in fact many people take alcohol and aspirin without disaster.

THE INTRODUCTION AND TESTING OF NEW DRUGS

The introduction of a new drug is usually a costly and protracted affair. It takes about 8–10 years from the time a chemical entity is discovered to its release for general use as a therapeutic agent and the process costs some £100 million. Many chemical compounds are screened for any action which might be useful in treating disease. This is done by testing them on animals, but on the whole animal in vivo, and on various organ preparations. The most usual species used are the rat and the dog.

A few drugs may appear promising and these have to be thoroughly tested for toxic effects. This is done in two stages. First, large doses of the drug are given to animals over a short period and the lethal and therapeutic doses are determined. The relationship between these doses is important, the lethal dose divided by the therapeutic dose being called the *therapeutic ratio*. It can be seen that the larger this ratio the safer the drug. The drug is then given in smaller doses to animals over long periods to see whether there are any toxic effects from prolonged administration. At this stage the drug is also tested to see if it produces any fetal abnormalities in pregnant animals or cancer after long-term use. Only if this testing shows satisfactory results is the drug given to humans. Animal toxicology has a limited predictive value and even if a drug appears to be

non-toxic in animals it may well cause an adverse reaction in man.

Phase 1. The first time a new drug is used in man it is given to normal volunteers. Small doses are used at first and then increased. The subjects are kept under close observation either in hospital or in some special unit. Measurements are made of the various actions of the drug and estimation of blood levels will determine the rate and degree of absorption and elimination.

Phase 2. If the preliminary studies are satisfactory permission must be obtained from the Committee on Safety of Medicines (CSM) for limited clinical trials of the new drug to find out whether, in fact, it is useful in treating disease (Fig. 22.1).

Phase 3. This is followed by larger trials involving about 2000 patients to confirm the safety and efficacy of the drug.

Only after this process will a *Product Licence* be given which allows the drug to be released for general use, though the CSM may still stipulate a limited period during which further information as to its effectiveness and possible dangers can be obtained.

This type of preliminary screening will usually discover serious and frequently occurring side-

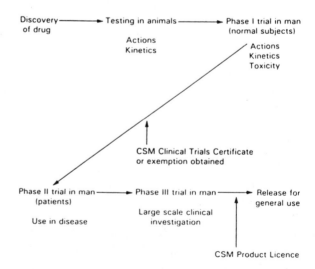

Fig. 22.1 Stages in introducing a new drug, indicating when the Committee on Safety of Medicines (CSM) licences are required.

effects but is of little use in picking up rare and unexpected adverse reactions. Other methods are being used to detect this type of adverse effect.

POST-MARKETING SURVEILLANCE

1. Voluntary adverse reaction reporting

Practising doctors and dentists are asked to fill in a *yellow card* and send it to the CSM if they suspect an adverse reaction to a drug. For older drugs only severe or unusual reactions should be reported but for recently introduced drugs, doctors should report any reaction. This method is limited by under-reporting and probably only 5–10% of these untoward reactions are recorded on the yellow cards.

2. A study of the national statistics

Statistics such as causes of death may rarely give a clue to some adverse reactions, an example being the rise in sudden deaths in young people suffering from asthma which was probably due to overuse of pressurized inhalers. This method usually requires an unacceptable increase in morbidity or mortality before the adverse effect becomes apparent.

3. Hospital-based systems

In a group of hospital patients all drugs given and their effects are carefully monitored, examples being the Dundee–Aberdeen Medicine Evaluation Group and the Boston Collective Drug Surveillance Scheme. Such schemes provide valuable information but are limited by the number of patients under surveillance. Nevertheless large collaborative studies provide a great deal of useful information not only about drug side-effects but also about other aspects of the use of drugs.

4. Monitored release and prescription event monitoring

When a new drug is released for the first time for general use it may be limited to certain doctors who are asked to report any untoward reactions. Alternatively the names of doctors who are using a certain drug can be obtained from prescription returns and they may be asked specifically whether they have noticed any untoward event which has happened to the patient. This method may become popular as a means of following up a newly introduced drug when it is released. It does depend on the collaboration of the doctors concerned who must be willing to fill in the appropriate reports.

5. Cohort studies

This method involves a large number of patients who are divided (randomly, if possible) into a group taking the drug and a control group. They are then monitored for a long period and the frequency of adverse effects compared between the two groups. Although the results can be useful, it is very expensive and laborious.

6. Case control studies

With this method the problem is approached in a different way. A watch is kept for a cluster of patients with similar symptoms which have occurred for no obvious reason, then the possible causes can be investigated. One problem with this technique is that even if taking a certain drug is a common factor, it does not prove that the drug actually caused the symptoms.

None of these methods is by any means perfect and in spite of much effort, adverse effects still pose a difficult problem. One of the most important factors in their early detection is that those who look after patients, especially nurses and doctors, are always on the look-out for something unexpected happening to a patient.

THERAPEUTIC TRIALS

In former times opinion as to the usefulness of a drug depended on impression and anecdote. As a result many drugs in common use were worthless, some of them having no therapeutic effect at all. One important advance in recent years has been the introduction of the clinical trial as a means of assessing the true value of a drug.

It is not always easy to assess the usefulness of a drug in practice and its trial requires careful planning. The usual way is to compare two groups of patients who are as nearly as possible similar. One group receives the drug under trial and the other group—the control group—receives a *placebo* (a placebo being an inert substance which must be similar in appearance to the drug which is being tested) or possibly another active drug against which the trial drug is being compared. This is because suggestion plays a considerable part in the relief of certain symptoms and may be responsible for some apparent therapeutic action of a drug. The usefulness of the active drug is then compared with the placebo by noting the beneficial effect in both groups. It is also important that the nurses and doctors who are looking after the patients during the trial do not know who is receiving the active drug and who the placebo, as even they may bias the result by unconsciously communicating their hopes and fears to the patients. This is known as a *double-blind trial*. The trial is designed so that the number of subjects involved is sufficient to give a clear answer as to the drug's efficacy. When completed the results are subjected to statistical analysis which will show the probability of the drug's therapeutic value.

Meta-analysis

Even with a well-designed controlled trial it is not always certain whether a particular new drug is more effective than those in current use. This is usually because the difference between the treated and control groups is quite small and the number of patients involved not large enough to give a clear result. To get round this difficulty the technique of meta-analysis has been introduced. This takes an overview of all properly controlled randomized trials of a particular drug or treatment. This technique has become very sophisticated and is giving useful information and guidance as to the best treatment in certain clinical circumstances. For example, meta-analysis of the trials in the use of the streptokinase in

coronary thrombosis has firmly established that it reduces mortality and it is now standard treatment.

ETHICS COMMITTEES

Experiments on human subjects, whether they be normal volunteers or patients, should be approved by an independent ethical committee before being started. This review is not statutory but any investigator would be most unwise to proceed without it and many journals will not accept articles if the work has not been approved by an ethical committee.

These committees have now been set up by most major medical institutions such as medical schools, research bodies and pharmaceutical companies. They have no approved constitution but should contain a wide medical representation and, in addition, nursing and lay members. Their main task is to protect the subject of an experiment from unnecessary risk and to ensure every safeguard is provided. They should also see that the subject will receive proper compensation if something goes wrong and some ethical committees take upon themselves the duty of criticizing, if necessary, the design of the experiment and ascertaining that the work is worth doing.

GENERIC PRESCRIBING

When a new drug is introduced it is given two names—a generic (approved) name and a brand name applied by the pharmaceutical manufacturer. If a drug is prescribed by its brand name the pharmacist must dispense that brand.

On introduction there is usually only a single brand of a drug so that the generic and brand names apply to the same product. However, when the patent expires (after 20 years) several manufacturers may produce a particular drug, each giving it a different brand name.

For many years there has been a move to use generic names only and to abolish brand names. This would eliminate the confusion due to a drug having several different names and would reduce the cost, particularly after the patent has expired. Against this it is argued that different brands may differ in quality and the doctor should know which brand is being dispensed. Also, it would reduce the profitability of the drug to the company which had introduced it and had spent many millions of pounds on its development.

FORMULARIES

The British National Formulary (BNF) lists the drugs and pharmacological preparations available in the UK together with indications for their use, dosage, adverse effects and cost. It also includes notes on the treatment of many conditions and useful guidance on a variety of problems encountered when using drugs. A copy should be available in every ward, outpatient department and doctor's surgery. It is updated twice a year. The BNF however, is not selective, for example, the current edition lists fifteen β blockers and it is obviously wasteful and extravagant for a hospital pharmacy to stock all these. A number of hospitals or districts and a few general practices have constructed their own formularies which list the drugs available in the pharmacy and chosen on the basis of efficacy and cost; these may also contain background information. Local formularies do seem to have reduced prescribing costs and have had some educational benefits by stimulating interest in rational and sensible prescribing.

THE PLACEBO RESPONSE

A placebo drug may be defined as a substance which has no pharmacological action but which, when used, produces a therapeutic effect.

There is now good evidence that in a wide variety of symptoms including pain, cough, headache, etc., the administration of an inert substance will produce marked improvement in about 30% of subjects. It is important to realize that this does not mean that the patient's symptoms were imaginary. The mechanism whereby this improvement is produced is not known but is obviously connected with the powers of suggestion.

The placebo effect has a number of important implications:

1. It is possible in some patients to control symptoms without using active drugs.
2. In assessing the effectiveness of new drugs, the placebo response must be remembered and as far as possible excluded. This is usually done by using controls who receive some inert preparation, thus producing the placebo response, who are compared with those taking the active drug (see above).
3. Further study of the placebo response might be useful in opening up new methods of treatment of symptoms by suggestion, thus making it possible to relieve symptoms without resorting to pharmacologically active drugs.

FURTHER READING

Bateman D N, Chaplin S 1988 Adverse reactions. British Medical Journal 296: 761

Brodie M J, Feely J 1988 Therapeutic drug monitoring and clinical trials. British Medical Journal 296: 1110

Brodie M J, Feely J 1988 Adverse drug interactions. British Medical Journal 296: 845

Davies D M (ed) 1991 Textbook of adverse drug reactions,

4th edn. Oxford University Press, Oxford

Editorial 1992 Clinical trials and meta-analysis. New England Journal of Medicine 327: 273

Systemic analysis of controlled trials (meta-analysis) 1992 Drug and Therapeutics Bulletin 30: 25

Symposium 1991 Drug development and clinical trials. Prescribers Journal 32: 219

23

Drug dependence (drug addiction)

Drug dependence may be defined as a state resulting from the interaction of a person and a drug in which the person has a compulsion to continue taking the drug in order to experience pleasurable psychic effects and sometimes avoid discomfort due to its withdrawal.

There are several groups of drugs of dependence:

1. Opioids
2. Cocaine
3. Amphetamines
4. Alcohol
5. Barbiturates
6. Cannabis
7. Hallucinogens (LSD, etc.)
8. Volatile solvents (glue sniffing).

It is usual to divide dependence into:

1. Psychic dependence where the drug produces a pleasant feeling, often relaxation, freedom from worry, or heightened awareness and increased energy and sexual drive. The patient suffers mental anguish when it is withdrawn.
2. Physical dependence where repeated administration produces biochemical changes in the subject taking the drug. If the drug is withdrawn, unpleasant symptoms and signs of a physical nature develop which may last for a varying period but will finally disappear. During this period there is an intense craving for the drug which, if given, will temporarily relieve the unpleasant symptoms. Tolerance, in which increasing doses are required to produce the

same effect, often develops with drugs causing dependence.

Drugs may be used intermittently for social or emotional reasons, for example, to relieve a stressful situation. Subjects who are truly dependent take drugs continually and may reach a state in which their whole life centres round obtaining and using drugs.

Dependence may not be confined to one drug or group of drugs. It is common to find dependent subjects who have escalated from more minor drugs (for example, cannabis) to hard drugs (for example, heroin) and some subjects may alternate or combine drugs; for example, cocaine and morphine would produce alternating stimulation and relaxation.

Why do people become dependent?

This is a very difficult question and the answer is still incomplete. It appears that there is no single cause for drug dependence, no single set of circumstances or special type of personality which becomes dependent. Among the motives which may be important are:

1. *Curiosity and wanting to belong.* Many young people start taking drugs because they want to know what it feels like. Pressure from peer groups may also play a part, particularly with drugs like alcohol and cannabis which are to some degree socially acceptable. This in turn may be tied up with the wish to belong to a group who have a common interest in drug taking and there may be an element of rebellion against accepted values. This need to achieve social acceptance may well be symptomatic of an underlying character disorder so that there are both social and psychological factors at work.
2. Some people take drugs to *relieve mental tension and worries* or to *give themselves more energy and confidence.* Most people have to face difficulties from time to time and look for a prop to help them. This may include advice from a friend, religion, a holiday, or the development of a psychiatric illness. The dependent person has taken what may be termed the 'chemical way out' and by altering his psychic state with drugs

partially escaped from reality. Unfortunately, this method brings only temporary relief as it does not solve anything and brings in its train further problems which are both physical and psychological.

3. It has long been suggested that people who become drug-dependent differ in their biochemical make-up from those who show no interest in drugs. This has been particularly suggested in alcoholism which might be regarded as a disease of metabolism, one facet of which is craving for alcohol. This is an attractive hypothesis because it takes the 'sin' out of dependence and puts it in a medical setting, but so far there is little evidence to support it.

4. *Availability.* There is little doubt that the availability and price of drugs of dependence influence both the amount and pattern of dependence. For example, countries where alcohol is cheap, such as France and South Africa, have a high incidence of alcoholism, cirrhosis of the liver, etc.

Opioids and their derivatives

There are probably more than 50 000 people dependent on opioids in this country at present. Most members of the opium group of drugs are to a greater or lesser extent drugs of dependence. The most frequently used is heroin which is extremely potent. It may be injected intravenously, taken orally or smoked. Dependence is both psychic and physical, and a few hours after withdrawal of the drug the person develops a craving for a further dose combined with increasing restlessness, anxiety and distress. After 48 hours physical symptoms such as nausea, vomiting and muscle cramps become prominent. Gooseflesh may develop ('cold turkey') and the patient may be pyrexial. The withdrawal symptoms last for about a week.

In addition to the hazards of withdrawal the patient runs further risks:

1. The possibility of overdosage.
2. The frequent occurrence of sepsis due to injection under nonsterile conditions. This may take the form of septicaemia or endocarditis. In addi-

tion, the sharing of injection needles greatly increases the risk of being infected with the virus of hepatitis B or the HIV causing AIDS. Between 15 and 60% of intravenous drug users are carrying the HIV and many will eventually develop AIDS.

3. Babies born to an addict may have a low birthweight and in addition, will suffer acute withdrawal symptoms after birth with a mortality of 50%.

4. An addict will go to any length, even serious crime, to obtain further supplies of the drug.

Management. Addicts must be registered and may then receive a supply of their drug from approved doctors. Attempts can be made to stop the narcotic; one method is the substitution of *methadone* (see p. 98) which is less addictive and which can be withdrawn at a later date. Alternatively, *clonidine* can be used. This drug which lowers blood pressure (see p. 58) prevents the rise of noradrenaline in the brain which occurs when opioids are withdrawn and is responsible for many of the unpleasant withdrawal symptoms. Its use in these circumstances requires careful monitoring combined with full support. It is important to tell the patient that the relief of symptoms may be delayed for 12–24 hours. Whatever method is used, the treatment of this type of dependence is difficult and disappointing.

Cocaine

Cocaine dependence is again on the increase. The drug produces a feeling of elation and appears to temporarily increase physical capacity. In South America the leaves of the coca tree which contain cocaine are chewed for this purpose. Cocaine can be given orally but it is absorbed through mucous membranes and may be sniffed, which can produce ulceration of the nasal septum. More rapid effects are obtained by giving cocaine intravenously when it may be mixed with heroin. *Crack* is the free 'base' of cocaine. If this is vaporized and the fumes inhaled the drug is absorbed through the lungs producing a rapid and intense effect. Because the action of cocaine is short-lived

it may be taken in repeated doses every 30 minutes or so and there is risk of dangerous overdose. Dependence is largely psychic and withdrawal symptoms are depression, sleepiness and increased appetite.

Amphetamines

For many years amphetamines were used as appetite suppressors and to treat mild depression and many people, mainly middle-aged women, became mildly dependent on them. In large doses amphetamines are powerful stimulants producing feelings of confidence but also sometimes, hallucinations and other mental disturbances. There is considerable psychic dependence but the withdrawal symptoms are not severe. Except for special circumstances (p. 34) amphetamines are now rarely used in medical practice.

'**Ecstasy**' is an amphetamine derivative producing a feeling of elation and 'togetherness'. It is largely used in the UK as a dance drug at 'rave' parties. The danger is that with vigorous dancing hyperpyrexia can develop with fits, collapse, renal failure and death. In addition, it can cause nausea and bruxism (spasm of the jaw muscles). It appears to have a low addictive potential but is far from safe. It has no medical use.

Barbiturates

Until some time after the Second World War barbiturates were the most commonly used hypnotic and sedative drugs. It is now realized that prolonged use, particularly in large doses, can lead to dependence. The addict is drowsy, ataxic and examination frequently shows nystagmus. Sudden withdrawal produces well marked symptoms with anxiety, vomiting and epileptic fits.

Cannabis (marihuana, hemp)

Cannabis is a resin obtained from a plant which is widely grown in America, Africa and Asia. It is usually smoked but can be taken by mouth. It produces mild excitement combined with a feeling of relaxation and peace. Perception of time is distorted and the passage of time is slowed ('spaced-out') and the subjects may be hungry ('the munchies'). The conjunctivae appear red due to vasodilatation.

Substances related to cannabis (cannabinoids) are used as an anti-emetic for patients who are being treated with cytotoxic drugs.

Cannabis is illegal in the UK but whether it is more addictive and socially more undesirable than alcohol is a matter of debate.

The main arguments against its legalization are:

1. Repeated use, particularly in high doses, can reduce motivation and interfere with the subject's life. Rarely, it can cause a psychotic state with hallucinations and disorientation.
2. The use of cannabis may lead a person on to take more seriously addictive drugs such as heroin. Although this happens infrequently, most heroin addicts have passed through a phase of using cannabis.
3. Cannabis is a drug of dependence in that there are withdrawal symptoms (anxiety and sleeplessness) and tolerance develops.

Volatile solvents

Various substances contain organic solvents which are volatile and highly fat soluble and therefore easily penetrate the brain causing depression of the cerebral function with euphoria and occasional hallucination.

The problem of 'glue sniffing' has become serious among teenagers and may prove difficult to control as the use of these solvents is widespread.

Hallucinogens

Some drugs cause severe disturbances of cerebral function. The best known of these is lysergic acid diethylamide (LSD). This drug causes hallucinations combined with a variety of mental abnormalities. A return to normal mental function usually occurs although in some subjects the symptoms persist and others do themselves seri-

ous damage while under the influence of the drug. It is very doubtful whether such substances have any place in medical treatment.

Alcohol

Alcohol presents a special problem as moderate amounts are taken for social reasons by many people. Dependence on alcohol is very common and its management is a very difficult medical and social problem. It occurs most often in those countries where alcoholic drinks are cheap, for instance the United States and France. Not only does it frequently lead to moral and financial breakdown for the patient but it is a tragedy for his/her family.

Alcohol causes both acute and chronic disorders. Acute consumption of excessive amounts of alcohol produces a deterioration of brain function with changes in behaviour progressing through slurred speech and unsteady gait to unconsciousness.

The relationship between blood concentration and effect is given below:

Blood level	Effect
20 mg/100 ml	Relaxed
30 mg/100 ml	Talkative
50 mg/100 ml	a little uncoordinated (knocks over glass)
100 mg/100 ml	Fall about, vomiting
300 mg/100 ml	Stupor

There is considerable interperson variation.

One half-pint of beer or one glass of wine or one single of spirits raises the blood alcohol level to about 10–20 mg/100 ml. Normally alcohol is rapidly absorbed from the gastrointestinal tract, though food may slow absorption. Peak blood levels are reached in about 1 hour. It is largely metabolized in the liver, though small amounts are excreted in the urine and breath.

Given the same dose of alcohol, women have a higher blood level and appear more prone to develop alcohol-related diseases. This is partly because they are generally smaller than men so the volume of distribution is less but also because, in women, less alcohol is broken down as it passes from the gastrointestinal tract via the liver to the circulation (greater bioavailability).

Chronic alcoholism damages several organs. In the *nervous system* abuse leads to failure of memory with ultimate dementia and peripheral neuritis.

The *liver* may be damaged leading ultimately to cirrhosis, the *stomach* may develop gastritis and alcohol can affect the *heart muscle* resulting in atrial fibrillation and cardiomyopathy. Chronic alcoholics are specially prone to *infection* and have a high incidence of tuberculosis.

It is now recognized that excessive consumption of alcohol during pregnancy causes the *fetal alcohol syndrome* with mild mental retardation, small head, turned-up nose and other facial abnormalities.

Alcohol intake. The intake of alcohol is usually measured in terms of units per day or per week.

One unit = Half pint of beer
           One glass of wine
           One glass of sherry or port
           One measure of spirits

Each of these contains about 8 g (10 ml) of alcohol.

A 'safe' level of daily alcohol consumption is very difficult to establish but a frequently quoted figure is three units per day for a man and two units per day for a woman.

Treatment. Withdrawal of alcohol from a dependent person leads to tremor, anxiety and tachycardia.

Sedation is best achieved with diazepam, starting with 40 mg daily and reducing the dose stepwise over 10 days. Chlormethiazole is excellent at relieving symptoms but has its own dependence risk. It is common practice to give large doses of vitamins (Parentrovite) in the early stages of treatment as deficiency of the vitamin B group may play a part in producing symptoms.

Delirium tremens is a more serious withdrawal disorder with hallucination and disorientation and the patient may be violent. In these circumstances diazepam (in the form of Diazemuls) may have to be given in 10 mg doses i.v. and repeated as required. Haloperidol 2–4 mg i.m. every 4–6 hours can be used but there is a risk of fits. Vitamins should be given as above.

Most alcoholics should give up drinking completely and this requires considerable supportive treatment. Occasionally they may be helped by giving *disulfiram.* This drug inhibits the breakdown of alcohol producing toxic substances which cause flushing, nausea and headaches, and thus the patient is discouraged from further drinking.

Alcohol and driving

Increasing doses of alcohol produce a progressive deterioration in physical and mental performance. This is particularly important as it may cause road traffic accidents. Drunk in charge of a car is a serious offence but the definition of drunkenness is difficult. In the UK it is an offence to have more than 80 mg of alcohol per 100 ml of blood while in charge of a car.

Nicotine

Nicotine is a constituent of tobacco smoke. It stimulates the autonomic nervous system (raised blood pressure and pulse rate) and has a mild cocaine-like stimulant action on the brain. It causes both psychic and physical dependence. Unfortunately, its use is associated with an increased incidence of several diseases, most notably:

- Cancer of the lung, lip and tongue
- Chronic bronchitis and emphysema
- Coronary artery disease
- Peripheral vascular disease.

Nursing point

Compared with other women nurses have a particularly high smoking rate, probably due to the stresses of their job. They should remember that in addition to the risks outlined above, heavy smoking causes:

- Some reduction in fertility
- Raised perinatal mortality
- Increased risk of thrombosis in those taking oral contraceptives.

The death rate among smokers is about twice that of non-smokers and the figure is higher for heavy smokers whose life expectancy is reduced by about 5 years. Stopping smoking results in a progressive improvement in prognosis.

Withdrawal symptoms include craving for nicotine, constipation and increased appetite.

Treatment is difficult and requires high motivation on the part of the patient. Subjects vary in their method of withdrawal, some preferring to stop suddenly, others to slowly reduce the number of cigarettes smoked. Various aids such as nicotine chewing gum (Nicorette) skin patches or hypnosis may be used. The success rate at 1 year is about 25%.

Caffeine

Although caffeine is not a serious drug of addiction transient symptoms of headaches, sleepiness and general depression occur when it is withdrawn from the diet. It is perhaps not generally realized that most people are taking caffeine regularly for, not only is it found in coffee but also in other articles of diet such as tea, chocolate, cocoa and coca cola.

Occasionally exclusion of caffeine from the diet will cure sleeplessness, anxiety and palpitations.

FURTHER READING

Editorial 1989 Cocaine and crack. British Medical Journal 299: 338
Editorial 1992 Ecstasy and the dance of death. British Medical Journal 305: 5

ISSD 1985 Drug misuse: A basic briefing. ISSD, London
Preston A 1992 Substance abuse: pointing the risk. Nursing Times 88 (13): 24
Rickard T 1984 Drug dependence. Nursing 2nd series, 24: 710

24

Drugs and the eye

The structure of the eye and orbit is shown in Figure 24.1.

The following types of drug are in frequent use in the treatment of eye conditions:

1. Antibiotics
2. Steroids and other anti-inflammatory drugs
3. Those which affect pupil size
4. Those used in the treatment of glaucoma
5. Local anaesthetics
6. Stains
7. Miscellaneous preparations.

Drugs can be administered to the eye either by local or systemic routes.

LOCAL USE OF DRUGS ON THE EYE

The following preparations are used in the local treatment of eye diseases: eye lotions, eye drops, eye ointments, subconjunctival injections or ampoules for injection into the anterior chamber at operation.

Whenever administering local preparations to the eye it is of paramount importance to ensure that the eye to receive treatment is clearly designated. Often only one eye is to be treated or the two eyes are to be treated differently. For example after an operation for angle closure glaucoma in one eye it may be necessary to dilate the pupil with drugs called mydriatics. Such treatment given to the other eye could be disastrous.

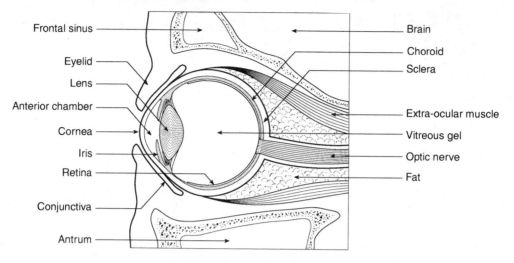

Fig. 24.1 Cross-section anatomy of eye and orbit.

Eye lotions prescribed as collyrium

These are used to wash foreign material from the eye and some have a mild antiseptic action. They are applied from an *undine* which is a small glass container with a fine spout and which resembles a miniature chemistry retort. In an emergency, however, if a little jug is at hand it will serve as well and may save vital minutes in treating a contaminated eye. The patient should lie back or sit in a chair with the head extended. The lotion should be warmed to 35°C (95°F) and before washing the eye it should be run up the cheek into the medial canthus, the lids being firmly separated by the fingers and a small basin held by the patient close to his face to catch the effluent. This is less unpleasant than pouring the lotion directly onto the cornea. The lotion should be steadily poured from the undine, the patient being instructed to move the eyes in all directions. There are many types of lotion but simple normal saline is very satisfactory for the removal of foreign material or dirt from the eye. In emergency cases, however, as in chemical contamination it is better to use plain cold tap water than to lose time in starting the treatment.

In cases of contamination by lime or cement an irrigation with *dihydrogen sodium versenate* is recommended. This substance is a chelating agent and has the action of converting an insoluble heavy metal salt, such as calcium hydroxide, into a soluble complex anion which can be removed in solution.

Eye drops prescribed as guttae

A number of drugs can be applied to the eyes by means of drops which should be instilled into the lower conjunctival sac. The patient is told to look upwards away from the dropper and the lower lid is held down with the finger. One drop only is instilled into the lower fornix and the patient is then told to close the eye for a short while and the excess is wiped away.

All drops and ointment should be sterile when supplied and once opened can no longer be considered so. There is an increasing tendency for them to be dispensed in single dose containers which can be discarded after use.

Eye ointments prescribed as oculentum

These can be applied similarly either on a glass rod or from a single dose container; the lower lid is pulled down and the ointment is placed in the lower fornix. About half an inch of ointment as squeezed from the tube should be used at each application. This should be delivered onto the end of a sterile glass rod or a prepacked plastic spatula. A separate applicator should be used for each eye if both are to be treated.

Subconjunctival injections

This method of application is used to obtain immediately a high concentration of a drug in the anterior chamber. This would be appropriate in the treatment of an acute intra-ocular infection.

This treatment is painful and the eye must first be thoroughly anaesthetized by the instillation of several drops of local anaesthetic. Injection is made with a hypodermic syringe and a fine needle.

Some drugs are manufactured in a depot form and are bound to a base substance from which they are released slowly. For example *Depo-Medrone* can be used as a steroid preparation for the local treatment of iridocyclitis. It is given as a subconjunctival injection and its action is continuous over a period of 3–4 days.

Ocusert preparations

Another way of effecting continuous administration of drugs in the eye is by means of these drug-containing dispensers. Here the active principle is absorbed into a small gelatinuous film which is slipped into the lower fornix and retained there for a period of some days after which it can be changed. This method is not often employed but can be useful in cases where prolonged administration is necessary, and especially in the elderly who may have glaucoma, arthritic hands and a poor memory. Ocuserts can be inserted by the nurse but many patients self-medicate.

ANTIBIOTICS

Antibiotics are used to treat a wide range of eye infections and they may be administered in three ways:

1. Drops are very satisfactory for superficial in-flammation such as conjunctivitis, but rapid dilution occurs because of the tears. The drops should be instilled at 2-hourly intervals at least if a reasonable concentration of antibiotic is to be maintained.

2. Ointments release the antibiotic more slowly and their action is helped by the eye being covered.

3. Subconjunctival injection is the best way of ensuring a rapid and high concentration of antibiotic within the anterior ocular segment. The maximum volume which can be injected at one time is 1.0–1.5 ml.

Although, owing to the accessibility of the eye, diseases of the anterior segment can usually be effectively treated by means of local administration of drugs, for those diseases which affect the posterior part, or the deeper intra-ocular structures, systemic administration is generally necessary.

Eye infections may be due to a variety of agents, both bacterial and viral. The correct antibiotic can be selected as a result of clinical observation and bacterial or viral studies.

The aminoglycosides and chloramphenicol are widely used in the treatment of superficial eye infections. They are active against a broad spectrum of bacteria and are particularly suitable for local administration as this avoids systemic toxicity. They include:

- Chloramphenicol 0.5% drops or 1.0% ointment
- Neomycin 0.5% drops and ointment
- Gentamicin 0.3% drops
- Ampoules of gentamicin sulphate 40 mg/ml for subconjunctival injection.

These drugs are active against both Gram-positive and Gram-negative organisms. Tobramycin is particularly useful in pseudomonas infections which are disastrous when they occur within the eye.

Norfloxacin (Noroxin), a member of the quinolone group, has a broader spectrum of antibacterial action than chloramphenicol and other commonly used antibiotics. It has fewer local side-effects than gentamicin and appears to have a similar spectrum of activity. It rivals chloramphenicol as a general prophylactic antibiotic.

The tetracyclines are wide spectrum antibiotics which also show activity against certain viruses and Rickettsia, particularly those causing trachoma. Tetracycline is available as a 1% ointment and its use together with systemic administration has helped to bring this widespread and blinding condition under control.

Two ocular conditions which respond well to prolonged administration of systemic tetracycline in low dosage are chronic staphyloccal blepharitis (inflammation of the eyelid margins) and ocular involvement in cutaneous acne rosacea. Here the usual dose is 250 mg daily for a period of up to 6 months.

Tetracyclines are contraindicated in young patients before eruption of the second dentition as the permanent teeth can be discoloured. The same caution must apply in administration during pregnancy.

Antibiotics of the penicillin group are rarely, if ever, used as local eye applications as they have a marked tendency to cause allergic reactions. However, they have an important place in the treatment of spreading infections of the eyelids, which are commonly of staphylococcal origin. In such cases the infection is deep in the tissues requiring systemic rather than local administration. In general, a broad spectrum penicillin is best, but if the infection is acquired in hospital one of the penicillinase-resistant type is preferable.

Sodium fusidate is particularly active against penicillin-resistant staphylococci. It has the property of being concentrated in bone and other connective tissues, including the sclera of the eye and the vitreous, and is therefore useful in treating intra-ocular infections, especially those acquired in the operating theatre which can often be due to resistant organisms. Dosage is 500 mg 8 hourly for 5 days.

Frequently after *major intra-ocular operations*, antibiotics are injected subconjuntivally. Prophylaxis against post-operative infection is gaining

importance in the face of a growing trend for major surgery, in particular for cataract, to be performed on an outpatient basis. For this purpose gentamicin 40mg is often used. This drug however causes a degree of toxic damage to the periocular tissues. **Cefuroxime** 125 mg has recently proved less troublesome in this respect.

Acute intra-ocular infections

In acute bacterial infection of the eye much of the damage occurs as a result of the inflammatory response rather than the direct activity of the bacteria. Consequently, it is important to use steroids at the same time as an effective antibiotic.

A particular problem exists in severe intra-ocular infections such as those following eye surgery. It is essential that vigorous antibiotic and anti-inflammatory treatment is started without delay. Otherwise, if the eye is not completely destroyed, it may well lose all useful vision. As time cannot be allowed for bacteriological studies, a combination of broad spectrum antibiotics and steroids are used by both subconjunctival and systemic routes together with a mydriatic.

A combination of *antibiotics, steroids* and *mydriatics* which has been found to be successful in this connection is now widely used as follows:

Locally: Framycetin 0.8 ml
(equivalent to
500 mg)   by
Methicillin 125 mg   subconjunctival
Gentamicin 20 mg   injection
Betnesol 4 mg
Mydricaine 0.3 ml

Orally: Fucidin 500 mg b.d.
Prednisolone 15 mg
q.i.d.

Systemic administration of antibiotics can be either orally or by injection. Their use may be indicated in spreading infections involving the eye, the eyelids and ocular adnexa such as the lacrimal sac. Sepsis around the eye, in particular, in the vicinity of the internal angular vein is of particular clinical importance as it may lead to a septic cavernous sinus thrombosis.

ANTIVIRAL AGENTS

Many eye infections are due to a virus. To mention some of the commoner ones, herpes simplex, adenovirus and herpes zoster are all infections that are frequently seen clinically. **Idoxuridine (IDU)** was the first generally available antiviral agent and it was and still is effective against the herpes simplex virus that causes dendritic ulceration of the cornea. This drug is available for ocular application under the name of *Kerecid.*

A similar preparation called *Herpid* is available for general cutaneous treatment, for example in herpes zoster (shingles). *One warning* however— Herpid also contains dimethyl sulphoxide which aids cutaneous absorption but which causes cataract if applied in the region of the eye. It must therefore *never* be used to treat the eyes or eyelids.

Idoxuridine acts as a competitive inhibitor in that it competes for DNA, an essential component of the virus. For this reason in order to be effective the concentration in the conjunctival sac must be maintained at a high level. Thus the recommended dosage when given in the form of eye drops is at hourly intervals. If ointment is used the intervals may be less frequent. Prolonged use of IDU may lead to unwanted toxic effects on the corneal epithelial cells.

As a treatment for herpes simplex infections the more recently developed **acyclovir**, is an excellent choice as it is effective and not likely to cause local toxicity. Its action can be supplemented by systemic administration. The recommended dose by mouth is 200 mg five times daily for 5 days and a 3% ointment may be applied five times daily. Absorption from the gastrointestinal tract is variable and uncertain and in the absence of a favourable response the course can be repeated at a higher dosage.

Herpes zoster may affect the eye when the ophthalmic branch of the trigeminal nerve is involved. Provided that treatment is commenced at the first appearance of the vesicular rash, acyclovir given orally can significantly reduce the severity of this distressing condition.

As an antiviral drug **trifluorothymidine (F3T)** shows good activity against herpes simplex. Its main use however is against the adenovirus which causes an unpleasant and prolonged acute conjunctivitis, often with corneal involvement which to some extent affects vision, albeit temporarily. In these cases it is the drug of choice as none of the other antivirals have an effect on this virus. It is not readily available but can often be obtained from the pharmacy of specialist eye hospitals. It is not a particularly stable preparation and must be freshly prepared and kept refrigerated.

STEROIDS AND OTHER ANTI-INFLAMMATORY DRUGS

The most commonly used steroid for local ophthalmic application is **betamethasone disodium phosphate (Betnesol)**. This can be used in 0.1% drops or ointment. In some preparations the steroid is combined with an antibiotic, for example *Betnesol-N* contains neomycin. Application can be as frequent as hourly and drugs of this type are used to suppress a wide variety of inflammatory processes within the eye. Steroids should not be used indiscriminately as their improper use may be followed by serious complications. This is particularly so for infective processes which may spread rapidly if steroids are given without a suitable antibacterial agent. For similar reasons they are rarely applied to virus infections of the eye and never in the presence of active *herpes simplex* (dendritic ulcer).

Administration of *dilute* steroid eye drops is, on the contrary and perhaps paradoxically, often beneficial in the treatment of herpetic corneal infection. This, however, is when corneal stromal opacification threatens and *when the viral activity has already been contained.* For this purpose prednisolone eye drops of 0.1% administered two or three times daily can, by suppressing the antibody–antigen reaction in the deeper layers of the cornea, prevent serious loss of vision. For local administration in the form of eye drops, **dexamethasone (Maxidex)** is often used. This drug has good penetration into the eye and is useful in the routine treatment of inflammatory conditions such as iritis. It is available in 1% solution and may be combined with neomycin; it is marketed as 'Maxitrol'.

In severe ocular inflammation a subconjunctival injection of **methylprednisolone acetate (Depomedrone)** produces a continuous level of steroids in the anterior chamber for several days.

In inflammation of the posterior uvea (choroiditis) it is necessary to administer steroids systemically as local applications do not readily reach the site of the disease. Here prednisolone may be used and is generally given in a very high dosage for a short period followed by a rapid reduction at first which is tailed off more slowly. A usual starting dose may be prednisolone 60 mg a day in divided doses, but on occasions as much as 80–100 mg may be given for a few days.

All steroid drugs, whether administered locally or systemically, can result in a rise in intraocular pressure. A steroid more recently developed and named **fluoromethalone** can be used for local administration. It has been shown to be relatively free of the unwanted side-effects that are characteristic of other steroid drugs. It has proved particularly useful in the management of chronic allergic conjunctival inflammations.

For superficial inflammation of allergic origin such as vernal conjunctivitis, a histamine antagonist like *sodium cromoglycate* is often useful. To be effective the concentration in the conjunctival sac must be maintained at a high level necessitating frequent or continuous administration. This must be done over the entire period of exposure to the antigen, i.e. throughout the pollen season.

Indomethacin. This nonsteroid anti-inflammatory agent is available as a suspension for ocular administration. Its value lies in its antiprostaglandin activity. In cataract surgery for example, prostaglandins are liberated as a response to tissue trauma. These mediators of inflammation can cause constriction of the pupil with con- sequent surgical difficulties. The local administration of indomethacin 1% suspension seems to protect against this effect. A suitable dose regime is every 2 hours by day for 24 hours before surgery.

There is also evidence that cases which receive indomethacin pre-operatively show a lower incidence of macular oedema following cataract removal.

DRUGS WHICH AFFECT PUPIL SIZE

These can be divided into those which enlarge the pupil (*mydriatics*) and those which constrict it (*miotics*).

Mydriatics

Mydriatics are of two sorts:

a. Those which cause paralysis of the muscular sphincter of the iris. The sphincter muscle is innervated by the parasympathetic nervous system and drugs which inhibit it are called parasympatholytic drugs (see p. 26).
b. Those which stimulate contraction of the radial dilator pupillae muscle which is sympathetically innervated. Such drugs are called sympathomimetics (see p. 27).

Type (a) Parasympatholytics

One of the earliest known drugs of this type is **atropine** which is the active principle in the poisonous berry of the deadly nightshade plant. Its mydriatic properties have been known for centuries and in the Middle Ages it was used as a cosmetic, hence the name belladonna. Today one of its main uses is to dilate the pupil in patients with iritis where the inflamed iris goes into spasm and adheres to the lens of the eye causing blindness. Because the ciliary muscle has the same nerve supply as the sphincter muscle of the iris, atropine can be used to paralyse the focusing of the eye (accommodation) for the sight testing of young children.

It is commonly used as eye drops of 1% or 0.5% strength and in the form of ointment. The action of this drug lasts for 18 days and it is not reversible by means of miotics. It is, therefore, unsuitable for dilating the pupil for fundal examination.

It is also dangerous as, in patients with narrow anterior chamber angles, a condition of acute angle closure glaucoma can result which will not respond to miotic therapy and will almost certainly require an emergency operation.

For most purposes a mydriatic with a shorter duration of action is appropriate. **Homatropine**, which is a homologue of atropine, can be used in 1% or 2% strengths. This has a rapid action, producing pupillary enlargement in 5–10 minutes and its effect rarely lasts for more than 24 hours and can be reversed with miotics.

A synthetic drug **cyclopentolate** is now commonly used and has a very short duration of action (about 4 hours). Its action is reversed by physostigmine eye drops.

Another short-acting mydriatic is **tropicamide** which, although it is a rapid pupillary dilator, is a weak cycloplegic and causes less blurring of vision. It is therefore useful for clinical fundal examination.

Type (b) Sympathomimetics

A typical one is **phenylephrine** which is used as eye drops in 10% strength. *Ephedrine* is another and also *cocaine* which can be combined with *homatropine* to make up 'guttae H and C'. The cocaine is in a concentration of 2% which is sufficient for it to be a Controlled Drug.

Sympathomimetics can be used synergically to assist those of the parasympatholytic group in cases where dilatation is difficult. A particularly useful preparation named Mydricain is available in two strengths. It contains atropine, adrenaline and procaine and is given by subconjunctival injection.

Miotics

Miotic drugs all act on the sphincter muscle of the iris, either directly or indirectly constricting the pupil. A typical one is **physostigmine (eserine)** which is used in 0.5% or 0.25% strengths or in oily suspension for prolonged action. It is powerful miotic and mainly used in the treatment of angle closure glaucoma. It is unsuitable for prolonged use as it tends to produce local skin hypersensitivity. It is also a powerful insecticide and is the drug of choice in treating pediculosis infestation of the eyelashes. It is applied as ointment or in solution dabbed on with a small cotton wool swab. Its effect is dramatic.

Pilocarpine which is used to treat chronic glaucoma is another. It is available in strengths of 1%–4% in the form of eye drops. It is slightly less powerful in action than physostigmine but less likely to cause irritation.

A synthetic miotic called **ecothiopate (phospholine iodide)** has been widely used when strong pupillary constriction is required. Unfortunately with prolonged use it produces cysts of the iris epithelium which may largely occlude the small, miotic pupil, thereby severely reducing vision.

During intra-ocular surgery such as cataract extraction, a rapid miosis may be required and can be achieved by the injection of *acetylcholine* directly into the anterior chamber. It is marketed as 'Miochol', a dry powder in a sterile ampoule containing its own diluent fluid. Mixing is done by breaking an inner seal but as the preparation has limited stability, it should be made up just before use. Its effect is dramatic but short-lived. After the insertion of an iris-supported acrylic lens replacement, a longer acting miotic is often advisable.

DRUGS USED IN THE TREATMENT OF GLAUCOMA

Primary glaucoma is of two types, the *chronic open angle type* and that due to *acute angle closure*. These are two entirely different diseases but the one common factor is that the eye pressure is raised above normal by the failure of the aqueous humour to pass through the outflow channels. The continuous secretion of aqueous by the ciliary body causes a build-up of pressure within the eye.

Drugs used in the treatment of glaucoma can be divided into two groups. Those which facilitate the outflow of the aqueous and those which reduce its production by the ciliary body. In angle closure the draining of aqueous into the canal of Schlemm through the trabecular meshwork is obstructed by the root of the iris. To treat this condition miotics are used to constrict the iris sphincter muscle and pull the root of the iris centrally thus relieving the obstruction. In patients with shallow anterior chambers and therefore narrow angles, both mydriatics and also strong miotics can precipitate acute glaucoma. These are termed either mydriatic glaucoma or, in the case of miotics, paradoxical glaucoma. In such subjects both groups of drugs should be used with extreme caution.

Drugs modifying the autonomic nervous system

In acute angle closure intensive administration **physostigmine** can be given in the form of oily drops of 0.5% strength. This means giving one drop a minute for 5 minutes, one very 5 minutes for half an hour and quarter-hourly thereafter. Because of the irritative action of *physostigmine*, **pilocarpine** in 4% strength may be preferred.

It is easy to see why miotics are effective in angle closure glaucoma as they help outflow by relieving the obstruction of the drainage angle. It is more difficult to understand why they should work in glaucoma of the open angle type. It has, however, been shown that they act by speeding up the passage of aqueous humour through the trabecular meshwork which is the band of specialized tissue which separates the anterior chamber from the canal of Schlemm, thus increasing the facility of outflow. In chronic open angle glaucoma pilocarpine is frequently used in strengths of between 1% and 4% applied from twice to four times a day.

Neutral adrenaline 1% (Eppy) has proved effective in controlling the intra-ocular pressure in cases of open angle glaucoma. It is, however, contraindicated in eyes with narrow angles where the pupillary dilatation could cause angle closure and precipitate an acute attack. It has two actions: that mediated by α receptors brings about an increase in the facility of aqueous outflow and that mediated by the β receptors causes reduction in aqueous secretion. These two actions thus combine to lower the intra-ocular pressure.

It is usually enough for the drops to be administered twice daily. They are normally clear and are best kept at 4°C as in a domestic refrigerator. They should be discarded if they turn amber or brown in colour as they are then inactive. As side-effects they can cause ocular irritation and reactive hyperaemia. This is annoying to the patient but not often dangerous.

A useful innovation to improve absorption is known as a *pro-drug* in which the drug is modified chemically so that it passes more readily into the eye. After absorption it is split, releasing the active constituent, an example being **dipivefrin hydrochloride** which is converted by intra-ocular enzymes to adrenaline.

Guanethidine is 5% or 10% concentration has also been used in open angle glaucoma. Its effect in lowering the pressure is often disappointing when used by itself. Recently, however, it has been found that when combined with neutral adrenaline there is a striking reduction of ocular pressure and a much weaker concentration of adrenaline can then be used. This helps to avoid the unwanted side-effects of the adrenaline. A preparation consisting of a mixture of guanethidine and adrenaline is now available and known as *'Ganda 305'*. This contains 3% guanethidine and 0.5% adrenaline. Other concentrations are also available.

Another drug which, acting as a β blocker, causes a reduction in aqueous secretion is **timolol**. This is marketed under the name of *Timoptol* in 0.25 and 0.5% strengths. It reduces the amount of aqueous humour that is formed and thereby lowers intra-ocular pressure. It has the advantage that is does not cause unwanted changes in pupillary size and is, therefore, a very useful drug in the treatment of open angle glaucoma. For this reason, however, it is not suitable for glaucoma of the closed angle type unless a miotic is used simultaneously. Another advantage of timolol is that, so far, it has been found not to have any irritative effects on the eye. It can, however, produce effects on the heart in certain patients and is contraindicated in asthmatics. **Betaxolol** is similar but is less likely to produce systemic effects. It seems to be less effective than timolol in lowering the intra-ocular pressure. There is, however, some evidence that its absorption via the conjunctiva results in a systemic effect which may increase the blood supply to the optic nerve.

Acetazolamide (see p. 193)

This has the action of inhibiting the enzyme carbonic anhydrase which is necessary for the secretion of aqueous humour. In acute glaucoma the drug is very useful, as by reducing the aqueous production the intra-ocular pressure can be at least temporarily lowered, and this may have the effect of allowing better penetration of locally applied anti-glaucoma therapy.

Acetazolamide may also be used to avoid having to operate on a hard and inflamed eye. It does, unfortunately, have some unwanted side-effects and its diuretic action may be inconvenient. It almost always causes paraesthesia of the extremities. Neither of these effects are permanent. Gastric irritation, nausea and depression are, however, more serious and if they occur the drug should be discontinued or an alternative, such as **dichlorphenamide (Daranide)**, substituted.

Acetazolamide is available in tablets of 250 mg and a full dose is 1 g daily in divided doses. Alternatively, a sustained release capsule of 500 mg can be used. This is known a *'Diamox Sustet'* and is given twice daily. It produces a more even action and, as it is absorbed in the intestine, avoids the gastric side-effects.

Dehydrating agents

Another method of reducing the pressure in acute glaucoma prior to surgery involves the intravenous infusion of certain hypertonic solutions which include such substances as *urea* and *mannitol*. These have the effect of producing a vigorous diuresis and cause dehydration of the bodily tissues including the eye and at the same time producing an inhibition in the secretion of aqueous. As an alternative to the use of intravenous infusion a similar, although less marked effect, can be produced by the ingestion of a strong *glycerine solution*.

ANAESTHETICS

Because the eye is a surface organ and covered with mucous membrane it is particularly amenable to topically applied anaesthetics which produce good operative conditions.

Cocaine has been in use for over a century, its application to ophthalmic surgery being first described in 1884. It is still widely used as a locally applied anaesthetic to the eye because it remains one of the most effective drugs of its kind. Besides being a local anaesthetic, it also potentiates the sympathetic nervous supply to the eye and causes dilatation of the pupil and vasoconstriction both of which actions may be useful during operations, for example, in cataract surgery. It does, however, have the tendency to cause clouding of the corneal epithelium and for this reason alternatives, for example, *amethocaine* in a 1% solution, may be preferred. For topical anaesthesia cocaine eye drops are used in 1–4% strength and at such a concentration, cocaine is a Controlled Drug and is subject to rigid regulations on storage and use.

Many local anaesthetics when used in the eye can cause quite severe stinging when first instilled. Consequently many prefer to use **oxybuprocaine (Benoxinate)**, especially in children. The action of this drug is rapid but less well sustained which makes it very useful for accident and emergency work as corneal sensitivity is regained relatively soon.

For the performance of eye operations under local anaesthesia, an injection is often given behind the eyeball and within the cone of muscles that surround the optic nerve. This is known as *retrobulbar injection* and may only be given by someone who is medically qualified and trained to do so. For this purpose lignocaine hydrochloride 1% can be used, up to a total volume of 2–4 ml. When a prolonged period of analgesia is required, a mixture of *lignocaine* and *bupivacaine* (*Marcain*) is very effective. All these anaesthetic agents can be combined with adrenaline, but these combinations are usually avoided by ophthalmic surgeons in view of the danger of injecting directly into an orbital vein.

To ensure rapid spread of the local anaesthetic agent, a proteolytic enzyme called hyaluronidase ('Hyalase') is often included in the injection.

In cases in which an eye is both blind and painful, a retrobulbar injection of 95% ethyl alcohol can be given. This substance destroys the branches of the 5th (trigeminal) nerve in the orbit and renders the eye permanently anaesthetic.

STAINS USED IN OPHTHALMOLOGY

Fluorescein

Fluorescein is applied locally to the eye to stain ulcers and abrasions of the cornea and thus allow them to be easily seen. It is usually dispensed dry in the form of impregnated paper strips, as in solution it tends to form a culture medium for infecting bacteria, especially *Pseudomonas.*

It can also be used in photographic investigations of patients with retinal diseases. Here it is injected rapidly intravenously using 5 ml of a 5% or 10% solution. As it passes through the retinal blood vessel it causes them to fluoresce and any leakage through blood vessel walls as, for instance, may occur in diabetic retinopathy, can be vividly demonstrated.

Rose bengal

This is a stain of carmine hue which is taken up actively by injured or infected cells. It is thus very useful to detect an active virus infection of the corneal epithelium, for example, in *herpes simplex.*

MISCELLANEOUS PREPARATIONS

There are many different eye drops designed to replace moisture when the tear film is deficient as in Sjögren's syndrome. These all contain a water binding substance, often a higher molecular weight organic sugar such as hydroxymethylcellulose, **hypromellose eye drops** being a typical product. As this preparation drips leaving a white deposit, one containing polyvinyl alcohol may be preferred.

5-Fluorouracil. The use of this cytotoxic drug has found a place in eye surgery as it exerts a delaying effect on the healing of scleral wounds. This is useful after drainage operations for glaucoma. The drug is given as a subconjunctival injection into the lower fornix, taking care that the bleb does not abut upon the cornea. 0.2 ml containing 5 mg is injected daily for 5 days. This dose is so small that the serious side-effects are avoided.

DRUGS WITH ADVERSE EFFECTS ON THE EYE

Many drugs in general use have an unwanted and often disastrous effect upon the eye. *Nurses in charge of patients receiving these drugs should be aware of the likely problems as their early recognition may help to avoid permanent ocular damage and possibly total blindness.* It should be remembered that where a drug is being administered systemically both eyes may be at risk. Some of the more important drugs are mentioned below.

Chloroquine was first used as an antimalarial drug and now plays a part in the management of rheumatoid conditions and tropical diseases. It can cause opacities in the cornea and a toxic effect in the retinae. The corneal condition is reversible when the treatment is stopped, but that in the retina is permanent and visual loss can be severe. The maximum safe dose is in the region of 250 mg a day over a period of 1 year. All patients receiving this drug should be under regular ophthalmic supervision.

Drugs affecting the autonomic nervous system. A variety of drugs have a sympathomimetic or anticholinergic action as their primary or secondary effects. These include bronchodilators such as ephedrine and others used in asthma and bronchitis, antidepressants of the tricyclic group and drugs used for Parkinsonism such as benzhexol or levodopa.

All these drugs have dangers when used in patients with glaucoma, but here a distinction must be made between the open and the closed angle types of disease. A patient with open angle glaucoma may merely show a relative increase in the resistance to aqueous outflow with the result that the ocular pressure becomes more difficult to control. One with narrow filtration angles, however, may suffer an acute attack which can be bilateral resulting in rapid and perhaps complete blindness. In the open angle type the use of such drugs may be justified provided the risk is recognized and the glaucoma therapy suitably adjusted. In the narrow angle patient these drugs should be avoided unless they are essential. When in doubt an ophthalmic opinion should be sought.

Corticosteroids which are widely used as inflammatory suppressants, for example in rheumatoid arthritis and in the collagen disorders, have three major side-effects on the eye. They can, as previously mentioned, precipitate a corneal infection with herpes simplex but with prolonged administration they can induce glaucoma of the open angle variety and can cause cataracts. The two latter effects can be produced by either local or systemic administration.

Practolol previously used as a β blocker in some cardiac conditions can cause drying of the tear secretion with a severe superficial inflammation of the conjunctiva and cornea. This is extremely painful, causes loss of vision and is difficult to treat. Fortunately, these cases are becoming less frequent owing to a very strict control on the use of the drug.

Ethambutol. This antituberculous agent can cause inflammation of the optic nerve with some visual disturbance. Fortunately, these effects regress spontaneously when treatment is discontinued and are less common if the dose of the drug does not exceed 15 mg/kg daily.

Amiodarone is very effective in treating some types of cardiac arrhythmias. It does, however, produce corneal deposits very similar in appearance to those caused by chloroquine. Fortunately, retinal side-effects are absent and the corneal changes do not affect vision.

Tamoxifen. This drug used in carcinoma of the heart has been reported to cause blurring of vision as the result of changes in the cornea, lens and retina. This occurs mainly after high doses.

Chemical toxicity. Ocular irritation may result from substances contained in ophthalmic preparations, either the active principle, the preservative or greasy base of ointments. Prolonged use can cause chronic and sometimes permanent pathological changes in the conjunctiva. This effect can also be seen with the proprietary cleaning and sterilizing fluids used in the care of hydrophilic contact lenses.

25

The local application of drugs

THE SKIN—DRUGS IN DERMATOLOGY

When drugs are applied to the skin the term *topical therapy* is often used. A topical application generally consists of an active application, the drug, in a base or vehicle. The type of topical application that is used depends on the type and stage of the skin disease and it is just as important to use the correct base as it is to use the correct active agent. The base consists of one or more of the following: powder, water and grease.

The most commonly used bases or vehicles are:

1. Ointments

The distinction between modern ointments and creams is no longer so obvious because of the wide range of bases that are used for both. Ointments are generally more 'greasy' and creams are thinner and consist of emulsions of various types. Ointments are of three types:

a. Water soluble ointments. These bases have the advantage that they do not stain.

b. Emulsifying ointments, that is those which emulsify with water. An example is *lanolin (hydrous wool fat)* which is still very commonly used, but prolonged use can lead to sensitization to the lanolin. These bases are useful for retaining active agents in contact with the skin for as long as possible.

c. Non-emulsifying ointments, that is those which

do not mix with water. The paraffins form the basis of most of the very greasy ointments. With the addition of a suitable active agent they are a good treatment of chronic, dry, skin disorders, such as chronic atopic eczema, psoriasis, ichthyosis (dry skin with fish-like scales) and for common conditions such as chapping of the hands.

2. Creams

Creams are emulsions which are either water dispersed in oil (i.e. oily cream), or an oil dispersed in water (i.e. aqueous cream). The latter are generally very acceptable to patients cosmetically and are used to moisten and soften the skin surface. Appropriate active agents can be added. Barrier creams protect the skin against physical agents such as water or sunlight.

3. Pastes

Pastes can be greasy or drying and they contain a large amount of powder. They are particularly useful for localized lesions, for example, in psoriasis. In this condition it is particularly important that the active agent should not be applied to the normal skin and therefore a paste is used for the abnormal areas. Pastes can also be used to protect inflamed or excoriated skin and can be applied very freely. A good example is *compound zinc paste.*

4. Lotions

Water lotions are used to cool acutely inflamed skin and may have to be frequently reapplied. *Potassium permanganate lotion* is very helpful for acute exuding lesions of the hands and feet. Lotions should generally not be used when the acute phase has subsided.

Shake lotions cool by evaporation and leave an inert powder on the skin surface. They are useful and safe for subacute lesions. *Calamine lotion* is a good example.

5. Dusting powders

These are drying agents and increase the effective evaporating surface. They are particularly useful in the folds of the skin. Talc, starch and zinc oxide are commonly used powders. Active agents can be added as needed, for example antiseptics for bacterial infections and antifungal agents for athlete's foot (tinea pedis).

ACTIVE INGREDIENTS IN PREPARATIONS

From this it will be seen that the first decision is the type of base that will be used, which will depend on the acuteness of the lesion. Many lesions in fact often derive more benefit from the base than from the active agent. A decision on the active ingredient to be added generally implies a diagnosis of the skin disorder. It is no longer useful to remember detailed prescriptions because the common ones can be found in the British National Formulary or equivalent publications. Ointments prepared by pharmaceutical companies have complicated formulae, but it is very important to know the active ingredients and their strength in these preparations.

1. Local corticosteroids

These are probably the most widely prescribed and useful ingredients to be added to the various bases. For this reason they are often over-prescribed and in particular *they should not be used alone where the cause of the skin disease is a bacterial, fungal or viral infection as they may cause spread of the infection by lowering local resistance.* They are very useful for acute and subacute conditions such as the eczemas and they are excellent for itching (pruritus). There are two main groups:

a. *Hydrocortisone ointment* (0.5–1%) is the most useful, standard preparation. Nothing stronger than this should ever be used in infants or on the face. These ointments need not be applied more than twice a day.

b. *The fluorinated corticosteroids (e.g. betamethasone valerate).* These can achieve a much more intense effect than hydrocortisone, but this may not be an advantage and can lead to atrophy of the skin. They are valuable for thick, dry skin conditions, such as the chronic eczemas, or with some special conditions such as lupus erythematosus. The absorption of these preparations is enhanced by occlusive dressings, for example, if they are covered with polythene. However, there is great danger of secondary infection with this method.

Sometimes corticosteroids are combined with an antibacterial or antifungal agent and used to treat dermatoses with superimposed bacterial or fungal infections.

2. Coal tar

Coal tar applied to the skin is an antimitotic and anti-inflammatory agent. A tar is the product of the destructive distillation of organic substances and coal tar is in many valuable preparations, although their use has been superseded by the corticosteroid preparations. For conditions such as psoriasis and chronic eczema they are preferred, because there are fewer side-effects. Cosmetically acceptable preparations are now available and a liquid form can be added to the bath for the treatment of some psoriatic patients. The National Formulary calamine and coal tar ointment contains the equivalent of 0.5% of tar. Coal tar pastes are also often used in eczemas. A useful preparation for psoriasis is betamethasone valerate ointment with liquor picis carb (tar) in yellow soft paraffin.

Dithranol is widely used to treat *psoriasis*. It is irritant and application must be limited to the psoriatic areas as it burns normal skin, particularly if the skin is fair or has previously been treated with steroids. It should not be used if there is evidence of infection.

3. Antibacterial agents

If a bacterial infection is suspected it is better to send a swab to the laboratory for culture and sensitivity tests first. In addition many infections of the skin are best treated with systemic rather than topical antibacterial agents. The prolonged use of most antibacterial agents (e.g. neomycin) on the skin carries a very high risk of sensitization to the agent so that a bacterial infection may be replaced by a contact dermatitis! Chlortetracycline is probably the best to add to an ointment. If topical antibacterial agents are used the treatment should be determined by the sensitivity of the organism. Sulphonamides and penicillin should *never* be used on the skin owing to the high risk of sensitization.

4. Antifungal agents

Skin scrapings to identify the fungus are best taken before commencing treatment.

Systemic treatment is used for widespread, unresponding fungal infections and nail (*tinea unguium*) and scalp ringworm. *Griseofulvin* is the drug of choice for widespread or intractable fungal infections of the skin. It is more effective in the skin than in the nails and needs to be continued for some months.

Topical treatments are usually adequate for most localized infections.

An acute fungal infection may need to be treated by *potassium permanganate* lotion 0.01% for the first few days. An ointment with salicyclic acid and benzoic acid is known as *Whitfield's ointment* and is widely used but tends to be cosmetically unacceptable. Effective preparations which are commonly used are the imidazoles (*clotrimazole, econazole, miconazole*). The *undecoanates* and *tolnaftate* are less effective in the treatment of ringworm infections.

Lotions and creams are usually the vehicle of choice. As ointments have occlusive properties they should be avoided on moist areas. Dusting powders are therapeutically ineffective in the treatment of fungal infections and liable to cause skin irritation and should be avoided except for toiletry purposes.

Infections with *Candida albicans* are common in patients with diabetes mellitus and those who have been treated with antibiotics and immunosuppressive drugs. Treatment may be with the broad-spectrum antifungal imidazoles. *Nystatin* is also equally effective and must be applied to the affected area, either as an ointment or a lotion.

5. Antiviral agents

Acyclovir cream is the treatment of choice for herpes simplex and herpes zoster of the skin. It is extremely important that the cream should be applied as early as possible, five times a day, for 5 days.

6. Emollients

These are used for dry skin (xeroderma) and especially for dry, scaly skin (e.g. ichthyosis, when the scale can be removed). They soothe and smooth the skin and a simple preparation such as aqueous cream is often a good treatment. Zinc cream is a traditional remedy and E45 a more recent one. With hyperkeratotic (i.e. thickened) and scaly conditions it is important to hydrate the skin first, that is with a bath or shower. The emollient should be applied immediately afterwards to keep the skin hydrated.

7. Miscellaneous

Many other agents can be applied to the skin for different, but sometimes very common, conditions. For example:

a. *Benzyl benzoate* or *malathion* is used for the treatment of scabies.
b. *Aminobenzoic acid lotion* protects the skin against sunlight.
c. *Cleansing agents* such as *cetrimide* are useful for removing adherent crusts or ointments.
d. *Sulphur* is used in rosacea.
e. *Salicylic acid* may be used to soften callosities, such as corns in the feet. These agents are called keratolytics.
f. *Aluminium chloride (20% lotion)* is an antiperspirant, often effective in the treatment of hyperidrosis, at any site. It is also used in many commercially available deodorants.
g. *Barrier creams* are used in industry to try and prevent damage to the skin. Most have been shown to be ineffective, but may be used for legal reasons.
h. *Calcipotriol* is a vitamin D derivative which has recently become available for treatment of mild to moderate psoriasis.

j. *Tretinoin,* a vitamin A derivative, may be used to treat acne.

APPLICATION OF SKIN PREPARATIONS

1. It must be remembered that drugs can be absorbed through the intact skin. It is therefore very important that the nurse wears gloves when applying any preparation to the skin, particularly those containing active ingredients.
2. Many patients will be required to apply their skin preparations over long periods so that it will be necessary that they are taught the correct technique. Adverse effects, such as redness and soreness and relapse, may require a change of treatment.
3. *Medicated baths:*
   - The bath water should be approx. 36°C.
   - Stir in the medication and mix well to ensure an even concentration.
   - The patient should soak for about 10 minutes.

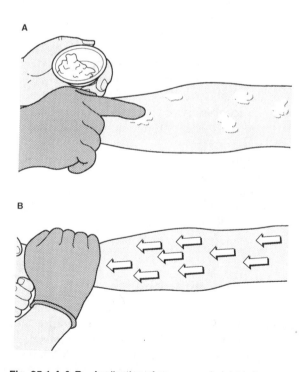

Fig. 25.1 A & B Application of creams and ointments: smooth on in the direction of the hair fall.

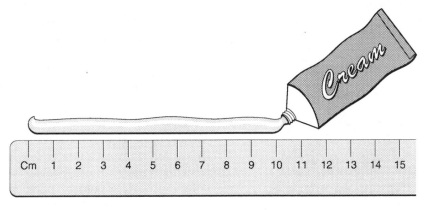

Fig. 25.2 Measuring ointment/cream.

4. *Creams and ointments:*
   - Apply sparingly.
   - Do not rub unless specifically prescribed.
   - Smooth the preparation on gently in the direction of the hair fall (see Fig. 25.1).
   - A 10 cm strip of cream or ointment from a standard nozzle of a tube of medication is the equivalent of 2 g (see Fig. 25.2).
5. *Steroid application:*
   - Steroids are best applied to hydrated skin.
   - Apply an emollient 20 minutes prior to the steroid to increase its effectiveness.
   - Care should be taken to apply only the prescribed amount of corticosteroid to avoid potential side-effects. The *Rule of Nines* is a recognized method for assessing the quantity of the preparation to be applied (see Fig. 25.3).
   - Patients may also be advised on how to use the *'Fingertip Method'* to apply their topical preparations in safe quantities (see Fig. 25.4).
6. *Dithranol application:*
   - Apply to affected areas only.
   - Palpate skin lesions (psoriatic plaques) to identify the edges of the lesion before applying dithranol.
   - Dithranol in Lassar's Paste is applied to the lesions with a spatula.
   - Starch powder or talc is patted on to Dithranol in Lassar's Paste to prevent spread of medication onto normal skin. The medication is removed with vegetable oil.

Rule of Nines

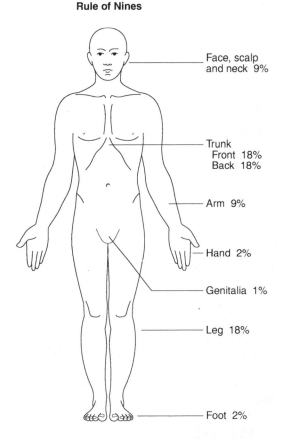

Face, scalp and neck 9%

Trunk
Front 18%
Back 18%

Arm 9%

Hand 2%

Genitalia 1%

Leg 18%

Foot 2%

Fig. 25.3 This shows the percentage of the total body surface area made up of the various parts of the body. It can be seen that the percentages are usually 9% or a multiple of 9%. In general, no more than 2 g of steroid ointment per 9% of body surface should be applied at any one time, i.e. 4 fingertips units per 9% of body surface (measured by the male finger) or 5 fingertips units per 9% of body surface (measured by the female finger).

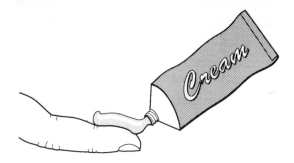

1g ointment/cream = 2 fingertip units (males)

2.5 fingertip units (females)

Fig. 25.4 Fingertip unit.

- Dithranol in cream or ointment base is rubbed into the skin lesion with a gloved hand (powder is not used).
- *Short contact therapy*—dithranol is left on the skin for 20 minutes or the prescribed time and then removed.

DRUG ERUPTIONS

A skin eruption due to drug therapy is now so commonly seen that this cause must always be considered whenever a patient is seen with an unusual rash. In addition, patients are often on more than one drug so that it is difficult or impossible to determine which one is responsible. All that can be done is to give an assessment of the possibilities.

The skin can only react in a certain number of ways, which are known as reaction patterns. A good example is *urticaria*, which can be provoked by a number of different drugs. If, however, the patient is taking aspirin or its derivatives, this is by far the most likely drug to provoke this reaction pattern. However, in practice, some drugs so commonly cause a particular eruption that this drug can be strongly suspected to be the cause if the patient is seen with a specific rash. For example, *frusemide* can cause a purpuric rash, *glutethimide* a generalized erythema and *sulphonamides* a measles-like rash.

Some drugs can cause many different types of skin eruption. *Gold* can provoke a generalized exfoliative erythroderma, which may be fatal, or a rash resembling pityriasis rosea or just a nondescript erythema associated with a stomatitis. *Penicillin* usually causes a severe erythema, and this may be so marked that a diagnosis of erythema multiforme may be considered.

Treatment is generally simple in that all drugs which are the likely cause should be withdrawn. Symptomatic treatment for symptoms may be called for, with calamine cream for pruritus or systemic antihistamines to make the patient more comfortable. It should be noted that the *topical* application of antibiotics, antihistamines and local anaesthetics should be avoided as they often cause sensitization rashes.

CONCLUSION

From this brief review it will be seen that practically anything can be applied to the skin and often is! Patients may have used a variety of unsuitable remedies before they see a doctor or nurse and your first duty is to apply a remedy that will not do any harm. This is why many dermatologists are very conservative in the treatment that they prescribe. Like any other part of the body, when it is inflamed the skin must be allowed to rest. If there is an external cause for the trouble then this must be removed and it is as well to remember that this may be an ointment which has been prescribed. If there is an infection it must be treated. The topical application of a suitable base may be all that the skin requires. The active agents, or drugs, should only be added if there is a definite indication for their use.

SKIN CARE

There is no doubt at all that good skin care needs soap and water, probably almost daily. Some individuals may prefer to use a soap substitute, such as an emulsifying ointment. Make-up should always be removed at night and aqueous cream can be used to prevent drying, and as a cleansing agent to remove make-up. The skin should always be protected from excessive exposure to the sun and if possible, excessive use of perfumes, hair dyes and so on. When it is said someone looks healthy, this means the skin is in good condition and looks normal.

FURTHER READING

Fincham-Gee C 1988 Safe use of topical steroids. Nursing, 29(3): 1043–1045
Fincham-Gee C 1990 Rule of Nines in steroid application. Soothing advice, Video, Healthcare Productions, London
Findlay A Y, Edwards P H, Harding K G 1989 The fingertip unit: a new practical measure. (Letter), The Lancet 2: 155
Greenhow M M 1983 Topical treatments—a simple guide. Nursing 2 (10): 281–284
Runne V, Kunze J 1982 Short duration ('minutes') therapy with dithranol for psoriasis: a new outpatient regime. British Journal of Dermatology 106: 135–139
Stone L A, Lindfield E M Robertson S 1989 A colour atlas of nursing procedures in skin disorders. Wolfe Medical, London.

THE NOSE

Medicaments may be instilled into the nose. It must be remembered, however, that their effect is very transient; the cilia lining the nasal cavities completely remove them in about 20 minutes. Furthermore, medication with strong solutions of antibiotics or vasoconstrictors will paralyse the cilia and thus impede rather than help the clearance of infected material from the nasal cavities.

Nose drops are best given as follows. The patient should lie back on a couch or bed with his head extended over the end. About 5 ml of the appropriate drops are instilled into each nostril, the patient being instructed to breathe through the mouth, thus closing the back of the nose and holding the nose drops in the nasal cavities. This position should be maintained for 3 minutes. This method of administration may be too strenuous for the elderly. There are a number of nose drops in use, amongst the most useful are:

Ephedrine nose drops 0.5%

Ephedrine	500 mg
Sodium chloride	500 mg
Chlorbutol	500 mg
Water to 100 ml	

Ephedrine nose drops are useful in sinus infection, for the ephedrine causes shrinkage of the swollen and inflamed mucosa and thus clears the nasal airway and allows proper drainage from the nasal sinuses. Over-use, however, may damage the delicate ciliated epithelium lining the nasal passages and the drops should not be used for more than a week.

Interaction. Ephedrine nose drops should not be given to patients taking monoamine-oxidase inhibitors or within 2 weeks of stopping these drugs, owing to the risk of a hypertensive crisis.

In allergic conditions of the nose (allergic rhinitis) several preparations are available which relieve congestion when applied locally. Corticosteroids (betamethasone 0.1%) can be given as nose drops two or three times daily or beclomethasone is available as a nasal spray, the dose being two sprays into each nostril twice daily. Sodium cromoglycate (see p. 222) can be given as a nasal spray, as drops or as an insufflation.

Local antibiotics have little place in the treatment of nasal infections but a cream containing *chlorhexidine* and *neomycin* (Naseptin) can be applied locally in patients who are carriers of the staphylococcus.

THE EAR

Although the instilling of drops into the ear may be useful in relieving symptoms, it is often done without any consideration of the underlying disease and thus proves fruitless and sometimes even dangerous.

The use of ear drops will be considered under individual disorders of the ear which can be helped by this method of treatment.

Instillation of drops

Warm ear drops to approximately blood heat.

The head is turned so that the affected ear is uppermost.

Discharge is gently mopped away.

Two or three drops are instilled and the head is held in position for a minute or two.

Wax in the ear

Wax may become hard and impacted in the ear and may resist efforts to move it by syringing. A 5.0% solution of sodium bicarbonate or warm olive oil instilled for a few days will usually soften it satisfactorily.

Otitis externa

Severe infection is best managed with expert guidance as regular aural toilet and medication are required.

Ear drops will only be effective if the meatus is cleared of debris. The following agents may be used three times daily if bacterial infection is suspected. Clioquinol 1% with flumethasone 0.02% (Locorten-Vioform) has a mild antibacterial and antifungal action but stains the skin and clothes. Gentamicin 0.3% with hydrocortisone 1% is anti-inflammatory and antibacterial.

Other combinations of antibacterials with steroids are available.

The following precautions should be observed:

1. Treatment with antibiotic ear drops should not be continued for longer than 1 week owing to the risks of drug sensitization and the development of fungal infection.
2. Gentamicin or neomycin ear drops should not be used if the eardrum is perforated as deafness may result.

In eczema or the ear, local steroids should be used to reduce irritation and inflammation. Prednisolone 0.5% or betamethasone 0.1% are satisfactory.

Otitis media

If the drum is not perforated the instillation of antibiotics into the external ear is useless as it will not reach the site of infection. Patients should be treated by systemic antibiotics. In adults, *benzylpenicillin* and in young children, *amoxycillin* will deal with most infections.

FURTHER READING

Symposium 1990 Ear, nose and throat disease. Prescribers Journal 30: 191

26

Disinfectants and insecticides

DISINFECTANTS

Disinfection is the destruction of vegetative bacteria but not necessarily their spores. Sterilization processes (e.g. autoclaving, gamma irradiation) destroy both vegetative bacteria and spores. However, in most circumstances (e.g. standard ward cleaning procedures, cleaning of bedpans and urinals), reduction in the total number of bacteria is sufficient to remove the threat of infection to the average patient and disinfection is the appropriate procedure. An exception to this rule is the severely immunocompromised patient nursed in protective isolation. Hospitals have their own protocols for the care of these very vulnerable patients. A good disinfectant is not necessarily a good cleaning agent and the two should not be interchanged.

There are two main types of disinfectant:

1. Environmental disinfectants which are used on non-living objects such as bedpans, urinal bottles, thermometers, etc.
2. Those used on living surfaces such as skin and mucous membranes—sometimes called antiseptics.

These two groups are not substitutes for one another. Environmental disinfectants are often potent chemicals which damage tissue, while antiseptics, which have been developed to prevent such damage, are not only too expensive for environmental use, but also tend to destroy a narrower range of bacteria.

ENVIRONMENTAL DISINFECTANTS

a. Phenolic derivatives. Phenol was one of the first disinfectants used and it killed bacteria by combining with their protein. It has now been replaced because it was not very effective, rapidly losing efficiency with dilution. It was very toxic causing local corrosion of the mouth, throat and stomach if swallowed and followed by kidney damage.

Commercially available derivatives include Hycolin which is used as a 2% or 1.5% solution and Clearsol which is supplied in sachets to be diluted before use. They are active against a wide range of bacteria but are unable to destroy most spores and are inactive against some viruses. Phenolics can damage the skin and should be used with protective gloves. They should not be used on food preparation surfaces.

b. Hypochlorite disinfectants. These disinfectants act by releasing chlorine, the amount released being measured in parts per million of chlorine which is available. They can be used both as environmental disinfectants and for wound cleaning.

Sodium hypochlorite solution is available in sachet form (Chlorasol) and diluted as required.

A 1% solution (10 000 parts per million) is used as an environmental disinfectant.

A 0.3% solution (3000 parts per million) is used for wound cleaning.

Hypochlorite disinfectants destroy hepatitis B and HIV in a 1% solution.

Diluted solutions decay rapidly and must be made up freshly before use.

Gluteraldehyde solution is used for sterilizing certain heat sensitive instruments. It is irritant and must be used in a well-ventilated room and gloves should be worn to prevent skin contact.

A freshly prepared 2% solution destroys HIV but is much more expensive than hypochlorites.

DISINFECTANTS USED ON THE SKIN AND MUCOUS MEMBRANES

Iodine is an effective disinfectant but is rapidly inactivated by the tissues. It can also cause skin sensitization. It is now used mainly in the form of *povidone-iodine*, a non-staining and less irritant complex available as:

- Povidone-iodine 10% alcoholic solution
- Povidone-iodine 10% (aqueous) antiseptic solution, used for pre-operative skin preparation
- 7.5% surgical scrub as a hand disinfectant.

Chlorhexidine is an expensive skin disinfectant and is most unsuitable for environmental use because it is effective mainly against Gram-positive bacteria (e.g. *staphylococci* and *streptococci*). It has little action against Gram-negative rods (e.g. *Pseudomonas, Klebsiella, Esch. coli*) and will destroy few spores or viruses.

It is used as:

- A 0.5% alcohol solution as a skin disinfectant
- A 0.2% solution of chlorhexidine gluconate as a mouthwash
- A 4% solution as a pre-operative scrub
- A 0.015% solution with cetrimide (Savlodil sachets, see below) for wound cleaning.

Hexachlorophane is similar and is available in several forms including:

- 1% soap and a 2% cream used for surface disinfecting.

It can penetrate the skin particularly if it is excoriated and the application is not followed by rinsing. It should therefore be used with special care in the new-born.

Hydrogen peroxide is used for irrigating infected wounds. It is not a very powerful disinfectant but when it comes in contact with damaged tissues, enzymes which are present release oxygen which bubbles up from the wound and helps to loosen debris thus cleaning the infected area.

Surface-acting agents lower surface tension and allow fats to be more easily emulsified. They are also bacteriocidal. This combined action is useful in that it cleans the infected area and allows the disinfectant to penetrate widely thus enlarging its range of antibacterial activity. One of the most widely used is *cetrimide* which is available as a cream or as a solution and may be combined with another disinfectant such as chlorhexidine (Savlodil).

Ethyl alcohol is used as a skin disinfectant and is most effective as a 70% solution but it may also be used as a vehicle for other disinfectants such as chlorhexidine, marketed as 'Hibisol'.

Hand decontamination

Hands can be decontaminated with soap from a wall container, a medical agent or alcoholic handrub. Trials have repeatedly shown the superiority of agents such as chlorhexidine over ordinary soap but such trials have not reproduced ward conditions where nurses hurry between patients and from clean to dirty tasks. Any hand hygiene will only be efficient if it is used frequently and appropriately, even between such manoeuvres as mouth care and patient feeding. Hands should also be washed when plastic gloves are removed as bacteria multiply in the warm, moist environment inside them.

Whichever agent is used, all hand and interdigital surfaces must be decontaminated and dried thoroughly as damp hands transfer bacteria more readily than dry ones. Although a thorough hand-washing technique may take longer, this is of value, particularly with medicated agents which need a minimum contact time with bacteria to be effective. When soap is used, evidence shows that the bacterial count is adequately reduced by the mechanical action of washing and thorough drying. The soreness which medicated agents are said to induce can be reduced by wetting the hands before application and rinsing thoroughly.

Use of disinfectants in various circumstances

The following recommendations are based on those given in the North Southwark and Lewisham District Formulary. Other hospitals will, no doubt, have their own procedures. It is necessarily incomplete.

Ampoules	Swab neck with 70% alcohol or use a Mediswab.
Bath water	For infected patients, add one Savlon Concentrate sachet to water, do not use soap.
Bed pans	Washer—Disinfector—NB these do not sterilize.
Bladder washouts	1. Normal saline or 2. Chlorhexidine 1:5000 aqueous solution.
Cleaning cuts and abrasion	Chlorhexidine 0.015% with cetrimide (Savlodil sachets).
Hand-washing (ward staff)	Liquid soap and water from a wall dispenser. In special circumstances, povidone-iodine surgical scrub.
Surgical scrubbing (surgeon)	Povidone-iodine surgical scrub or chlorhexidine scrub if iodine sensitive.
Operating theatres (walls, floors, etc.)	1. Neutral detergent. 2. Infected material—Hycolin 1.5% or hypochlorite (0.1%) with detergent.
Skin preparation (injection)	70% alcohol or 0.5% chlorhexidine in 70% alcohol.
Skin preparation (pre-operative)	Povidone-iodine 10% alcohol solution or chlorhexidine 0.5% in alcohol solution. Surgeons have their preferences and may require a coloured solution to delineate the disinfected area.
Thermometers (clinical)	Individual—wipe with 70% alcohol swab after each use and store dry.

After discharge—wash with detergent and soak in fresh 70% alcohol for 10 minutes and store dry.

HIV and hepatitis B

These virus carried diseases now present a special problem and local guidelines will be available in most districts and are also available from the Royal College of Nursing, 20, Cavendish Square, London. All blood and body fluids should be regarded as potentially infectious.

Contamination should be immediately treated with 1% hypochlorite solution or in the community—1 part of bleach in 10 parts of water, freshly made. Gloves should be worn whenever handling blood or body fluids, and the hands washed afterwards.

INSECTICIDES

Some knowledge of insecticides is important to the nurse for these substances are widely used in the disinfection of patients' bedding and houses, etc., and some of them are highly poisonous substances which produce side-effects unless used properly.

Anticholinesterases

Malathion is commonly used. It paralyses the nervous system of the parasite. If correctly used, it is not toxic but the alcoholic solution should be avoided in asthmatics and very young children.

Carbamates

Carbaryl is similar to the above.

Lindane

This substance is a useful insecticide and has been used as a 1% application in the treatment of scabies, and infestation by lice. However, it does not kill the ova of the lice and as it is only effective for a short time, relapses will occur.

Large doses in animals cause convulsions, but provided it is used carefully it appears safe, although it should be avoided in pregnancy and young children.

Pyrethroids

This group of insecticides is obtained from the pyrethrum flowers which belong to the chrysanthemum family. They are quick-acting insecticides used in many insecticidal sprays. They are effective and if used properly are safe, although sensitization can occur.

Nursing point

Patients often ask the nurse about the use of topical preparations such as skin disinfectants and medical insecticides. With the advent of nurse-prescribing the nurse will not only be expected to provide practical help and reassurance but to assess the circumstances in which such preparations are needed.

MEDICAL USES OF INSECTICIDES

The two commonest uses for insecticides in medical treatment are:

Scabies

Scabies is due to a mite, the female of which burrows into the skin at certain sites, namely between the fingers, wrists, hands, buttocks and skin folds.

Therapeutics. A number of substances have been used in the treatment of scabies.

1. Malathion 0.5% aqueous solution (Derbac). This is very effective and the least toxic of the applications available. The solution is applied to the entire body from the neck downwards. It is very rare for the face or hair to be involved in adults. If the solution is applied to the face, avoid the eyes and around the mouth. It is left on for 24 hours. All close contacts are treated whether they have symptoms or not. The mite dies very quickly away from the skin but it is worth laundering sheets and clothes. Itching takes about a month to subside and calamine lotion or 1% hydrocortisone ointment are useful for symptomatic treatment.

2. Permethrin (a pyrethroid) is available as a cream (Lyclear) which is applied over the whole body except the head. The body should be washed 12 hours later. It appears to be effective but occasionally causes itching and erythema.

Benzyl benzoate has now been largely superseded.

Pediculosis (lice)

It is necessary to prevent the development of strains of lice which are resistant to treatment, therefore the preparations used should be rotated every 3 years. Effective preparations include:

- *Carbaryl 0.5% in alcohol (Carylderm).*
- *Malathion 0.5% in alcohol (Prioderm)* for head pediculosis.
- *Malathion 0.5% in aqueous solution (Derbac)* for pubic pediculosis or for those with abrasions or sensitive skin.
- *The pyrethroids, permethrin cream* and *phenothrin 0.2%* lotion in alcohol are used for head lice. In asthmatics and very young children alcoholic solutions should not be used.

Preparations are rubbed into dry hair, scalp or other affected areas. They are allowed to dry naturally; direct sunlight or heating should be avoided as they break down the drug and could ignite the alcohol. After 12 hours the hair is washed in the normal way using soap. Special medicated shampoos are unnecessary as the lice are already dead. The hair can be combed with a Secker comb to remove nits and treatment should be repeated after 1 week to kill lice emerging from the eggs.

It is important to treat the whole family.

FURTHER READING

Collins B J 1982 The use of chemical disinfectants in hospital. Nursing 2nd series 7: 190
Gould D 1991 Hygienic hand decontamination. Nursing Standard 6 (32): 33–36
Gould D 1991 Skin bacteria. What is normal? Nursing Standard 5(52): 26–29
Hoffman P 1986 Disinfection in hospitals. Nursing 3rd series 3: 106
Hoyland B 1981 Infestation. Nursing lst series 23: 988
Lowbury E J et al 1992 Control of hospital infection. A practical handbook, 3rd edn. Chapman and Hall, London.
Maunder J W 1991 Strategic aspects of insecticide resistance in head lice. Journal of the Royal Society of Health III 1: 24–26
Maurer I M 1985 Hospital hygiene, 3rd edn. Edward Arnold, London
Smith F, Ross F 1992 Prescribing topical agents. Community outlook 2(7): 29–32
Ward K 1992 The management of skin infestations. Nursing Standard 26 (6): 28–31

27

Poisoning and its treatment

The treatment of acute poisoning has of recent years become increasingly important. About 10% of acute medical admissions to hospital are due to an overdose but 80% of these only require observation until the effects of the poison wear off. Most of the section on general treatment below applies to the more severely poisoned patient. This may be due to attempted suicide, less often to accidental poisoning and very rarely to homicide. Perhaps the commonest cause of overdosage is an attempt by the patient to draw attention to or modify some intolerable situation. In these circumstances he is not seeking death but merely trying to shock relatives or friends into realization of his problems.

In children poisoning occurs most commonly in the 1 to 5 year age group as the child becomes mobile and is inclined to put everything in his mouth. Drugs and other harmful substances must be kept not only out of reach but also out of sight as children are adept at reaching 'impossible' places. Occasionally poisoning may be due to accidental overdose of a drug.

The most frequently used suicide agents are centrally-acting drugs including sedatives, hypnotics and antidepressants, analgesics including aspirin, paracetamol and opioids and a mixed bag which includes cardiovascular drugs. Coal gas, although still used, is less common than formerly since methane has replaced it for domestic use. In addition, poisoning can occur, particularly in children, from various chemicals used domestically or in the garden and from a number of berries.

GENERAL MANAGEMENT

When a patient is admitted to hospital suffering from poisoning the first step is to decide if life is at immediate risk from airway obstruction or respiratory arrest. If so, the appropriate measures should be taken at once.

The next steps are to assess the severity of the poisoning, the nature of the poison used (overdose by more than one drug is common) and to institute appropriate treatment.

Severity of poisoning

The severity of the poisoning will be based largely on three criteria.

1. Level of consciousness. This is usually classified in four grades:

- Grade I. Drowsy but responds to light stimulation
- Grade II. Unconscious but responds to light stimulation
- Grade III. Unconscious but responds to severe stimulation
- Grade IV. Unconscious with no response to stimulation.

2. Circulation. Many drugs cause circulatory failure. The nurse is frequently asked to measure the blood pressure at intervals and a low blood pressure is indicative of failing circulation. However, it must be realized that what really matters is the perfusion of vital organs such as the brain and kidney. It is possible to have a reasonable blood pressure maintained by intense constriction of blood vessels, but organ perfusion will be poor. In such a situation the hands and feet will be cold and blue and this may be a useful sign. In addition, certain drugs (particularly antidepressants) can cause cardiac arrhythmias so that ECG monitoring is necessary.

3. Respiration. Depression of respiration so that oxygen reaches the lungs is a common cause of death in overdosage. Respiratory rate should be charted at regular intervals. Cyanosis is a useful sign of under-ventilation of the lungs, and if facilities are available the respiratory minute volume and blood gases must be measured.

Nature of poison used

The identification of the poison used will depend on circumstantial evidence, on clinical signs and on analysis of gastric aspirate, blood and urine. Samples should be collected, carefully labelled and analysed as soon as possible. The results may not only be useful in the management of the patient but they may have medico-legal implications.

TREATMENT

The treatment of poisoning can be divided into:

1. Non-specific measures
2. Specific measures which are considered under individual poisons.

Non-specific measures

1. Maintenance of ventilation. In the unconscious patient the reflexes which protect the airways may be lost so there is danger of respiratory obstruction by the tongue and the aspiration of vomit. These patients should be nursed in the coma position with an airway in place until it is possible to insert a cuffed endotracheal tube which can be kept in place for up to 72 hours. Secretions should be aspirated regularly.

With severe respiratory depression, oxygen and/or assisted ventilation will be required.

2. Reducing absorption of poisons. It is obviously desirable to minimize the absorption of poison from the gut and this can be achieved in two ways:

1. Emptying the stomach by emesis or washouts.
2. Giving substances which bind to the poison in the gut and thus prevent its absorption.

Emptying the stomach. If the patient is conscious, vomiting can be induced by stimulation of the posterior pharyngeal wall, or, more effectively, by giving *ipecacuanha emetic mixture (paediatric)* 30 ml for an adult or 10–15 ml for a child, followed by a glass of water. This drug stimulates both the stomach and vomiting centre and acts in 90% of subjects within 30 minutes.

In the unconscious patient lavage is the most efficient measure and should be performed:

a. When dangerous amounts of poison have been taken within the previous 2 hours. A longer period is reasonable with certain drugs e.g.

Salicylates	24 h
Tricyclic antidepressants	8 h
Opioids	8 h

b. After a cuffed endotracheal tube has been inserted as there is considerable risk of inhalation of vomit in these patients.

Lavage is carried out via a 30 English gauge Jaques catheter lubricated with Vaseline, and a 50 cm length should be adequate. Great care is needed to ensure that the tube is in the stomach and not the trachea. 300–500 ml of warm water should be used for each wash which is repeated three or four times. At the end the stomach should be empty except in the case of iron poisoning when 5 g of desferioxamine should be left in situ. Although gastric lavage and emetics have been used for many years in the treatment of poisoning their efficacy is under critical review and it seems probable that, except when very large amounts have been taken, they have little effect on the prognosis unless carried out within an hour or two of ingestion.

Absorption can also be reduced by giving *activated charcoal* by mouth. The dose is 25–100 g and it is usually given via a nasogastric tube. It prevents absorption throughout the gut and in some circumstances is more effective than gastric lavage.

3. Maintenance of blood pressure. Some patients will have a low blood pressure and failing circulation. Adequate ventilation (see above) will often improve matters. Raising the foot of the bed is simple and is usually successful in mild poisoning. With severe hypotension the infusion of volume expanders such as dextran may be required.

4. Increasing elimination of poisons. This can be achieved by increasing elimination via the kidneys or by haemoperfusion. Renal elimination of some drugs can be increased by altering the pH of the urine and an example is in the treatment of salicylate poisoning (see p. 308).

In haemoperfusion the blood is passed through a column of charcoal or some other substance which removes the poison. This method undoubtedly removes poisons but there is a risk of damaging platelets and blood cells so it is rarely used.

A similar effect can be more easily achieved by giving repeated oral doses of activated charcoal; the poison passes from the gut wall and binds to the charcoal in the lumen.

5. Nutrition, hydration and electrolyte disturbances. In comatose patients the problems of *nutrition, hydration* and *electrolyte disturbances* will require consideration although intravenous infusion will not usually be necessary unless the coma is prolonged.

6. Follow-up. When the patient has recovered it is important that the social and psychiatric background to a suicide attempt is investigated and most of these patients will require continued supportive treatment.

INDIVIDUAL POISONS

Benzodiazepines

These drugs are widely used so it is not surprising that overdose is common. They produce coma without any specific features and cardiorespiratory depression is minimal. It should not be forgotten, however, that they may have been combined with other more sinister agents. Some of this group of drugs have long half-lives and/or active metabolites and full recovery may take several days.

Treatment. It is usually sufficient to maintain a clear airway and give general nursing care. *Flumazenil* is a specific antidote which reverses the actions of this group of drugs but it is only rarely required in severe overdose.

Salicylates (aspirin)

Aspirin has long been a common cause of poisoning although in recent years its place has been partially taken by paracetamol. In addition to suicide attempts, it is particularly dangerous as a cause of accidental overdosage in children who are more sensitive to its toxic effects than adults.

Symptoms. Nausea, vomiting, tinnitus, increased respiration, and with severe overdose confusion, convulsions and coma.

Aspirin also produces complicated changes in the acid–base state of the body. Early on it causes increased respiration and thus washes carbon dioxide out through the lungs and causes an alkalosis. The aspirin itself is an acid and tends to produce an acidosis after some hours.

Treatment:

1. Wash out the stomach with water. This is worth doing up to 24 hours after ingestion of the drug.
2. If the patient is conscious, give 5% sodium bicarbonate solution by mouth together with a high fluid intake.
3. In severely ill and unconscious patients (serum salicylate > 600mg/litre for adults and > 300 mg/litre for children) intravenous fluid and electrolyte replacement is essential and forced alkaline diuresis and/or haemodialysis should be considered.
4. Equally effective is oral charcoal 100 g followed by 50 g 4 hourly, although vomiting may make this difficult.

Paracetamol

Overdosage with paracetamol produces liver damage which may prove fatal. This is due to abnormal breakdown products which do not occur with normal dosage but only when excess has been taken. As little as 10 g (20 of the usual tablets) can be dangerous. Early symptoms, usually nausea and vomiting, are minimal and it is only after 2 or 3 days that jaundice with hepatic failure and/or more rarely renal failure develop. Patients in whom the blood level of paracetamol is above 200 mg/litre 4 hours after ingestion, or 30 mg/litre 15 hours after ingestion of the drug, are likely to develop severe liver damage.

Treatment. The stomach should be washed out. There are several drugs available which alter metabolism of the drug and prevent liver damage:

- Methionine 2 g 2 hourly for 5 doses, *or*
- N-acetylcysteine 150 mg/kg in 200 ml of 5% dextrose over 15 minutes followed by 50 mg/kg infused over 4 hours, and finally 100 mg/kg infused over the next 16 hours.

This treatment is not effective if given more than fifteen hours after ingestion of paracetamol. It should therefore be given *immediately* to all patients in whom there is good evidence of overdose without waiting for the results of a blood level estimation. When this becomes available treatment can be modified if necessary.

Otherwise, treatment is symptomatic.

Opioids

Morphine and related substances are common causes of poisoning. This may occur as a suicide attempt or because an addict has misjudged his/her 'fix'. Although morphine and heroin are the best known of this group, serious overdosage can occur with so-called weak narcotics such as codeine, dihydrocodeine and dextropropoxyphene (see below), provided a big enough dose is taken.

Symptoms. The classic symptoms are coma, depressed respiration and pin-point pupils. The patient sweats and is liable to develop hypothermia. The pulse is slow. Pulmonary oedema may develop rapidly and is often fatal.

Treatment. Respiratory depression is reversed by naloxone (p. 100) 800 micrograms–1.2 mg given intravenously. It is, however, short-acting and repeated doses may be required. Respiratory arrest will require full resuscitation with assisted ventilation. Hypothermia should be treated in the usual way.

Dextropropoxyphene

This requires special mention. In the UK it is usually taken combined with paracetamol as co-proxamol (Distalgesic) tablets and is one of the commonest causes of fatal poisoning. In relatively small doses, i.e. more than 20 tablets, it can produce marked respiratory depression and circulatory collapse. If the patient survives this there is a danger of paracetamol liver damage. The effects of dextropropoxyphene but not paracetamol are reversed by naloxone.

The central effects of all opioids are increased by concurrent consumption of alcohol.

Tricyclic antidepressants (imipramine, amytriptyline)

The older tricyclic antidepressants are very dangerous in overdose, largely because of their effects on the heart. The more recently introduced drugs, however, are less toxic.

Symptoms. With small overdosage the patient is flushed, agitated with some blunting of consciousness and has a rapid pulse. The pupils are dilated and accommodation paralysed. The QRS interval on the ECG becomes progressively longer with increasing severity of poisoning. Larger doses cause fits, coma, depression of respiration and blood pressure and various cardiac arrhythmias.

Treatment. There is no specific remedy and diuresis and dialysis are no help. Wash out the stomach up to 8 hours after ingestion and leave 100 g of activated charcoal in the stomach. Further doses of charcoal, 50 g 4 hourly, should be given orally to minimize absorption. Cardiac arrhythmias are treated along the usual lines. Hypotension can be reversed by raising the cardiac output with dopamine and fits controlled by diazepam. Systemic acidosis may require correction by infusion of sodium bicarbonate.

Alcohol

The patient may be conscious but mentally disorientated or may be unconscious. There is a smell of alcohol on the breath.

Treatment. Most patients will recover if kept warm and allowed to sleep it off. In severe cases, the stomach should be washed out if the alcohol has been taken recently and treatment continued as in barbiturate poisoning except that forced diuresis is not used. It is very important to remember that patients who are drunk may have received injuries of which they are not aware. *It should also be remembered that patients may have taken other drugs in addition to alcohol.*

Barbiturates

These are no longer the commonest cause of fatal poisoning in Great Britain.

Symptoms. The patient is confused or in coma. The respirations are depressed and the blood pressure is low. Skin blistering is quite a common feature.

Treatment. In barbiturate poisoning death is usually due to respiratory depression, circulatory failure, or pneumonia at a later date.

1. The airway must be kept clear and if the cough reflex is absent an endotracheal tube should be inserted, particularly for gastric lavage in the unconscious patient.
2. Gastric lavage is only justified if the drug has been taken within the previous 3 hours.
3. Ventilation is important and if there is respiratory depression some form of mechanical ventilation is required.
4. Fluid and calories must be given intravenously.
5. Forced alkaline diuresis (only for phenobarbitone).

The appropriate antibiotic should be given if pulmonary infection develops.

Carbon monoxide

Symptoms. Confusion or coma usually combined with cyanosis or pallor. The classical bright red colour of the skin and mucous membranes due to carboxyhaemoglobin is rare.

Treatment:

1. Get the patient out of the poisonous atmosphere.
2. Ensure a clear airway.
3. Give oxygen (not oxygen and CO_2).
4. Artificial respiration may be necessary.

Phenothiazines (chlorpromazine, etc.)

Symptoms. These drugs produce coma, with hypotension and sometimes hypothermia. Chronic intoxication causes a Parkinson-like state.

Treatment is largely symptomatic although it is worth trying gastric lavage up to 6 hours after ingestion. Parkinson-like states and other forms of dystonia respond to orphenadrine (see p. 151).

Iron compounds

These substances, particularly ferrous sulphate, are sometimes taken by children—because of their colour and sugar coating.

Symptoms. Vomiting with haematemesis; pallor, collapse and tachycardia. Fatal collapse sometimes occurs after apparent recovery. *Iron overdose in children must always be taken very seriously.*

Treatment:

1. Wash out the stomach with 5% sodium bicarbonate solution (1 oz per pint).
2. The iron chelating agent desferrioxamine which combines with iron and prevents absorption should be used in severe cases. 5 g in 100 ml of water is given orally, and 2 g is given intramuscularly twice daily. In severe poisoning desferrioxamine can also be given intravenously to a maximum dose of 80 mg/kg of body weight in 24 hours.

Table 27.1

	Plasma concentration producing severe overdose	Upper limit of therapeutic plasma level
Hypnotics		
Barbiturates	50 mg/l	5 mg/l
Diazepam	5 mg/l	1 mg/l
Anticonvulsants		
Phenobarbitone	100 mg/l	30 mg/l
Phenytoin	35 mg/l	20 mg/l
Analgesics		
Salicylates	600 mg/l	250 mg/l
Paracetamol	200 mg/l (4 h after ingestion) 30 mg/l (15 h after ingestion)	20 mg/l
Miscellaneous		
Amitriptyline	1 mg/l	0.2 mg/l
Ethanol	3 g/l	0.8 g/l is the legal limit for driving

Paraquat

Paraquat is a weed killer. The granules available for domestic use contain only 5% of the substance and are not lethal. However, the pure substance used in agriculture is very dangerous—30 mg may be fatal. Death usually occurs after 1–2 weeks and is due to progressive lung failure, sometimes combined with kidney and liver damage. Treatment is nearly always ineffective, although if administered soon after ingestion, an oral suspension of fuller's earth has proved valuable in preventing absorption of paraquat.

CHELATING AGENTS

These substances combine with metals and thus render them inactive. They are used in treating heavy metal poisoning.

Dimercaprol (BAL). Some heavy metals produce their toxic effects by combining with a chemical grouping found in living tissues and called SH groups. Their toxic effects can be prevented by giving dimercaprol which also contains SH groups and thus combines with and inactivates heavy metals.

Therapeutic use. Dimercaprol is useful in poisoning by arsenic, mercury and gold. The initial dose of 3 mg/kg body weight is repeated 4 hourly on the first and second days of treatment and reduced thereafter. It should be given by deep intramuscular injection.

Penicillamine is used in treating Wilson's disease which is due to the excessive deposition of copper in the brain and liver. It chelates the copper which is then excreted. It can be given orally in doses of 0.5–2.0 g daily. It is also used in treating rheumatoid arthritis (see p. 109).

FURTHER READING

Henry J, Volans G 1984 ABC of poisoning. BMA, London
Davis J E 1991 Activated charcoal in acute drug overdosage. Professional Nurse 6(12): 710

28

The nurse and the pharmaceutical service

Introduction

In hospital the overall responsibility for the care and supply of drugs lies with the pharmacist, and he will be the central point for advice on their handling and use. The nurses' responsibilities for the handling of drugs fall into seven areas: they will **obtain drugs**, **possibly prescribe them**, **store them**, **prepare and administer them to patients**, **record the administration**, and **observe their effects**, in accordance with the requirements of the law and with hospital rules and procedures. In all of these activities they are able to call upon the pharmacist for help and advice.

In recent years, a much closer working relationship has been built up between pharmacists and nurses by the pharmacist emerging from his department and providing a ward pharmacy service. Such services are provided in most large and many small hospitals, and although the precise form varies from hospital to hospital, the usual practice is for the pharmacist to visit the ward once or twice a day, in order to see the prescription sheets, initiate the dispensing of any drugs required, raise any queries on dosage, availability or incompatibility with the doctor, and form the first point of contact for drug information required by the doctor or nurse. By doing this, the pharmacist very quickly becomes familiar with the requirements of the ward both in terms of supply and information, and can play a considerable part in ensuring the safe handling and use of drugs.

Drug selection and dosage

The selection of a drug is the responsibility of the doctor, advised as appropriate by senior colleagues or the pharmacist. Many hospitals are now extending these practices by the preparation of Drug Formularies, which aim to recommend a 'best-buy' drug from the often bewildering range available, and to give information on dosage, routes of administration, costs, contraindications, and side-effects. Hospital pharmacies usually stock only those drugs listed in the Formulary.

Nurses are now permitted to prescribe some preparations as a further development of their extended role (see p. 21).

Drug supply

Drugs in frequent use in a ward, or likely to be required in an emergency, are usually supplied as ward stock. Traditionally, the nurse has been responsible for ordering stock drugs, either by writing out a list of items required or by using a pre-printed order form, in each case basing her requirements on the empty containers in the cupboard or trolley. In many hospitals the pharmacy now operates a top-up system with a pharmacy technician checking and supplying drugs to an agreed stock level on a weekly basis, thus removing the responsibility of ordering from the nurse. Whichever system is used, the aim must be to avoid both wasteful overstocking and running out at times when the pharmacy is closed.

Individual patient dispensing is used for less frequently required drugs and in cases where the preparation is tailored to the patient's particular requirements. Although most drugs are manufactured by industry, hospital pharmacies are always able to prepare different dose-forms or strengths, for example a mixture for a patient unable to take solids, a paediatric mixture where the child needs a lower dose, or a suppository if the oral route is contraindicated. Some hospitals are able to prepare injections of novel or little-used chemicals, or formulate a chemical substance into preparations suitable for administration by a variety of routes. These more expert services, although concentrated in a few hospitals, are available to all through the district pharmaceutical organization. The ward pharmacist will always be pleased to advise on a suitable preparation and arrange for it to be made available.

The law requires that drugs of addiction, known as Controlled Drugs, must be supplied only against the signature of the sister or nurse in charge of the ward, and that the requisitions for these drugs must state precisely the name, form, strength, and quantity of the drug required. Controlled Drugs most likely to be met by the nurse include *morphine, diamorphine (heroin), papavertum ('Omnopon'), cocaine, pethidine, methadone, dextramoramide, buprenorphine* and the *barbiturates* and *amphetamines*. In addition some hospitals place similar controls on other drugs liable to misuse, such as *night sedatives, tranquillizers,* and *antidepressants,* and on spirits such as *whisky* and *brandy*.

Drug storage

All drugs are potentially dangerous, and all must be stored in locked cupboards reserved specifically for drugs. The ward sister is legally authorized to possess Controlled Drugs for use in her ward (but not for any other purpose) and these and all other drugs issued to the ward are in her custody. Keys to the drug cupboards must be held by a sister, staff nurse, or nurse in charge of the ward at the time. Drugs in current use may be stored in drug trolleys provided that these are locked and immobilized between drug rounds. Topical preparations such as ointments, lotions and disinfectants are also dangerous if misused, and these too must be locked in cupboards. This has been mandatory for many years in children's wards. More specific local rules on drug storage may be made.

Storage conditions are important for most drugs, and it is the pharmacist's responsibility to ensure that the label on the container bears adequate instructions such as 'store in a refrigerator'. Drugs which need cool or cold storage will begin to deteriorate if left at room temperature for more than a few hours, and if this happens the pharmacist's advice must be sought —it is not sufficient to put the drug in the fridge after 2 days and hope for the best.

All injections and many tablets have expiry dates assigned by the manufacturer, and if a nurse notices that a drug is nearing this date she should mention the fact to the ward pharmacist, who may be able to arrange for it to be used elsewhere. Special care should be taken to check infrequently-used drugs such as those contained in emergency kits. A nurse should not administer a drug which has passed its expiry date unless she has sought the advice of the pharmacist who, in the light of his knowledge of the drug, may authorize its use. Similar constraints apply if the nurse feels that the condition or appearance of the drug is unusual or unsuitable.

Drug preparation

Nurses are required to do little in the way of preparation of drugs except for reconstituting injection solutions and making additions to intravenous infusion fluids. The practice of crushing tablets and mixing them with jam or sugar in order to get a child to take them, or of crushing tablets to put down a nasogastric tube, should be used only on specific pharmaceutical advice since many tablets are carefully formulated to give a sustained release of the drug, while others have the drug protected by a film, sugar, or enteric coating to disguise a bitter taste or prevent gastric irritation: these characteristics will be destroyed if the tablet is crushed. The pharmacist will always prepare a suitable formulation for a particular patient.

Reconstitution of injection solutions from vials of sterile powder is taught as a nursing procedure. Reconstitution of certain drugs, such as the cytotoxic agents, can be hazardous to the nurse, and local precautions, including the use of protective clothing, must be obeyed. Only specially trained nurses undertake this activity, and increasingly, cytotoxic injections are being reconstituted centrally by pharmacy staff in cabinets designed to protect the product from microbial contamination and the operator from the drug. Such centralized services can save money by avoiding wastage of residues from reconstituted vials. Repeated contact with antibiotics can cause skin sensitization, and care must be taken to avoid skin or mucous membrane contact when these are being handled (see p. 216). Reconstitution of any drug should be carried out immediately before use, using the diluent recommended in the package leaflet or advised by the pharmacist, and in general any reconstituted solution remaining should be discarded. In the case of very expensive preparations it may be possible to store and re-use the residue, but great care must be paid to storage conditions and expiry, both of which will differ from those of the dry powder. Local rules and procedures must be followed. Limitations on re-use are that the reconstituted solution must never be stored in a syringe, must not be used for intravenous or intrathecal injection, and must be used within 6 hours. In cases of doubt, the pharmacist will advise.

Most drugs are injected intramuscularly but where a very rapid effect is required, or the drug is too irritant for intramuscular injection, or if it is desired to give the drug at a constant rate over several hours, the intravenous route may be used, either by direct intravenous injection, by injection as a bolus into the intravenous giving set, or by addition to an intravenous infusion fluid.

The addition of drugs to intravenous infusion fluids has become an acceptable procedure for nurses who have been specially trained and authorized. Authorization is restricted to registered or enrolled nurses with practical experience, but requirements will differ between hospitals. Problems which may arise in this procedure are microbial contamination of the infusion fluid, incomplete mixing of the drug and the fluid, and chemical incompatibilities (not always visible) between the drug and the fluid or between two drugs added to the same fluid. The first two are a result of faulty technique, while the third may be prevented by reference to an incompatibility chart provided by the pharmacy. In cases of doubt, the pharmacist should be asked. Some hospitals provide a 24-hour advisory service from the pharmacy, a few have a resident pharmacist, while others have an on-call service for information or advice on this or any drug-related matter.

Drug labels

The style and content of labels will vary from hospital to hospital, but some typical labels for drugs dispensed for inpatients are shown in Figure 28.1. In each case the name of the patient and the ward are put first in order to aid selection of the container during a medicine round, followed by the drug name, strength and quantity. In addition the date of dispensing, and the initials of the pharmacist are shown, although these are of less importance to the nurse. Warning labels, on precautions and storage conditions, are also shown. In addition labels for outpatient or take home prescriptions will contain specific instructions to the patient on the frequency or method of administration.

Drug administration

Drugs are administered under the supervision of the ward sister or staff nurse, and great responsibility rests on the nursing staff to ensure that there are no errors. The principles behind the rules are that the right patient must receive the right dose of the right drug in the right form by the right route at the right time, and that the fact is duly recorded. Local policies and rules must be obeyed. A full discussion of the nurse's role may be found on page 14.

It is important that the precise directions for dose, time and frequency are followed. With some potent modern drugs, variations in times of dosing may lead to a loss of effect.

Many hospitals are rewriting their drug policies to permit administration of drugs by a nurse without this being checked. A few hospitals are developing computer systems on which the doctor will prescribe and the nurse record the administration of drugs, avoiding the traditional medicine sheets. This will provide an excellent tool for audit and costing purposes.

Drug doses prescribed by the doctor are checked by the pharmacist, but if a nurse thinks

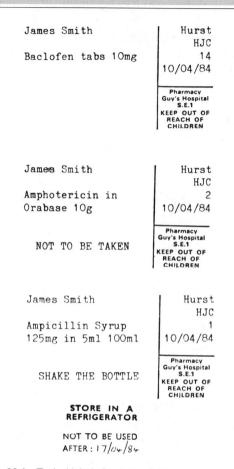

Fig. 28.1 Typical labels for drugs dispensed for inpatients.

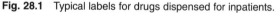

a dose is unusually high (or low) she should draw this to the attention of the nurse in charge, who should check in the British National Formulary and if necessary contact the doctor. When there is any doubt about the drug, the nurse must seek advice before giving the dose: it may be too late afterwards.

Doctors and nurses often assume that once a patient leaves the ward he will continue to take the drugs provided in accordance with the directions: but this is frequently not the case. There should be an ongoing preparation of the patient for discharge, including an explanation of how drugs should be taken or used, the importance of following the dosage instructions, and details of any precautions which should be observed. This can result in a significant improvement in patient compliance.

Patients receiving steroid, insulin or anticoagulant therapy or being treated for depression with monoamine oxidase inhibitors must be issued with cards describing precautions to be taken, and instructed to show the card to their doctor, dentist or pharmacist when receiving treatment or purchasing proprietary medicines. Such cards are usually available on the wards or from the pharmacy.

Some hospitals now issue patients with cards detailing their medication, which are shown to the patient's general practitioner and amended by him if therapy changes. In this way, any practitioner treating the patient will be presented with an up-to-date medication profile.

Observing the effects of drugs

Having given the drug, the nurse may be required to observe its effect by taking measurements, such as recording temperature, monitoring pulse rate or blood pressure, measuring urine output or testing urine for glucose, proteins, etc. Such measurements are part of the ward routine and contribute to the building up of a picture of the patient's condition and progress. However, the nurse can play a greater part in the observation of a drug's therapeutic action and of its side-effects by her observation of the patient throughout the day, and by making notes of the patient's condition in the nursing record. She is in an ideal position to do this, since she alone of the health team is with the hospital patient continually. However, to be effective in this vital role she must know the desired effect of the drug, its side-effects, its possible interaction with other drugs, and how its effect might be modified by the patient's condition: and it is in this area that the pharmacist can play an important part.

Information needs of the nurse

During training the nurse will acquire a basic knowledge of therapeutics and pharmacology which will probably have been extended by reading textbooks. It is possible, however, that she will be very familiar with only a limited number of drugs, usually those in widespread use in the hospital wards on which she trains. It is certain that during her professional career she will meet new drugs—either those which have been recently introduced, or those which are only occasionally used for common disease, or those which are used to treat rare conditions. Likewise she will not know the doses, availability and presentation of all the drugs which she will be expected to handle and administer. She will therefore need a source of information about drugs, and this should be the ward pharmacist whom she meets daily.

Most large hospital pharmacies have **drug information units**, which provide information on request to doctors, nurses, and other health workers on drugs, their choice, use, effects, doses, side-effects, and precautions. Nurses are encouraged to contact these units through the ward pharmacist, and the answers given will always be appropriate to the nurse's understanding and needs. Some hospitals are also providing information cards or files which are kept on the wards and contain concise nurse-oriented information on drugs likely to be encountered, although the range of drugs covered in this way will not be complete. In addition, ward pharmacists are always pleased to spend a few minutes talking to small groups of nurses about any aspect of drugs and their use. Nurses who are given projects involving drugs during their training are also encouraged to seek the help of the pharmacy, specifically the drug information unit.

Legal responsibility of the nurse as regards drugs

The laws affecting drug supply and use are the Misuse of Drugs Act 1971 and the Medicines Act 1968, together with Regulations made under these Acts. The Misuse of Drugs Act governs the drugs of addiction, termed 'Controlled Drugs' whereas the Medicines Act governs the manufacture, marketing, and supply of all drugs. The Secretary of State for Health is empowered under the National Health Services Act to make regulations concerning aspects of practice, including the prescribing and administration of drugs.

Under the Misuse of Drugs Act and Regulations, the **sister** or **acting sister** for the time being in charge of a ward, theatre, or other department in a hospital or nursing home may possess Controlled Drugs supplied to her by the pharmacist, and may administer them in accordance with the directions of a doctor or dentist. A midwife has additional authority under the Act to obtain, possess and administer *pethidine* in the practice of her profession. A doctor may not prescribe diamorphine (heroin) or cocaine for the treatment or relief of addiction unless he is licensed to do so by the Home Office.

Drugs may not be marketed without a product licence, which is granted by the Secretary of State on the advice of the Committee on Safety of Medicines, an expert body which considers evidence on the safety and efficacy of each new product.

Since April 1985, doctors, whether in hospital or general practice have not been able to prescribe certain black-listed drugs and drug preparations on a National Health Prescription. This restriction was imposed by the Secretary of State for Health in order to reduce public expenditure on drugs which were considered by his advisors to be unnecessary, or for which a cheaper alternative was available. The drugs banned included some antacids, laxatives, vitamins and cough and cold remedies, and are listed in the Drug Tariff (HMSO, published monthly).

The Medicines Act and its Regulations permit a **hospital nurse** to obtain and possess 'prescription only' medicines, i.e. those which are only available to patients on the prescription of a practitioner, for use on her ward, and to administer them in accordance with the directions of a doctor or dentist. Hospital rules usually extend this control to all drugs whether they are legally 'prescription only' or not. **Midwives** are permitted under the Act to administer a specified range of drugs in the practice of their profession. **Nurses in hospitals** have no authority to administer drugs except on the directions of a doctor or dentist, whether these are in the form of a specific prescription for a patient or as part of a written procedure accepted by the hospital authority. Any nurse doing so may face disciplinary action;

and if harm comes to the patient, may render herself liable to civil action. Hospital rules are based on *Guidelines for the safe and secure handling of medicines* (The Duthie Report, Dept of Health, 1988).

Certain procedures in the administration of drugs which were formerly performed by doctors only, are now regarded as part of the extended role of the nurse. Policy varies from hospital to hospital, but two examples are the addition of drugs to intravenous infusion fluids and the intravenous injection of drugs as a bolus via an intravenous line, which are sometimes undertaken by nurses who have been specially trained and authorized.

In the community

Today nurses have considerable experience in the community before they are qualified. The new roles of the district nurses and health visitors are discussed on page 21. In the community, the local pharmacist has the same role as in hospital, supplying prescribed medication and ensuring the safety and appropriateness of the drugs. Many pharmacists become well acquainted with their regular clients and some maintain their records on a computer. This means that the pharmacist can check new prescriptions against current medication and other details such as known adverse effects. Nurses who prescribe should develop good relationships with pharmacists who often provide advice about over-the-counter medication and their knowledge and records may also be of value to the prescriber nurse in preventing possible interactions.

Nurses working in the community, and private nurses, have authority to possess Controlled Drugs only in order to administer them in accordance with the directions of a doctor or dentist. Unlike nurses in hospitals, they may not hold a 'stock' of Controlled Drugs, but may obtain them only on prescription for a specific patient.

Similarly **nurses in community or private practice** have no authority to obtain or possess 'prescription only' medicines except on prescription, or to administer them to patients except in accordance with the directions of a doctor or dentist.

Dosage calculations

Patients may be prescribed doses of a drug which are not precisely equivalent to a single tablet, ampoule or 5 ml spoonful. In this case, it is necessary to calculate the quantity of drug preparation which will contain the dose prescribed, and this is a common source of error in drug administration. *The ward pharmacist should always be asked to annotate the prescription with the precise quantity of drug preparation which will contain the prescribed dose.* If the dose must be given before the ward pharmacist has seen the prescription, then any calculation made must be checked by a second person, and if there remains any doubt, advice must be sought before the drug is administered. Remember that the most common error when calculating drug dosage is a misplaced decimal point, i.e. the patient receives 10 times too much or only 1/10 of the dose.

Dosage calculation is a worry to nurses (and others!) and they may find it helpful to read *Maths for Nurses* by S. Pirie, published by Balliere Tindall, Eastbourne, 1985.

Summary of pharmaceutical services available to the nurse

Supply of drugs for use on the ward.

Preparation of unusual formulations or doses of drugs.

Advice on storage conditions and expiry dates.

Advice on legal responsibilities.

Ward pharmacy services providing a ready point of contact and enquiry.

24 hour service or on-call service.

Advice on preparation and reconstitution of drugs.

Advice on addition of drugs to intravenous infusion fluids.

Information on physical, chemical and pharmacological properties of drugs.

Information on dose, method of administration, effects, side-effects, precautions and contraindications associated with drugs.

Information on drug costs and drug usage in a particular hospital.

Seminars and discussions on drugs and their uses.

Information to assist with drug projects.

Advice about prescribing in the community.

Appendix 1

Weights and measures

WEIGHTS AND MEASURES

METRIC SYSTEM

Weight

1 kilogram (kg)	=	1000 grams (g)
1 gram (g)	=	1000 milligrams (mg)
1 milligram (mg)	=	1000 micrograms (μg)

Capacity

1 litre (l)	=	1000 milliliters (ml) or 1000 cubic centimetres (cc)

1 litre of water at 4°C weighs 1 kilogram.

Domestic measures

1 teaspoonful	=	about 5 ml
1 dessertspoonful	=	about 10 ml
1 tablespoonful	=	about 20 ml
1 tumblerful	=	about 250 ml

Glossary of terms used

Types of drugs referring to mode of action

Anaesthetics

General anaesthetics depress cerebral function, induce unconsciousness and prevent all sensation.

Local anaesthetics interfere with the function of a nerve or nerve ending and prevent all sensation from a localized area without loss of consciousness.

Analgesics relieve pain without interfering with consciousness.

Anthelmintics kill or aid the removal of worms from the intestines.

Antiepileptics prevent fits.

Antipyretics reduce body temperature when it is raised above normal.

Antibiotics are prepared from living organisms and kill or prevent multiplication of bacteria in the body. Many antibiotics are now prepared synthetically.

Aperients loosen the bowels.

Carminatives promote belching.

Chemotherapeutic agents are prepared synthetically to kill or prevent the multiplication of bacteria within the body.

Contraceptives prevent conception.

Cytotoxic agents are drugs which damage or kill malignant cells and are used in treating cancers.

Diaphoretics induce sweating.

Disinfectants kill bacteria.

Diuretics increase the secretion of urine by the kidneys.

Emetics produce vomiting.

Expectorants make the bronchial secretion more liquid and therefore more easily expelled.

Hypnotics produce sleep.

Hypotensive drugs lower blood pressure.

Mydriatics dilate the pupil.

Myotics constrict the pupil.

Neuroleptics are anti-psychotic drugs.

Opioids have a similar action to opium.

Pro-drug a substance which is inactive but is converted into an active drug in the body.

Sedatives soothe but may also cause drowsiness.

Styptics stop local bleeding.

Tonics are said to restore general well-being but are of doubtful value.

Tranquillizers promote mental relaxation without drowsiness.

Terminology referring to administration

Although many hospitals now have special prescription forms which have eliminated the use of the following terms, they are still widely used when prescribing in outpatients departments and general practice. It would be better if they were eliminated from prescription writing as they are a potential source of error.

a.c.	—before meals
ad lib	—as much as required
b.d.	—twice daily
b.i.d.	—twice daily
gutt.	—drops
inj.	—injection
o.h.	—every hour
o.m.	—every morning
o.n.	—every night
p.c.	—after meals
p.r.	—per rectum
p.v.	—per vaginam
q.d.	—four times daily
q.h.	—four hourly
rep	—repeat
s.o.s.	—if necessary
t.d.s.	—three times daily

Appendix 3

Proprietary and other drug names

The following list of proprietary names of drugs with the non-proprietary equivalent or similar preparation is not intended to be complete but merely to include drugs which are often prescribed under their proprietary names.

Proprietary or trade name	Non-proprietary name of drug or similar preparation
AT 10	Dihydrotachysterol
Acepril	Captopril
Achromycin	Tetracycline
Acthar Gel Injection	Corticotrophin gelatin injection
Actilyse	Alteplase
Actinomycin D	Dactinomycin
Acupan	Nefopam
Adalat	Nifedipine
Adcortyl	Triamcinolone
Adifax	Dexfenfluramine
Adriamycin	Doxorubicin
Albucid Eye-drops	Sulphacetamide eye-drops
Alcobon	Flucytosine
Alcopar Granules	Bephenium granules
Aldactone	Spironolactone
Aldomet	Methyldopa
Alimix	Cisapride
Alkeran	Melphalan
Aludrox	Aluminium hydroxide
Alupent	Orciprenaline
Amikin	Amikacin

Proprietary or trade name	Non-proprietary name of drug or similar preparation	Proprietary or trade name	Non-proprietary name of drug or similar preparation
Amoxil	Amoxycillin	Canesten	Clotrimazole
Anafranil	Clomipramine	Capoten	Captopril
Antabuse	Disulfiram	Cardura	Doxazosin
Antepar	Piperazine citrate	Catapres	Clonidine
Anthisan	Mepyramine	CCNU	Lomustine
Anturan	Sulphinypyrazone	Cedocard	Isosorbide dinitrate
APD	Disodium pamidronate	Celevac	Methylcellulose
Apresoline	Hydralazine	Centyl	Bendrofluazide
Aprinox	Bendrofluazide	Ceporin	Cephaloradine
Artane	Benzhexol	Ceporex	Cephalexin
Ativan	Lorazepam	Chloromycetin	Chloramphenicol
Atrovent	Ipratropium	Choledyl	Choline theophyllinate
Augmentin	Amoxycillin + potassium clavenulate	Ciproxin	Ciprofloxacin
		Cidex	Glutaraldehyde
Aureomycin	Chlortetracycline	Claforan	Cefotaxime
Avomine	Promethazine theoclate	Colofac	Mebeverine
Azactam	Aztreonam	Co-proxamol	Paracetamol + dextropropoxyphene
AZT	Zidovudine		
Bactrim	Co-trimoxazole	Cordarone X	Amiodarone
Becotide	Beclomethasone	Cordilox	Verapamil
Benadryl	Diphenhydramine	Corgard	Nadolol
Benemid	Probenecid	Corlan	Hydrocortisone pellets
Berkdopa	Levodopa	Corsodyl	Chlorhexidine mouthwash
Beta-Cardone	Sotalol		
Betadine	Povidone iodine	Coversyl	Perindopril
Betaloc	Metoprolol	Crystopen	Benzylpenicillin
Betnesol	Betamethasone	Cyclospasmol	Cyclandelate
Betnovate	Betamethasone	Cytamen Injection	Cyanocobalamin injection
Biogastrone	Carbenoxolone		
Bioral	Carbenoxolone	Cytosar Injection	Cytarabine injection
Blocadren	Timolol	Cytotec	Misoprostol
Bolvidon	Mianserin	Cytoxan	Cyclophosphamide
Bricanyl	Terbutaline	Daktarin	Miconazole
Brietal	Methohexitone	Dalacin C	Clindamycin
Brocadopa	Levodopa	Dalmane	Flurazepam
Brufen	Ibuprofen	Daraprim	Pyrimethamine
Burinex	Bumetanide	Deltacortril	Prednisolone
Buscopan	Hyoscine butylbromide	Demerol	Pethidine
Butazolidin	Phenylbutazone	De-Nol	Bismuth chelate
Cafergot	Ergotamine + caffeine	Depixol	Flupenthixol
Calpol	Paracetamol paediatric elixir	Depo-Medrone	Methylprednisolone
		Depo-Provera	Medroxyprogesterone
Calsynar	Salcatonin	Deseril	Methysergide
Camcolit	Lithium carbonate	Dexedrine	Dexamphetamine

Proprietary or trade name	Non-proprietary name of drug or similar preparation	Proprietary or trade name	Non-proprietary name of drug or similar preparation
DF118	Dihydrocodeine	Fortral	Pentazocine
Diabinese	Chlorpropamide	Fortunan	Haloperidol
Diamox	Acetazolamide	Frumil	Co-amilofruse
Dianabol	Methandienone	Fucidin	Sodium fusidate
Diazemuls	Diazepam injection	Fungilin Lozenges	Amphotericin lozenges
Diconal	Dipipanone + cyclizine	Furadantin	Nitrofurantoin
Difflam	Benzydamine	Furosemide	Frusemide
Diflucan	Fluconazole	Genticin	Gentamicin
Dilantin	Phenytoin	Glibenese	Glipizide
Dindevan	Phenindione	Glucophage	Metformin
Dioctyl-Medo	Docusate sodium	Heminevrin	Chlormethiazole
Diprivan	Propofol	Herpid	Idoxuridine
Disipal	Orphenadrine	Hibiscrub	Chlorhexidine
Distalgesic	Paracetamol + dextroproproxyphene	Hibitane Gluconate	Chlorhexidine gluconate
Dixarit	Clonidine	HRF-Ayerst	Gonadorelin
Dolobid	Diflunisal	Hypnovel	Midazolam
Dramamine	Dimenhydrinate	Hypovase	Prazosin
Dromoran	Levorphanol	Hytrin	Terazosin
D.T.I.C.	Dacarbazine	Ilosone	Erythromycin
Dulcolax	Bisacodyl	Imferon	Iron Dextran
Duogastrone	Carbenoxolone	Imigran	Sumatriptan
Duphalac	Lactulose	Imodium	Loperamide
Durabolin	Nandrolone phenylpropionate	Imuran	Azathioprine
		Inderal	Propranolol
Dytac	Triamterene	Indocid	Indomethacin
Edecrin	Ethacrynic Acid	Innovace	Enalapril
Elantan	Isosorbide mononitrate	Intal	Sodium cromoglycate
Eminase	Anistreplase (Apsac)	Isoket	Isosorbide dinitrate
Endoxana	Cyclophosphamide	Isordil	Isosorbide dinitrate
Entero-vioform	Clioquinol	Istin	Amlodipine
Epanutin	Phenytoin	Jectofer	Iron sorbitol
Epilim	Sodium valproate	Kabikinase	Streptokinase
Erythrocin	Erythromycin	Keflex	Cephalexin
Eppy	Adrenaline eye-drops	Keflin	Cephalothin
Esidrex	Hydrochlorothiazide	Kemadrin	Procyclidine
Euglucon	Glibenclamide	Kloref Tablets	Potassium chloride effervescent tablets
Euhypnos	Temazepam	Lanoxin	Digoxin
Fansidar	Sulfadoxine + pyrimethamine	Largactil	Chlorpromazine
		Larodopa	Levodopa
Feldene	Piroxicam	Lasix	Frusemide
Fentazin	Perphenazine	Ledermycin	Demeclocylcline
Flagyl	Metronidazole	Lentizol	Amitriptyline (sustained release)
Fluothane	Halothane		

Proprietary or trade name	Non-proprietary name of drug or similar preparation	Proprietary or trade name	Non-proprietary name of drug or similar preparation
Leo-K Tablets	Potassium chloride slow tablets	Negram	Nalidixic acid
Leukeran	Chlorambucil	Neo-Epinine	Isoprenaline
Librium	Chlordiazepoxide	Neo-NaClex	Bendrofluazide
Lincocin	Lincomycin	Nephril	Polythiazide
Lindane	γ Benzene hexachloride	Netillin	Netilmicin
Lioresal	Baclofen	Nipride	Sodium nitroprusside
Livial	Tibilone	Nobrium	Medazepam
Lomotil	Co-phenotrope	Nolvadex	Tamoxifen
Lopresor	Metoprolol	Normison	Temazepam
Losec	Omeprazole	Norval	Mianserin
Madopar Capsules	Co-beneldopa	Novocaine	Procaine
Maloprim	Dapsone + pyrimethamine	Nuelin	Theophylline Liquid
		Nurofen	Ibuprofen
Marcain	Bupivacaine	Omnopon	Papaveretum
Marplan	Isocarboxazid	Oncovin	Vincristine
Maxolon	Metoclopramide	One alpha	Alfacalcidol
Medomet	Methyldopa	Oramorph	Morphine solution
Melleril	Thioridazine	Orbenin	Cloxiacillin
Meptid	Meptazinol	Palfium	Dextromoramide
Merbentyl	Dicyclomine	Paludrine	Proguanil
Metopirone	Metyrapone	Palaprin Forte	Aloxiprin
Midamor	Amiloride	Panadol	Paracetamol
Minocin	Minocycline	Paramol 118	Co-dydramol
Mithramycin	Plicamycin	Parentrovite	Vitamin B and C injection
Mitoxana	Ifosfamide		
Modecate Injection	Fluphenazine decanoate injection	Parlodel	Bromocriptine
		Penbritin	Ampicillin
Moduretic	Co-amilozide	Pepcid PM	Famotidine
Mogadon	Nitrazepam	Persantin	Dipyridamole
Molipaxin	Trazodone	Petrolagar	Liquid paraffin emulsion
Motilium	Domperidone		
Mycardol	Pentaerythritol tetranitrate	Phenergan	Promethazine
		Phyllocontin	Aminophylline slow release
Myleran	Busulphan		
Mysoline	Primidone	Physeptone	Methadone
Mynah	Ethambutol + isoniazid tablets	Picolax	Sodium picosulphate
		Pipril	Piperacillin
Naprosyn	Naproxen	Piriton	Chlorpheniramine
Narcan	Naloxone	Ponderax	Fenfluramine
Nardil	Phenelzine	Ponstan	Mefenamic acid
Natrilix	Indapamide	Praxilene	Naftidrofuryl
Natulan	Procarbazine	Premarin	Conjugated oestrogens
Navidrex	Cyclopenthiazide	Prepulsid	Cisapride
		Pripsen	Piperazine

Proprietary or trade name	Non-proprietary name of drug or similar preparation
Priscol	Tolazoline
Pro-Banthine	Propantheline
Prostigmin	Neostigmine
Prothiaden	Dothiepin
Prozac	Fluoxetine
Pyopen	Carbenicillin
Questran	Cholestyramine
Rastinon	Tolbutamide
Redoxon	Ascorbic Acid
Rifinah	Rifampicin + Isoniazid
Rivotril	Clonazepam
Rogitine	Phentolamine
Rynacrom	Sodium cromoglycate nasal spray
Rythmodan	Disopyramide
Salazopyrin	Sulphasalazine
Saluric	Chlorothiazide
Sando K Tablets	Potassium chloride effervescent tablets
Saventrine Tablets	Isoprenaline slow release
Scoline	Suxamethonium
Scopolamine	Hyoscine
Seconal Sodium	Quinalbarbitone
Securopen	Azlocillin
Selexid	Pivmecillinam
Selexidin	Mecillinam
Septrin	Co-trimoxazole
Serc	Betahistine
Serenace	Haloperidol
Serenid D	Oxazepam
Serevent	Salmeterol
Serpasil	Reserpine
Sinemet Tablets	Co-careldopa
Sinequan	Doxepin
Sinthrome	Nicoumalone
Slow K Tablets	Potassium chloride slow release
Soneryl	Butobarbitone
Sotacor	Sotalol
Sparine	Promazine
Stelazine	Trifloperazine
Stemetil	Prochlorperazine
Streptase	Streptokinase

Proprietary or trade name	Non-proprietary name of drug or similar preparation
Stugeron	Cinnarizine
Surmontil	Trimipramine
Sustac	Glyceryl trinitrate sustained release
Symmetrel	Amantadine
Synacthen	Tetracosactrin
Syntometrine	Oxytoxin + ergometrine
Synalar	Fluocinolone
Tagamet	Cimetidine
Tambocor	Flecainide
Tanderil	Oxyphenbutazone
Tegretol	Carbamazepine
Temgesic	Buprenorphine
Tenormin	Atenolol
Tensilon	Edrophonium
Terramycin	Oxytetracycline
Tetracyn	Tetracycline
Theo-Dur	Theophylline slow release
Ticar	Ticarcillin
Tildiem	Diltiazem
Tofranil	Imipramine
Trandate	Labetalol
Transiderm-Nitro	Glyceryl trinitrate patch
Trasicor	Oxprenolol
Tridil	Glyceryl trinitrate injection
Tridione	Troxidone
Triludan	Terfenadine
Tryptizol	Amitriptyline
Uniphyllin Continus	Theophylline slow release
Valium	Diazepam
Vallergan	Trimeprazine
Velbe	Vinblastine
Ventolin	Salbutamol
Vepisid	Etoposide
Vibramycin	Doxycycline
Visken	Pindolol
Voltarol	Diclofenac
Welldorm	Dichloralphenazone
Xylocaine	Lignocaine
Yomesan	Niclosamide

Proprietary or trade name	Non-proprietary name of drug or similar preparation	Proprietary or trade name	Non-proprietary name of drug or similar preparation
Zantac	Ranitidine	Zofran	Ondansetron
Zarontin	Ethosuximide	Zovirax	Acyclovir
Zestril	Lisinopril	Zyloric	Allopurinol
Zinacef	Cefuroxime		

Information about drugs

There are now many books and articles about drugs. Three important publications which should be available in every School of Nursing library give clear and up to date information about drugs and treatment:

Prescribers journal (published monthly)
Enquires to: HMSO
               PC 11B/2
               51 Nine Elms Lane
               London SW8 5DR

Drug and Therapeutics Bulletin (published fortnightly)
Enquires to: Dept. DTB
               Consumers Association
               Castlemead
               Gascoyne Way
               Hertford SG14 ILH

The British National Formulary (BNF) which is published twice a year is a very useful book of reference. It contains essential details of all drugs currently available in the UK with brief sections on treatment. A copy should be kept on every ward.

Pharmaceutical companies provide a Data Sheet for each of their products. These sheets contain information as to the nature and action of the drug, its dose and therapeutic use, adverse effects and contraindications. They are also published annually as a compendium and are a useful source of information.

There are several good textbooks of clinical pharmacology. The most prestigious and arguably the best is:

The Pharmacological Basis of Medical Practice by A. G. Goodman and L. S. T. Gilman, Pergamon Press, New York, 1990.

It is extensive and expensive.

Index

W

Warfarin, 69
Whitfield's ointment, 293
Wolfe–Parkinson–White syndrome,
    treatment of, 53

X

Xamoterol, 48

Z

Zidoyudine, 215
Zinc undecenoate, 293
Zopiclone, 115